ESSENTIAL OILS

FOR MEN'S

HEALTH

1st Edition

Published by 2050 Institute

3602 John Ct. Annandale, VA 22003

www.2050i.org

Phone: 202-538-6798

ISBN: 978-1-963938-00-5

Printed in USA

Contents

Introduction

For centuries, the minarets of ancient Baghdad were brushed first by dawn's light as apothecaries and herbalists set up stalls in the lively markets. On all types of rare spices, resins, and herbs, on the shelves and tables, in the wide-angle bins and glass jars, bottles of sparking liquid take their place of honor—these are precious essential oils. This speaks to a time past in which people from all walks of life, be they noble lords or desert nomads, understood and revered the potency of these distilled wonders. The threads of this rich tapestry between man and essential oils frayed to become all but forgotten. Today, we aim to rethread this tapestry and renew these deep connections between essential oils and many facets of men's health.

Essential oils are the wonders discussed by dealers who roar with hunger at the scent of spices and the noise of barter among the ancient markets of Damascus. The distillates of these plants were not mere luxuries or perfumes; they were from the very fabric of ancient health care. But within this age-old story, one voice is often smothered out: the voice of men's health. Nowadays, our attention is directed to this theme, and we embark on a powerful world of essential oils that immensely influence male health.

From the deep and rich scent of grounding cedar wood warriors had once used before taking the battlefield to the bright scent of peppermint that had even caught the notice of ancient Greek scholars. Essential oils carry with them many stories: stories of strength, clarity, and rejuvenation.

The book aims to break myths, bust stereotypes, and reintroduce modern people to the world of healing with essential oils. Not that it's about being a follower or anything, but rather getting back to our basics, the ancient wisdom, and basically realizing that nature at its most unadulterated form always has a reason for our joy.

For many, essential oils conjure images of fragrant spas, beauty rituals, or the allure of exotic perfumes. Few people will spontaneously juxtapose them with the tough, grimy hands of a warrior, the thoughtful gaze of a scholar, and the everyday slogs of modern man. And yet, somewhere within the annals of history, there lie whispers of Roman soldiers who refreshed themselves with rosemary before the battle and of ancient Egyptian pharaohs who, while bathing, suffused themselves with frankincense to make the heart bolder.

People hardly expect that a world with a whole array of essentials lined up in little, delicate bottles and emanating fragrant smells could have any room for men. But looking back even further, it was actually men who turned to the healing power of botanicals for vitality, resilience, and balance. Essential oils were the purest extract of these plants and were, and still are, a powerful tool for men's health.

This is the Odyssey. The kind of voyage into the heart of forests, where sandalwood trees would whisper ancient secrets, on past sun-drenched Mediterranean coasts, where the citrus groves glow, and the wild, crisp mint would dance in the wind within the coves. After all, it is a journey that follows in the footsteps of our forebears, catches the essence of their wisdom—quite literally—and breathes it back into modern life.

But as you dig in deeper, there is the complex science behind these oils. You get to know how lavender molecules calm a racing heart or how components in sage will help hormonal balance. It's not only the aromatic pleasure but also about one's physical, emotional, and mental health.

You will get access to experts from different areas of expertise—botanists, aromatherapists, and doctors—who will summarize their research and underline the many advantages of essential oils. They will guide you toward using these oils in your fitness, food, sleep hygiene, and even the emotional way of caring for yourself.

So, dear reader, if you are an experienced enthusiast or only an interested beginner, welcome an invitation: an invitation to explore, experiment, and experience the power that Essential Oils bring to transform men's health. Welcome to a world where nature meets nurture and health is truly within your reach.

Every drop of essential oil unmasks a story in the coming chapters—ancient traditions, hard science, and then personal transformation. It is a story asking every modern to understand, try, and ultimately rejuvenate.

The tale here unfolds page after page as the rest of our enlightening journey towards reconciling nature's essence with the essence of manhood. Welcome to the world of pure and empowering essential oils. For men.

We underscore every time what should be given attention when using essential oils. We bother to underscore these at the end of each chapter, each use, or each usage. Just don't think that is repetition or verbosity. We do this so that we can see and follow these precautions when we see that every part is ensuring our safety.

The best ways to use this book are:

1. Browse: Get to know new knowledge and master new skills in advance to prepare for the emergency.

2. Find relevant chapters according to your physical discomfort.

3. This book first analyzes the physical conditions and hazards, starting from a number of circumstances men usually meet in life, what essential oils can help improve, and the mechanism of their effects. Then, they will be given the recipes for blending the essential oil but recommended the use of methods and procedures.

Finally, there will be reminders of the various safety matters to which we must pay attention.

Essential oils belong to ancient legends, but this is quite a new thing to us modern people! Especially to men. Through reading the book, you'll find ways to praise the great and practical gift given to us by nature even more, and, what's more, learn how to use it properly to alleviate the sub-health conditions of men!

Chapter 1

Essential Oils and Men's Health

In today's world, essential oils are beginning to be used daily by a few people, but essential oils are usually associated with women. This chapter explores the benefits of essential oils for men's health and well-being. We will work to address common concerns and misunderstandings to provide a solid foundation for understanding the power of essential oils.

1.1 Plants and Essential Oils

Plants and essential oils have a deep and interconnected history. For centuries, humans have recognized and utilized the powerful properties of plants, especially in the form of essential oils, for countless purposes ranging from spiritual rituals to medicinal treatments. Plants are used directly to form ancient and mysterious traditional Chinese medicine; after refining their essence, essential oils are produced. This book will not discuss traditional Chinese medicine but will focus on plants and essential oils, so let's delve deeper into this relationship.

A. Plants: Can Only Protect by Themselves

1. Origin and evolution: Plants have graced our planet for over 500 million years. Long before humans took their first steps, plants established vast forests, laying the foundation for the ecosystems we know today. Over thousands of years, they have faced countless challenges, from dramatic climate changes to invasive species. Yet they not only survived, but they also thrived. Without human interference, plants still have a long history. Although they have experienced countless destructions and fatal blows, they continue to survive and thrive! Young humans need plants, but plants do not necessarily need humans.

2. Natural defense mechanisms: Plants cannot escape danger, unlike animals. Compared with humans, their living environment is even worse! This immobility means they must develop numerous defense mechanisms to protect themselves. Some of these defenses are obvious, while others are subtly complex.

* Physical barriers: To protect themselves, many plants develop thorns, spikes, and tough leaves to deter herbivores. The bark on the tree isn't just for support; it also serves as a protective layer against pests and diseases.

* Chemical warfare: Besides physical barriers, plants produce a surprising array of chemicals to protect themselves. Some of the toxic chemicals they produce can deter animals from eating them. Other compounds are more subtle, such as attracting pest predators or interfering with the reproduction of harmful fungi or bacteria. Through these, plants receive additional levels of protection.

* Camouflage and imitation: After hundreds of millions of years of tempering, some plants have evolved to look like other more dangerous plants or the surrounding environment, making natural enemies fearful and avoid them! This makes them less likely to be eaten or disturbed.

* Symbiotic relationship: Plants form beneficial alliances with other living things. For example, some provide nectar or shelter to insects and, in return, protect the plant from herbivores.

3. Adapt to environmental stress: Plants can defend themselves against more than just living threats. They have developed complex mechanisms to withstand environmental stresses such as droughts, floods, and extreme temperatures. Cacti, for example, can store water in their tissues and have thick outer layers to reduce evaporation, allowing them to thrive in desert condi-

tions.

4. Signaling and communication: Recent research shows that plants can communicate with each other, often using chemical signals. When a plant is attacked, it may release chemicals to warn neighboring plants. These neighbors can then reinforce defense mechanisms in anticipation.

5. Essential oils as defense tools: Essential oils are the essence of plants. Essential oils play a vital role in the countless chemical defenses plants use. These concentrated compounds serve multiple purposes: deter pests, prevent fungal and bacterial infections, and attract beneficial insects. These oils become valuable for their therapeutic properties to humans, but their primary purpose in plants is usually defense.

6. A legacy of resilience: Plants' endurance is a testament to their resilience and adaptability. They have withstood challenges that have led to the extinction of countless other species. Their persistence is a testament to the power of evolution and the delicate balance of life on Earth. Humans especially need this endurance of plants!

When appreciating the beauty and utility of plants, it is crucial to recognize the depth of their evolutionary processes and the complex defenses they weave into their existence. In a world increasingly defined by change, there is much to learn from these silent, steadfast guardians of the Earth. We must learn how to survive and use their power, essence, and value well!

B. Nature's Lessons: How Humans Harness the Power of Plant Essential Oils

The relationship between plants and humans is ancient, deeply symbiotic, and rich in knowledge. As humans observed, revered, and interacted with plants over thousands of years, they began to decipher their secrets, especially the power contained in essential oils. The origin and development of ancient Chinese medicine and traditional Chinese medicine are the best examples of humans learning from animals and plants. Here's how this beautiful relationship evolved and the wisdom we glean from plants:

1. Observe nature's patterns: ancient civilizations observed the effects of plants on animals before science could explain their mechanisms. Animals that rub against certain plants appear to be healthier or exhibit strange behaviors, observations that pique human curiosity. Before human beings had

science and developed thinking, to survive better, they had to observe their surroundings to see if they could find useful things and methods.

2. Ancient uses of essential oils: Historical records from civilizations such as ancient Egypt, China, and India show that distilled plant extracts were used in religious rituals, medical practices, beauty treatments, and even mummification. Thousands of years ago, they recognized the powerful nature of plants and applied them to every aspect of life.

3. Learning through trial and error: Our ancestors did not have the same scientific methods as we do today. They rely heavily on trial and error. They would note the effects of different plant extracts on the human body, leading to the development of early herbal medicine. China's " Shen Nong Tasted a Hundred Herbs" is a story that will last forever!

4. Essential oils for healing: As humans began to understand plants better, they began to use essential oils more systematically. For example:
    * Lavender is recognized for its calming and healing properties and is often used for burns, wounds, and relaxation.
    * Mint is used to aid digestion and refresh the senses.
    * Tea tree is known for its powerful antiseptic properties, especially against wounds and infections.

5. Cooking and preservation purposes: Spices were scarce and popular commodities in ancient times. Plants such as rosemary, oregano, and thyme are used not only for their aromatic qualities in cooking but also for their ability to preserve food due to the antimicrobial properties of their essential oils.

6. Mental and Emotional Health: In addition to physical health, humans have also discovered the profound effects of essential oils on emotional and mental health. For example, for centuries, frankincense and myrrh have been closely intertwined with religious and meditative practices. Burning frankincense during religious ceremonies can create an environment of evaluation, tranquility, and peace, making believers more confident and pious.

7. Modern research and verification: Today, scientists invest a lot of time and energy in research, verifying many ancient uses of essential oils and trying to discover deeper uses. Research into essential oils' antibacterial, anti-inflammatory, and stress-reducing properties is powerful, bridging the gap between ancient wisdom and modern understanding.

8. Sustainably and Ethically Harvested: As we rely more and more

on essential oils, it's crucial to remember the lessons of balance and respect. Overharvesting and unsustainable practices threaten to harm the plants that were once our mentors. It is our responsibility to ensure that essential oils are harvested, respecting the cycles of nature.

The journey to understanding and harnessing the power of plant essential oils is a testament to human curiosity, adaptability, and the deep-rooted connection we share with the natural world. As we look to the future, the wisdom of the past reminds us to treat nature with reverence, gratitude, and stewardship.

1.2 Benefits and Uses for Men.

Essential oils have many benefits and uses that cater specifically to men's health and well-being. Here are some of the key benefits and applications of essential oils for men:

1. Boosts energy and vitality: Certain essential oils, like peppermint and rosemary, are known for their uplifting properties, helping to increase energy levels, mental alertness, and overall vitality.

2. Support muscle recovery: After physical exertion or strenuous exercise, essential oils like eucalyptus and lavender can be used topically or in a massage blend to soothe muscles, reduce inflammation, and promote faster recovery.

3. Enhance focus and mental clarity: Essential oils like lemon, basil, and frankincense are thought to enhance cognitive function, improve concentration, and promote mental clarity, making them valuable for work, study, and concentration.

4. Promotes relaxation and stress relief: Many essential oils have calming properties that help men relax, reduce stress, and promote relaxation. Lavender, chamomile, and sandalwood are often used for their soothing effects.

5. Supports male hormonal health: Essential oils like sage, geranium, and ylang-ylang are known for their potential to balance hormones and support male reproductive health and well-being.

6. Helps with shaving and aftershave: Essential oils like tea tree, ce-

darwood, and chamomile can be used to soothe skin irritations, prevent razor burn, and provide natural antiseptic properties during shaving and aftershave.

7. Solve skin problems: Essential oils like tea tree, lavender, and frankincense are often used to address common skin issues that men face, including acne, blemishes, and dryness.

8. Promote scalp and hair health: Essential oils like rosemary, cedarwood, and peppermint are beneficial in maintaining a healthy scalp, supporting hair growth, and solving dandruff or scalp problems.

9. Boost confidence and mood: Certain essential oils, including citrus oils like bergamot and uplifting oils like vetiver, can enhance mood, boost confidence, and promote a positive mindset.

10. Natural fragrances and personal care: Essential oils provide a variety of naturally pleasant aromas and can be used in colognes, body care products, and homemade personal care products, allowing men to embrace natural fragrances and avoid synthetic fragrances.

Remember that individual experiences with essential oils may vary, and it is important to consider personal preferences and sensitivities and consult with a qualified aromatherapist or healthcare professional when incorporating essential oils into your daily routine.

1.3 Common Concerns and Misunderstandings

There are some common concerns and misconceptions we may have when it comes to essential oils. Addressing these concerns or misconceptions is critical to provide accurate information and help individuals make informed decisions. Here are some of the significant questions and misconceptions surrounding essential oils for men:

1. Attention: Essential oils are only suitable for women

Clarification: The application of essential oils is not gender specific. People of any gender can use and enjoy them. The benefits and applications of essential oils are not limited to a specific gender.

2. Concern: Essential oils are ineffective or just a placebo

Clarification: Essential oils have been used for centuries by various cultures and have a long history of traditional use. While scientific research on essential oils is ongoing, many studies have shown their potential therapeutic benefits. However, it is essential to note that individual responses may vary.

3. Attention: Essential oils can replace medical treatment

Clarification: Essential oils should not be used as a substitute for professional medical advice or treatment. While they can supplement and support overall health, consulting a healthcare professional regarding specific health concerns or conditions is important. Essential oils are not a replacement for modern medical treatments but a compliment.

4. Attention: Essential oils can be used undiluted on the skin

Clarification: Most essential oils are highly concentrated and should be diluted before skin application. Undiluted use may cause skin irritation or sensitization. Diluting with an appropriate carrier oil or following recommended guidelines ensures safe and effective use. Moreover, dilution will reduce the effectiveness of essential oils and their volatilization, resulting in less absorption by the human body.

5. Concern: All essential oils are the same

Clarification: Essential oils come from a variety of different plants or different parts of the same plant and have different chemical compositions, resulting in different properties and potential benefits. Each essential oil has its unique properties, scent, and potential applications.

6. Attention: Essential oils are safe to take

Clarification: Essential oils should be taken with caution and under the guidance of a qualified professional. Not all essential oils are safe to take internally, and improper use can cause adverse effects. It is essential to follow proper dosage and safety recommendations, and internal use is recommended under the guidance of a professional.

7. Concern: Essential oils are regulated like drugs

Clarification: Essential oils are now generally classified as cosmetic or perfume products rather than as drugs in countries worldwide. Regulations can vary from country to country, so choosing a high-quality, reputable brand that prioritizes safety and transparency is essential.

8. Focus: Essential oils can cure or treat specific illnesses

Clarification: While essential oils exhibit potential therapeutic properties, they are not intended to cure or treat a specific disease. They can be used to support overall health, promote relaxation, and solve specific problems, but medical conditions require professional medical advice.

Handling essential oils with an understanding of their benefits, limitations, and proper use is crucial. Consulting with a reputable source, aromatherapist, or healthcare professional can help clarify questions and provide tailored guidance for safe and effective essential oil use.

Chapter 2

Precautions for Using Essential Oils

Essential oils require careful consideration and compliance with safety guidelines to ensure a safe and effective experience. Here are some important safety precautions to keep in mind.

2.1 Safe selection and use of essential oils

We'll delve into the topic of choosing and using essential oils safely. We discuss the importance of understanding essential oil safety guidelines and potential risks associated with improper use and provide practical advice on selecting, handling, and applying essential oils to ensure a safe and enjoyable experience.

A. Understand Essential Oil Safety

Essential oils are highly concentrated plant extracts, and their potency is one of their defining characteristics. These oils come from various parts of the plant, such as leaves, flowers, stems, and roots, and they contain concentrated aromatic compounds that give each plant its unique scent and healing properties. Due to their potency, essential oils should be used with caution and respect for their concentrated nature.

Here are a few key points to keep in mind:

1. Small amounts often: A little bit of essential oil goes a long way. Just a few drops contain many of the plant material's aromatic and therapeutic qualities. This is why they are usually diluted before use.

2. Safe dilution: In some cases, applying undiluted essential oils directly to the skin can cause skin irritation, sensitization, and even allergic reactions. Diluting with a carrier oil (such as coconut, jojoba, or almond oil) can help mitigate these risks while allowing for safe use.

3. Potential for sensitization: Excessive use of essential oils or without proper dilution increases the risk of sensitization, where the body becomes sensitive to a specific oil, resulting in adverse reactions upon subsequent exposure.

4. Variability in sensitivity: People vary in their sensitivity to essential oils. What works for one person may not work for another. Factors such as skin type, age, and health can affect oil tolerance.

5. Precautions for Internal Use: In most cases, it is not recommended to ingest essential oils without the guidance of a qualified aromatherapist or healthcare professional. Some oils can be toxic if ingested; internal use requires specific knowledge and expertise.

6. Pets and Children: Pets, especially cats and dogs, may be sensitive to certain essential oils. Additionally, children's skin is more delicate and more sensitive to essential oils. Be especially careful when using essential oils around them.

7. Pregnancy and Medical Conditions: Pregnant women, people with certain medical conditions, or people taking certain medications should consult a health care professional before using essential oils, as some essential oils can interact with medications or pose risks during pregnancy.

The concentrated nature of essential oils offers tremendous therapeutic potential when used safely and appropriately. To enjoy their benefits while avoiding potential risks, it is important to understand each oil, its properties, and recommended uses. When in doubt, seek guidance from a qualified aromatherapist or healthcare professional who can provide personalized advice based on your specific needs and circumstances.

It is important to be aware of the potential risks associated with using essential oils. While they offer many benefits, there are certain risks and caveats to keep in mind:

1. Skin sensitivities and allergic reactions: Essential oils are powerful substances that can cause skin irritation, redness, itching, or allergic reactions in some people. Conduct a patch test before using any new essential oil topically. Apply the diluted oil solution to a small skin area and wait 24 hours to check for any adverse reactions.

2. Photosensitivity: Some citrus essential oils, such as bergamot, lemon, and lime, can cause skin sensitivity when exposed to sunlight. Avoiding sunlight on the treated area for 12 to 24 hours after applying these oils topically is recommended.

3. Pregnancy and breastfeeding: Pregnant or breastfeeding women should exercise caution when using essential oils. Some oils are contraindicated during pregnancy, while others may be safe when properly diluted and used in moderate amounts. In the meantime, it's best to consult a healthcare professional before using essential oils.

4. Drug interactions: Essential oils can interact with certain medications. If you are taking any prescription medications, consult your healthcare provider before using essential oils to ensure there are no potential interactions.

5. Children and babies: Children's skin is more delicate and generally more sensitive to essential oils. Certain oils should be avoided or used in extremely diluted forms with children. Some oils are not suitable for babies. Before using essential oils on children, consult a pediatrician or certified aromatherapist.

6. Internal use: Extreme caution should be exercised when ingesting essential oils, preferably under the guidance of a trained professional. Some oils may be toxic or cause adverse reactions when ingested.

7. Asthma and Respiratory Problems: People with asthma or other respiratory problems should be cautious when using essential oils, especially those with high menthol (such as peppermint) or eucalyptol (such as eucalyptus) content. Strong aromatic oils may cause respiratory discomfort.

8. Pet Safety: Pets, especially cats and dogs, may react adversely to certain essential oils. Some oils can be toxic to pets whose sense of smell is much stronger than ours, making them more susceptible to the scent.

9. Quality issues: Inferior or adulterated essential oils increase the risk of adverse reactions. Choose a reputable brand that offers pure, high-quality oils.

10. Allergies: If you are allergic to certain plants or pollens, be careful when using essential oils extracted from these plants, as they may trigger allergic reactions.

11. Individual variability: People can respond differently to essential oils based on their personal health, genetics, and sensitivities.

To minimize risk and ensure a safe experience, always dilute essential oils correctly, follow recommended usage guidelines, and be aware of your body's reactions. Conducting a patch test before applying new oil to a larger skin area is also wise. If you experience any adverse reactions, discontinue use and seek medical advice if needed. Consulting with a certified aromatherapist or healthcare professional can provide personalized guidance based on your health and specific needs.

B. Quality and Purity of Essential Oils

Sourcing high-quality, pure essential oils from reputable suppliers is critical to ensuring safety and effectiveness. Here are some reasons why sourcing is important:

1. Purity and Potency: Reputable suppliers adhere to strict quality standards and use steam distillation or cold-pressed extraction methods to ensure the oil is pure and potent. High-quality oils contain the required therapeutic compounds, making them effective for various uses.

2. No additives or contaminants: Pure essential oils should not contain additives, synthetic fragrances, or contaminants. Low-quality or adulterated oils may not provide the expected benefits or cause adverse reactions.

3. Safety: Authentic essential oils come from natural compounds in plants. However, low-quality oils or oils with additives may contain harm-

ful substances that can cause skin irritation, allergic reactions, or other health problems.

4. Consistency: Reputable suppliers maintain consistent quality from batch to batch. This consistency ensures you get the same therapeutic benefits every time you buy the oil.

5. Ethical and sustainable sourcing: Trustworthy suppliers typically source raw materials from sustainable and ethical sources. This supports both the environment and the local community.

6. Transparency: Reputable suppliers provide detailed information about the oil's botanical name, extraction method, country of origin, and relevant test results. This transparency allows you to make informed choices.

7. Education: Established suppliers often provide educational resources and information on proper use, dilution ratios, and safety precautions. This is especially helpful for those who are new to using essential oils.

To ensure you are getting high-quality essential oils, consider the following:

* Research: Look for suppliers with a strong reputation in the aromatherapy and natural health community.

* Testing: Reputable suppliers often provide third-party test results for their oils, indicating the oil's purity and chemical composition.

* Botanical Name: Make sure the oil you purchase lists the botanical name of the plant species. Different species can have different healing properties.

* Price: Extremely low prices may indicate poor quality or adulteration. High-quality oils require large amounts of plant material to produce, which increases their cost.

* Reviews and Recommendations: Review reviews and recommendations from trusted sources, such as certified aromatherapists or natural health practitioners.

* Certifications: Some suppliers may carry certifications demonstrating their commitment to quality, sustainability, and ethical practices.

Remember that the term " therapeutic grade " is not regulated in the essential oil industry, so it's important to focus on the supplier's reputation and transparency rather than marketing claims. Investing in high-quality essential oils from reputable sources ensures a safe and effective aromatherapy experience.

Recognizing quality standards when purchasing essential oils is critical to ensuring you get a pure and effective product. Here's how to identify quality essential oils:

1. Certified organic: Look for essential oils certified by a reputable organization. Organic certification ensures that the plants are grown without synthetic pesticides or chemicals, which could affect the oil quality.

2. Third-party testing: Reputable suppliers often provide third-party testing reports for their essential oils. These reports detail the oil's chemical composition, purity, and potential contaminants. Look for oils with readily available test results.

3. Botanical name and country of origin: Quality essential oils will be clearly labeled with the botanical name of the plant species and country of origin. This information will ensure you get the right essential oil with your desired properties.

4. Extraction method: The extraction method used to obtain the oil should be mentioned on the label or product description. High-quality essential oils are usually extracted through methods such as steam distillation or cold-pressed extraction.

5. Proper labeling: The label should include the essential oil's common name, botanical name, extraction method, and volume. Avoid products with unclear labels or missing information.

6. Pure ingredients: High-quality essential oils should contain only essential oils from specified plants, with no additions or dilutions. Be careful if it's labeled " Fragrance Oil " products or products that list synthetic additives.

7. Aromatherapy Grade: Although "Therapeutic Grade" is not regulated, some reputable suppliers may use " aromatherapy grade " and other terms to express their commitment to quality standards.

8. Price: High-quality essential oils require large amounts of plant material and careful processing, which increases their cost. Be wary of unusually low prices, which may indicate poor quality or adulteration.

9. Supplier Reputation: Research the supplier's reputation in the aromatherapy and natural health community. Look for a supplier with positive reviews, recommendations from certified aromatherapists, and a history of ethical practices.

10. Transparency: Reputable suppliers provide information about their purchasing practices, testing procedures, and quality control measures. They may also provide educational resources to help you use oils safely and effectively.

11. Packaging: Essential oils are sensitive to light and air, which can degrade their quality over time. Premium oils are often packaged in dark glass bottles to protect them from light.

Remember, the quality of an essential oil plays an important role in its safety and effectiveness. Prioritize sourcing from established and trustworthy suppliers who adhere to high-quality standards and provide transparent product information.

C. Overview and Properties of Essential Oils

Here are some common essential oils, along with their properties, properties, potential benefits, and precautions:

1. Lavender:

* Characteristics: floral, sweet, herbal aroma.
* Properties: Calming, soothing, and balancing.
* Benefits: Promotes relaxation, reduces stress and anxiety, aids sleep, and soothes skin irritation.
* Note: Generally safe, but some people may be sensitive. Avoid during the first trimester of pregnancy.

2. Mint:

* Features: Fresh, minty, uplifting scent.
* Characteristics: energizing, cooling, and analgesic.

* Benefits: Relieves headaches, relieves muscle tension, aids digestion, and clears congestion.
* Note: Strong oil, use at low dilution. Avoid closing your eyes and sensitive skin.

3. Eucalyptus:

* Characteristics: Strong camphor aroma.
* Properties: Decongestant, expectorant, and antiseptic.
* Benefits: Clears respiratory congestion, supports respiratory health, and refreshes your mind.
* Precautions: Avoid use by children under 6 years of age and do not ingest.

4. Frankincense:

* Characteristics: Woody, earthy, and slightly sweet aroma.
* Properties: Relaxing, centering, and immune boosting.
* Benefits: Enhances meditation, reduces stress, supports skin health, and promotes a sense of peace.
* Caution: Generally safe, but sensitive individuals may experience skin irritation.

5. Tea tree:

* Characteristics: Medicinal, fresh, slightly spicy aroma.
* Properties: Antiseptic, antibacterial, and immune stimulant.
* Benefits: Treats skin problems (acne, cuts, bites), supports the immune system, and freshens the air.
* Note: Do not ingest. Dilute before applying to the skin.

6. Bergamot:

* Characteristics: Citrusy, uplifting, slightly floral aroma.
* Properties: Calming, mood-enhancing, and antispasmodic.
* Benefits: Relieves anxiety and stress, enhances mood and supports digestion.
* Note: Bergamot oil is photosensitive, so avoid sunlight after applying it to the skin.

7. Chamomile:

* Characteristics: Sweet, fruity, and herbal aroma.
* Properties: Relaxing, anti-inflammatory, and soothing.
* Benefits: Relieves tension, promotes relaxation, and supports digestive health.
* Note: People with ragweed allergies may be sensitive to chamomile.

8. Lemon:

* Features: Bright, citrus, and uplifting fragrance.
* Properties: Energizing, detoxifying, and antiseptic.
* Benefits: Elevates mood, cleanses surface, supports the immune system.
* Note: It is photosensitive; please avoid sun exposure after use.

9. Sandalwood:

* Characteristics: Woody, earthy, and grounding.
* Properties: Relaxing, grounding, and aphrodisiac.
* Benefits: Calms the mind, promotes meditation, and supports skin health.
* Note: Sandalwood is considered safe but should be used in moderation.

10. Ylang-Ylang:

* Features: Sweet, floral, and exotic fragrances.
* Properties: Relaxation, aphrodisiac, and emotional balance.
* Benefits: Reduces stress, promotes relaxation, enhances mood, and supports emotional well-being.
* Cautions: Strong aroma; use in moderation as it can cause headaches in some people.

Remember that individuals may react differently to essential oils, and it's crucial to do a patch test before using any new oil on your skin. Additionally, if you have certain health conditions or are pregnant, consult a healthcare professional before using essential oils.

Understanding the essential oil profile before use is crucial to a safe and effective aromatherapy experience; here's why it's important:

1. Safety: Different essential oils have varying degrees of potency and potential sensitivities. Some oils can cause skin irritation or allergic reactions

if used incorrectly. Knowing the specific safety precautions for oils can help prevent adverse reactions.

2. Allergies and Sensitivities: Certain essential oils, especially those from plants in the same plant family, can trigger allergic reactions in sensitive individuals. Understanding the botanical family and ingredients of oils can help avoid potential allergens.

3. Dilution: Essential oils are concentrated substances that should dilute before direct skin application. Knowing the recommended dilution ratio for each oil can help prevent skin irritation and sensitization.

4. Photosensitivity: When applied to the skin and exposed to sunlight, some citrus oils can cause skin discoloration or burns due to their photosensitizing properties. Knowing which oils are photosensitive and their safe use can help prevent skin damage.

5. Contraindications: Certain essential oils are not recommended for use by pregnant women, children, or individuals with certain health conditions. Knowing the contraindications can ensure you avoid essential oils that may be harmful in these situations.

6. How to use: Different oils suit different application methods. Some oils are safe to use topically, while others are better for inhalation. Understanding recommended application methods can maximize benefits and minimize risks.

7. Aromatic characteristics: Essential oils have unique aromas that can affect mood and emotions. Understanding the aroma of oil can help you choose an oil that resonates with the effect you want, whether that's relaxation, alertness, or mood enhancement.

8. Blends: Essential oil blends are often formulated for specific purposes, such as relaxation or immune support. Understanding the individual properties of oils can help you create a balanced and effective blend. In Chapter 9, we will introduce some theories and methods of blending essential oils and some DIY recipes for blending essential oils.

9. Personal Reaction: People's reactions to essential oils may vary based on factors such as skin type, health, and personal preference. By understanding the profile of your motor oil, you can better predict how it might affect you.

10. Quality and Authenticity: Essential oils should be sourced from reputable suppliers to ensure purity and quality. Understanding the characteristics of motor oil can help you identify genuine oil from synthetic or adulterated oil.

To get an overview of essential oils, consult reliable sources such as essential oil reference books, reputable aromatherapy websites, and information from trusted essential oil brands. Also, before using new oils on your skin, do a patch test and watch for any reactions. If you have specific health concerns, please consult a qualified aromatherapist or healthcare professional for personalized guidance.

D. Diluting Oil and Carrier Oils

Proper dilution is critical to ensuring the safe and effective use of essential oils; here's why it's important:

1. Skin Sensitivity: Essential oils are highly concentrated extracts that may be too potent to be applied directly to the skin. Diluting them in a carrier oil reduces the risk of skin irritation, redness, and allergic reactions, especially for people with sensitive skin.

2. Prevent skin damage: Some essential oils, if used undiluted, can cause chemical burns, blisters, or other adverse skin reactions. Dilution creates a protective barrier and allows for controlled and gentle application.

3. Absorption and Even Application: Carrier oil helps the essential oil spread evenly on the skin, promoting better absorption. This ensures that the benefits of the essential oil are effectively delivered.

4. Children and Vulnerable Groups: Children, the elderly, and individuals with certain health conditions are more susceptible to adverse reactions from undiluted essential oils. When using essential oils with these populations, proper dilution is critical.

5. Photosensitivity: Some essential oils, such as citrus oil, are photosensitive and can cause skin damage when exposed to sunlight. Dilution helps mitigate this risk and avoids sun exposure after topical application.

6. Maximize Benefits: Dilution will not reduce the therapeutic effects

of essential oils. Dilution enhances absorption and provides longer-lasting benefits due to slower evaporation.

7. Stretching Resources: Dilution helps make essential oils more economical and extend their use. A small amount of essential oil goes a long way when diluted properly.

8. Safe use over time: Long-term and undiluted use of certain essential oils can cause allergies, where the body develops an allergic reaction to the essential oil. Dilution reduces this risk, allowing safe and sustainable use.

9. Blending and Customizing: Essential oils are often combined to create blends for specific purposes. Dilution provides the right medium for mixing different oils to achieve the desired effect.

10. Aromatherapy Safety: In aromatherapy practices such as inhalation, undiluted essential oils can be overwhelming and irritate the respiratory system. Dilution is the key to creating a comfortable and safe aromatic environment.

The most common dilution for adults is about 2 to 3% (about 12 to 18 drops of essential oil per ounce of carrier oil). For children, the elderly, and those with sensitive skin, a lower dilution ratio is recommended. Always use pure, high-quality carrier oils and reputable essential oils. Before widespread use, a patch test must also be performed on a small area of skin to ensure there are no adverse reactions. If you are unsure about appropriate dilution or have specific health concerns, it is recommended to consult a certified aromatherapist or healthcare professional.

Carrier oils play a vital role in diluting essential oils to ensure safe and effective use. They are vegetable oils derived from seeds, nuts, or the fatty parts of fruits. Here's why carrier oils are important and some commonly used carrier oils:

Importance of carrier oil:

1. Dilution: Carrier oils dilute the concentration of essential oils, reducing the risk of skin irritation or adverse reactions.

2. Skin barrier: Carrier oil forms a protective barrier on the skin, helping the essential oils diffuse evenly and gradually absorb.

3. Skin Nourishing: Many carrier oils contain nutrients that nourish and moisturize the skin, enhancing the overall benefits of the blend.

4. Stability: Carrier oil helps stabilize essential oils, which are volatile and will evaporate quickly if used directly.

5. Safe to use: Carrier oils are safe to apply directly to the skin, making them an ideal medium for essential oil use, especially topical applications.

Common carrier oil:

1. Jojoba oil Similar to the skin's natural sebum, jojoba oil is easily absorbed and suitable for most skin types.

2. Coconut oil is solid at room temperature and needs to be melted before use. It nourishes the body and hair.

3. Sweet almond oil is rich in vitamins and suitable for all skin types. It is often used for massage and general skin care.

4. Grape seed oil is light and not greasy. Grape seed oil is good for massage and skin moisturizing.

5. Avocado oil is rich, highly moisturizing, and beneficial for dry skin.

6. Olive oil is a common kitchen oil used in skincare, but it has a strong aroma that may affect the fragrance of the mixture.

7. Almond oil is light and gentle, suitable for sensitive skin and facial care.

8. Sunflower seed oil is rich in vitamin E. Sunflower seed oil has a moisturizing effect and can be used for massage and skin nourishment.

How to dilute essential oils with a carrier oil:

1. Choose a carrier oil based on your skin type, intended use, and your preferred scent.

2. The common dilution ratio is 2 to 3% of adult essential and carrier oils. This means approximately 12 to 18 drops of essential oil per ounce (30ml) of carrier oil. For children, the elderly, or those with sensitive skin, use

a lower ratio.

3. Mix the desired amount of essential oil with the carrier oil in a small glass bottle. Shake and mix well.

4. Patch test Before using the diluted mixture on a larger area, perform a patch test on a small skin area to check for sensitivity or allergic reaction.

5. Application: Apply the diluted mixture to the desired area as needed. For facial applications, use a milder oil and a lower dilution rate.

Using a carrier oil ensures the safety of your essential oil blend and allows you to enjoy its therapeutic benefits without the risk of skin irritation or adverse reactions.

E. Patch Testing and Sensitivity

Patch testing is essential before using a new essential oil or blend on your skin. This simple test can help you determine if you may have any adverse reactions or sensitivities to oils. Here is why patch testing is important:

1. Skin sensitivities vary. Everyone's skin is different, and what works for one person may not work for another. Some people are more sensitive to certain essential oils than others.

2. Allergic Reactions Essential oils are highly concentrated extracts from plants and may contain compounds that may trigger allergic reactions in some people.

3. Skin Irritation Certain essential oils, when used undiluted or in high concentrations, can cause skin irritation, redness, itching, and even rashes.

4. Photosensitivity: some essential oils can increase the skin's sensitivity to sunlight and can cause sunburn or other skin reactions if exposed to ultraviolet rays after use.

5. Undesirable Effects: If essential oils are unsuitable for your skin type or specific condition, they may exacerbate existing problems.

How to perform a patch test:

1. Dilute the oil. Mix a small amount of essential oil (1 to 2 drops) with a carrier oil. A carrier oil helps reduce concentration and prevent direct contact with the skin.

2. Select a test area; choose a small, inconspicuous area of skin, such as your wrist or the inside of your forearm.

3. Apply the mixture, dabbing a small amount of the diluted mixture onto the test area. Let it absorb.

4. Wait and watch for 24 hours without cleaning the area. Watch your skin for any signs of redness, itching, irritation, or discomfort.

5. Check for reactions, and if you notice any adverse reactions during this period, discontinue use and avoid using that specific oil or mixture. If there is no reaction, the oil is probably safe for you.

Additional tips:

* Please be patient: some reactions may not appear immediately. Waiting 24 hours may cause delayed reactions to become apparent.

* Repeat for mixture: If you are testing a mixture, make sure to patch-test the entire mixture, not just the individual oils.

* Photosensitivity: If the oil is known to be photosensitive, perform a patch test on an area that will not be exposed to sunlight.

* Test with caution. If you have sensitive skin or a history of skin allergies, consider testing essential oils you have used before.

Remember that patch tests are not foolproof, but they are useful for minimizing the risk of adverse reactions. If you're unsure about an oil or blend, consulting a qualified aromatherapist or healthcare professional is a wise approach, especially if you have a pre-existing skin condition or sensitivity.

Performing a patch test is a simple process involving applying a dilute mixture of essential oils and carrier oils to a small skin area. This will help you evaluate whether the oil may cause any adverse reactions. Here's how to perform a patch test and interpret the results:

Perform a patch test:

1. Choose an Essential Oil Choose an essential oil to test and make sure it is of good quality and comes from a reputable source.

2. Select a test area. Choose a small, inconspicuous area of skin, such as the inside of your wrist, forearm, or behind your ear.

3. Dilute the Oil. Mix one drop of selected essential oil with one teaspoon of carrier oil. Common carrier oils include jojoba, coconut, almond, or grapeseed oil.

4. Apply the mixture: Gently apply a small amount of the diluted mixture to the test area. Spread it in a thin layer and let it absorb.

5. Wait and watch: Leave the test area uncovered for 24 hours. Avoid washing the area or exposing it to excessive moisture during this time.

Patch-testing results:

24 hours, you can evaluate the test area for any signs of adverse reactions. Here's what to look for:

1. No reaction: If you don't experience any redness, itching, irritation, or discomfort, this indicates that the essential oil is probably safe for you.

2. Redness or Irritation: If you notice redness, itching, or irritation in the test area, this may be a sign that you are sensitive to the essential oil. Discontinue use and avoid using this oil.

3. Delayed Reaction: Sometimes, reactions may appear after the first 24 hours. If you notice any problems within 48 hours of the patch test, this is still a sign of sensitivity.

Additional tips:

* Choose an area to clean: Make sure the test area is clean and free of other products that could interfere with the results.

* Labeling: If you are testing multiple essential oils, label the test area to keep track of which essential oil is used.

* Reactions may vary: Remember, everyone's skin is different. Anoth-

er may well tolerate an essential oil that causes a reaction in one person.

* Photosensitivity: If the oil is known to be photosensitive, ensure the test area is not exposed to sunlight during testing.

* Seek professional advice: If you have a history of skin allergies, sensitive skin, or any concerns, please consult a qualified aromatherapist or healthcare provider before using essential oils.

Remember that patch tests provide guidance but don't guarantee that you won't react when using the oil on larger areas of your body. Always use essential oils cautiously and be aware of your body's reactions. Get medical advice if you have severe or prolonged reactions.

F. How to Use

Essential oils can be used in a variety of ways, each with its benefits and considerations. Here's a breakdown of the different application methods:

1. Local application:

* Dilute essential oils with a carrier oil before applying them to the skin. This helps prevent skin irritation and allows for safe use.
* Apply the diluted mixture to pulse points, temples, neck, or desired area of the body.
* This method is suitable for massage, relaxation, skincare, and targeted relief.

2. Inhalation:

* Inhale essential oils directly from the bottle for quick aromatherapy effects.
* Add a few drops of essential oil to a bowl of hot water. Place a towel over your head and bowl and inhale the steam.
* Use a personal inhaler stick, a diffuser necklace, or a tissue dipped in a few drops of oil for on-the-go relief.
* Inhalation effectively promotes relaxation, improves concentration, and supports respiratory health.

3. Diffusion:

* Use an aromatherapy diffuser to disperse essential oils into the air to create a pleasant, therapeutic atmosphere.
* Add water and a few drops of essential oil to your diffuser according to instructions.
* Diffusion is great for creating a calming environment, improving air quality, and enhancing mood.

4. Massage:

* Dilute essential oils in a carrier oil and use the mixture for massage.
* Massage can help with relaxation, muscle tension relief, and overall well-being.

5. Bathing:

* Add a few drops of essential oil to a warm bath.
* The steam produced by bathing releases fragrance, provides relaxation, and benefits the skin.

6. Apply:

* Add a few drops of essential oil to a warm or cold water bowl.
* Soak a cloth or towel in water, wring it out, and place it on the affected area.
* Dressings can help relieve local pain, inflammation, and relaxation.

7. Direct inhalation:

* Put a drop of essential oil on a tissue or cotton ball and inhale directly.
* Direct inhalation helps quickly relieve stress, nausea, or congestion.

8. Steam inhalation:

* Add a few drops of essential oil to a bowl of hot water.
* Cover your head with a towel and lean over the bowl to inhale the steam.
* Inhaling steam can help with breathing problems and relaxation.

9. Indoor spray:

* Mix water and a few drops of essential oil in a spray bottle.

* Use as a natural air freshener or to create a calming atmosphere.

Please remember the following general tips:

* Start with small drops and increase if needed, especially when using strong oils.
* Consider personal preferences and sensitivities.
* Store essential oils in a cool, dark place away from direct sunlight.
* Use only high-quality, pure essential oils.
* If you are pregnant, nursing, or have a specific medical condition, consult a healthcare professional before using essential oils.

Always listen to your body and adjust your use based on your comfort and response.

Here's a breakdown of the benefits, considerations, and suitability of each essential oil application method in specific situations:

1. Local application:

* Benefits: Provides targeted relief, skin nourishment, and relaxation. It can be used in massage and skin care routines.
* Note: Dilution is essential to prevent skin irritation. Perform a patch test before applying it to a larger area. Some oils are photosensitive, so avoid sunlight after use.
Best for: Muscle tension, skin care, relaxation, local discomfort.

2. Inhalation:

* Benefits: Experience the benefits of fragrance quickly and effectively. Supports respiratory health, relaxation, and mood improvement.
* Caution: Direct inhalation may be strong for some people. Use with caution if you have respiratory sensitivities.
Best for: Stress relief, respiratory support, quick mood boost.

3. Diffusion:

* Benefits: Create a soothing atmosphere, improve air quality, and promote relaxation. Provides long-lasting aromatherapy benefits.
* Note: Choose a well-ventilated area. Use the appropriate dilution for your diffuser. Some oils may not be safe for pets.
Best for: Creating a calm environment, improving sleep quality, and

enhancing mood.

4. Massage:

* Benefits: Combines the benefits of aromatherapy and physical contact. It relieves muscle tension, promotes relaxation, and improves blood circulation.
* Note: Dilution is essential to prevent skin irritation. Ensure proper technique to avoid stress.
Best for Muscle tension, relaxation, and promoting emotional well-being.

5. Bathing:

* Benefits: Provides a relaxing and aromatic experience. It helps nourish skin and relieve stress.
* Note: Essential oils should not be mixed with water alone; use a dispersing agent like Epsom salts or a carrier oil.
* Suitable for relaxing after a long day, promoting sleep, and enhancing the bathing experience.

6. Apply:

* Efficacy: Topical relief of pain and discomfort. Can help relieve inflammation and muscle tension.
* Note: Use appropriate oil according to the situation. The temperature of the dressing (warm or cold) can be chosen as desired.
* Suitable for Helping muscle soreness, reducing swelling, and relieving dysmenorrhea.

7. Direct inhalation:

* Benefits: Quick and portable aromatherapy method. It can help provide immediate relief from stress or nausea.
* Caution: Inhaling strong oils directly can be overwhelming. Use with caution.
Best for: Quick stress relief and nausea relief.

8. Steam inhalation:

* Benefits: Provides respiratory support, clears congestion, and relaxes.

* Caution: Be careful to avoid hot water burns. Close your eyes when inhaling to avoid irritation.
* Great for Respiratory congestion, sinus relief, and relaxation.

9. Indoor spray:

* Efficacy: Freshen the air, cover up odors and create a pleasant atmosphere.
* Caution: Avoid spraying directly on furniture or delicate surfaces. Shake well before each use.

It is best for Creating a welcoming environment, promoting relaxation, and freshening the air.

Keep in mind that personal preferences and sensitivities vary. Always start with a low dilution and listen to your body's reaction. If you are new to essential oils, consult a certified aromatherapist or healthcare professional for personalized guidance.

2.2. Emergency Preparedness

If you experience an adverse reaction to an essential oil, it is important to take prompt and appropriate action. Here are the steps to consider:

A. Irritation to skin

1. Stop using: If you develop skin irritation, redness, itching, or a rash after applying an essential oil, stop using the oil immediately.

2. Dilution: If the irritation is mild, you can try diluting the affected area with a carrier oil such as coconut, jojoba, or sweet almond oil. Do not use water, as it will diffuse the oil and possibly worsen irritation.

3. Cleaning: Gently clean the area with mild soap and water to remove any residue of the essential oil.

4. Cold compress: Cold compresses can help soothe the skin and reduce inflammation.

5. Seek medical treatment: If irritation persists, worsens, or severe reactions occur (such as blistering or difficulty breathing), seek immediate medical attention.

B. Accidental Ingestion

1. Do not induce vomiting: If you accidentally swallow essential oils, do not attempt to induce vomiting. Some oils can be harmful if breathed into the lungs.

2. Drink milk or water: If you feel discomfort, drink a glass of milk or water to help dilute the oil and relieve any burning sensation.

3. Contact Poison Control: If you experience serious symptoms such as nausea, vomiting, dizziness, difficulty breathing, or any other unusual reactions, contact your local poison control center or seek immediate medical help.

C. Prevent Adverse Reactions

1. Patch Test: Always perform a patch test before applying any essential oil to a large area of skin. Apply a small amount of the diluted oil to the inside of your forearm and wait 24 hours to check for any adverse reactions.

2. Proper dilution: Follow proper dilution guidelines and avoid using undiluted essential oils directly on your skin, especially on sensitive areas.

3. Place it out of reach: Keep essential oils out of the reach of children and pets to prevent accidental ingestion or contact.

4. Consult a Professional: If you have any underlying health conditions, are pregnant or nursing, or are taking medications, please consult a healthcare professional before using essential oils.

Remember that everyone's body reacts differently to essential oils, and what works for one person may not work for another. If you are unsure about the effects of oil or are concerned about its safety, it is best to consult a medical professional.

If you or someone you know has a serious adverse reaction to an essential oil, it is important to seek medical help immediately. In the case of accidental ingestion or severe skin irritation, contacting a poison control center or seeking medical help can make a difference. Here are some resources and contact information:

USA:
Poison Control Hotline: 1-800.222.1222
Website: https://www.poison.org/

Canada:
Poison Control Hotline: 1-844-POISON-X
Website: https://infopoison.ca

U.K:
NHS 111 (24-hour medical help): Dial 111
Website: https://www.nhs.uk/conditions/poisoning/

Australia:
Poison information hotline: 13 11 26
Website: https://www.poisonsinfo.nsw.gov.au/

Chapter 3

Essential Oils for Physical Health

and Performance

This chapter focuses on how essential oils can enhance men's physical fitness and performance. We'll delve into improving energy and endurance, supporting muscle recovery, and relieving joint and muscle discomfort.

3.1 Enhance Energy and Endurance

First, explore how essential oils can help improve men's energy levels and stamina. We discuss their invigorating properties and various ways to incorporate them into your daily life to promote energy and stamina.

A. Understanding Fatigue and Low Energy

First, fatigue and low energy levels can stem from many factors, including lifestyle choices, nutritional deficiencies, hormonal imbalances, sleep disorders, mental and emotional health, chronic illness, medications, environmental factors, age-related changes, and even chronic fatigue syndrome disease. By identifying the root cause of fatigue, men can take proactive steps to improve their energy levels and overall health. It is crucial to address these issues through lifestyle changes, proper nutrition, adequate sleep, stress management, medical counseling, and creating a supportive environment. Through a holistic approach and understanding of why, men can regain their energy and vitality and live more fulfilling and vibrant lives.

Addressing the underlying factors is critical to long-term physical fitness enhancement. By taking a holistic approach and considering various aspects such as lifestyle changes, targeted nutrition, hormonal balance, stress management, sleep optimization, regular physical exercise, and managing underlying health conditions, men can contribute to sustained energy levels and overall health. Pave the way. It is essential to individualize the approach and seek professional guidance when necessary. By addressing the root causes of fatigue and low energy, men can experience lasting improvements, increase energy, and enjoy a more energetic and fulfilling life.

B. Vitality Essential Oils

Essential oils like peppermint, rosemary, eucalyptus, and citrus oils can be valuable allies in boosting energy levels and promoting a sense of vitality and well-being in men. These essential oils can provide a natural and aromatic lift to combat fatigue, improve focus, and improve mental clarity by harnessing their uplifting and uplifting properties. It's important to explore different application methods, such as inhalation, topical use, and diffusion, to find what works best for your personal preferences and needs. As with any essential oil use, it is crucial to take safety precautions and consult an expert when necessary. With the support of these energizing essential oils, men can tap into their natural energy reserves and experience new vitality and energy in their daily lives.

Peppermint essential oil

* Uplifting and refreshing fragrance
* Stimulates mental clarity and focus
* Increase energy levels and fight fatigue
* Can be used by inhalation, topical application, or diffusion

Rosemary essential oil

* Uplifting and stimulating aroma
* Enhance mental alertness and cognitive function

* Combats mental fatigue and promotes clarity
* Can be used by inhalation, massage, or blending.

Eucalyptus essential oil

* Uplifting and energizing scent
* Promote respiratory health and purify the mind
* Increase alertness and rejuvenate the senses
* Can be used by inhalation, vapor, or diffusion

Citrus essential oils (orange, lemon, grapefruit)

* Uplifting and refreshing aroma
* Lifts mood and promotes positivity
* Improve energy levels and fight fatigue
* Can be diffused, inhaled, or used topically

The uplifting and stimulating effects of essential oils such as peppermint, rosemary, eucalyptus, and citrus can be attributed to their unique chemical composition and interaction with our senses. Here's a brief explanation of the science behind how these oils stimulate and revitalize the senses:

1. Aromatic Compounds: Essential oils contain volatile aromatic compounds that are responsible for their characteristic smell. When these compounds are inhaled, they interact with the olfactory system in our noses, which is made up of olfactory receptors. These receptors detect odor molecules and transmit signals to the brain, specifically the olfactory bulb and limbic system.

2. Olfactory bulb and limbic system: The olfactory bulb is the structure in the brain that receives signals from olfactory receptors. It plays a crucial role in processing and transmitting odor information to other areas of the brain, including the limbic system. The limbic system is associated with emotion, memory, and emotion regulation.

3. Stimulating and uplifting effects: When we inhale the aromatic compounds of essential oils, they stimulate olfactory receptors and activate the olfactory bulbs. This activation triggers the release of neurotransmitters and chemicals in the brain, such as serotonin and endorphins, which are known to enhance mood, increase alertness, and promote a sense of well-being.

4. Cool and refreshing feeling: Essential oils such as peppermint and eucalyptus contain menthol, which has a cooling effect on the skin and mucous

membranes. When applied topically or inhaled, menthol activates cold-sensitive receptors called TRPM8 receptors, which are responsible for the cooling sensation. This cooling sensation can create a refreshing and uplifting experience.

5. Cognitive and mental effects: Some essential oils, such as rosemary, have been studied for their cognitive-enhancing properties. These oils may interact with certain neurotransmitter systems in the brain, such as acetylcholine. They play a role in memory and attention. Inhaling or applying topically rosemary oil has been shown to improve cognitive performance, increase alertness, and reduce mental fatigue.

Overall, the science behind how these oils stimulate and revitalize the senses involves activating olfactory receptors, releasing neurotransmitters and chemicals in the brain, and interacting with specific sensory receptors. These effects can help increase a sense of alertness, improve mood, and an overall uplifting experience when using these essential oils.

C. Inhale for a Quick Energy Boost

The inhalation technique using essential oils is a quick and effective way to uplift and stimulate your senses instantly. Inhalation allows the aromatic molecules of essential oils to interact directly with your olfactory system, triggering a rapid response in the brain and promoting alertness and energy. Here are some inhalation techniques you can use with essential oils:

1. Direct inhalation

Place a few drops of desired essential oil on a tissue or handkerchief.
Hold the tissue close to your nose, breathe deeply and slowly, and inhale the aroma directly.
This technology allows for immediate and concentrated inhalation of the aromatic molecules of the oil.

2. Aromatherapy bath

Add a few drops of your chosen essential oil to a warm bath.
Relax and inhale deeply while enjoying the steam and aroma of the oil.
Combining warm water and essential oils creates a soothing and energizing experience.

3. Steam inhalation

Fill a bowl with hot water and add a few drops of essential oil.

Place your face over the bowl, close your eyes, and cover your head with a towel to create a steam tent.

Breathe deeply and allow the essential oil-infused vapor to enter your respiratory system.

This technique can help clear your sinuses, promote respiratory health, and provide energy benefits.

4. Aromatherapy Diffuser

Use an aromatherapy diffuser to disperse essential oils into the air.

Follow the manufacturer's instructions for the specific diffuser you are using.

Inhale the diffuse aroma as it fills the room, creating an uplifting and energizing environment.

5. Personal inhaler

Use a personal inhaler or aromatherapy inhaler wand.

Add a few drops of the desired essential oil to your inhaler and keep it with you.

Breathe in from your inhaler whenever you need a quick boost of energy or rejuvenation.

Remember to choose essential oils known for their uplifting and energizing properties, such as peppermint, citrus, rosemary, or eucalyptus. Each inhalation technique offers a unique experience; you can experiment to find what resonates best with you. Inhaling essential oils can provide instant refreshment, increase alertness, and promote a sense of vitality and well-being.

Use inhalation as a convenient energy boost throughout the day to help you stay alert, focused, and rejuvenated. Here are some practical tips for incorporating inhalation technology into your daily life:

1. Portable Inhaler: Purchase a personal inhaler or aromatherapy inhaler stick that you can easily carry with you. Use energizing essential oils like peppermint, citrus, or rosemary. Take a few deep breaths from your inhaler whenever you need a quick boost of energy.

2. Desk Diffuser: Place a small aromatherapy diffuser at your desk or workspace. Add a few drops of an energizing essential oil or essential oil blend and let it diffuse throughout the day. Whenever you feel low on energy or need a pick-me-up, inhale the aroma.

3. Inhalation breaks: Take short inhalation breaks throughout the day. Find a quiet space, close your eyes, and deeply inhale a few drops of the energizing essential oil using a tissue or cup of hand. Please focus on the aroma and let it rejuvenate your senses.

4. Morning Ritual: Start your day by inhaling an energizing blend of essential oils. Place a few drops on a tissue or cotton ball and take a few deep breaths to let the scent awaken your senses and set a positive tone for the day.

5. Afternoon pick-me-up: Fight the afternoon slump by inhaling uplifting essential oils like citrus or peppermint. Keep a small oil bottle in your desk or bag, and take a moment to inhale its aroma whenever you feel your energy waning.

6. Commuting Companion: If you have a long commute, inhale this uplifting blend of essential oils to feel more energized. Use a car diffuser or put a few drops on a paper towel or cotton ball and place it in your car. Take deep breaths while driving to help stay alert and focused.

7. Exercise Boost: Enhance your workout routine by inhaling energizing essential oils before exercise. Choose oils like eucalyptus or peppermint, which can increase alertness and refresh your workout.

Remember to choose quality essential oils and use them safely. Please consult a qualified aromatherapist or healthcare professional if you have any sensitivities or health concerns. Incorporating inhalation techniques into your daily routine can be a convenient and effective way to boost energy levels, improve focus, and lift your mood throughout the day.

D. Essential Oil Blends that Create an Energy Boost

Here are some recipes and blending suggestions for creating a personalized energy-boosting blend using essential oils:

1. Vibrant Citrus Blend

* 3 drops of orange essential oil
* 2 drops of lemon essential oil
* 2 drops of grapefruit essential oil

2. Refreshing Mint Blend

* 2 drops of peppermint essential oil
* 2 drops of spearmint essential oil
* 2 drops of eucalyptus essential oil

3. Focus and Clarity Blending

* 3 drops of rosemary essential oil
* 2 drops of lemon essential oil
* 1 drop of frankincense essential oil

4. Uplifting Woody Mix

* 2 drops of pine essential oil
* 2 drops of cedar essential oil
* 2 drops of bergamot essential oil

5. Herbal Energy Blend

* 2 drops of basil essential oil
* 2 drops of peppermint essential oil
* 2 drops of rosemary essential oil

To use these blends, you add the recommended number of drops to a diffuser, personal inhaler, or aromatherapy jewelry. Alternatively, you can create a roller blend by diluting the essential oils in a carrier oil (such as jojoba or sweet almond) and applying the blend to your pulse points or temples for a quick boost of energy.

Feel free to adjust the number of drops based on your personal preference and the desired strength of the mixture. Remember to patch test and use essential oils safely by following the recommended dilution guidelines.

Experiment with different essential oil combinations and ratios to find the blend that resonates best with you and provides the energy boost you need. Everyone's preferences and reactions to essential oils may differ, so it's important to customize the blend to meet your individual needs.

Here are some combinations of essential oils known for their energizing and mental alertness-enhancing properties:

1. Mint and Rosemary

Peppermint essential oil is refreshing and refreshing, while rosemary essential oil is known for its ability to increase focus and mental clarity. Together, they create a potent mixture of energy and alertness.

2. Lemon and Eucalyptus

The lemon essential oil has a bright and uplifting aroma, while eucalyptus essential oil provides refreshing and stimulating effects. This combination can help awaken the senses and promote mental alertness.

3. Grapefruit and Basil

Grapefruit essential oil has an uplifting and energizing scent, while basil essential oil is known for its ability to enhance focus and mental stamina. This blend provides a balanced energy boost and mental clarity.

4. Bergamot and Frankincense

Bergamot essential oil has a citrusy and uplifting aroma that promotes positivity and energy. Frankincense essential oil is grounding and can help reduce mental fatigue. Together, they create a harmonious blend of sustained energy and mental focus.

5. Orange and Ginger

Orange essential oil is known for its energizing and mood-boosting properties, while ginger essential oil provides warming and stimulating effects. This combination provides an instant energy boost and mental alertness.

To create a synergistic blend, start with the exact proportions of each essential oil and then adjust the proportions to your liking. For example, you can use 2 drops of peppermint, 2 drops of rosemary, 2 drops of lemon, and 2 drops of eucalyptus in a diffuser or personal inhaler. Please consider personal sensitivities and consult a qualified aromatherapist if you have any questions.

Try different combinations to find what works best for you. Everyone may react differently to essential oils, so exploring and discovering a blend that gives you the energy and mental alertness boost you need is important.

E. Local Application of Sustained Energy

Applying essential oils topically can be a beneficial way to maintain energy throughout the day. When applied to the skin, essential oils can penetrate the bloodstream and provide ongoing benefits. Here are some of the benefits of topical application of sustained energy:

1. Absorption: The skin can absorb essential oils, allowing their beneficial properties to enter the bloodstream and provide ongoing support. When used topically, energizing essential oils are released gradually throughout the day, promoting sustained energy levels.

2. Stimulate blood circulation: Essential oils applied to the skin can help improve blood circulation, which can increase energy levels. Improved blood circulation can better deliver nutrients and oxygen to cells, helping to fight fatigue and promote vitality.

3. Targeted application: You can target its energetic effects by applying essential oils to specific areas, such as your pulse points or the back of your neck. These areas are rich in blood vessels near the skin's surface, allowing for efficient absorption and topical benefits.

4. Personalized Blend: The topical application allows you to create a personalized blend tailored to your specific energy needs. Mix energizing essential oils with a carrier oil or lotion to create a custom energizing moisturizer or body oil.

5. Aromatherapy effects: Besides being beneficial to the body, the aroma of essential oils can also psychologically impact energy levels. When used topically, the uplifting scent of energizing essential oils can help uplift the mind and increase mental alertness.

To use essential oils topically for sustained energy, consider these tips:

Dilute the essential oil in a carrier oil before applying it to your skin. This helps prevent skin irritation and allows for safer use. A common dilution ratio is 2 to 3% of essential oil and carrier oil.

Choose a skin-nourishing carrier oil such as sweet almond, jojoba, or coconut oil.

Apply diluted mixture to pulse points, back of the neck, or soles of feet for maximum absorption and sustained release of energy properties.

Before applying the mixture to a larger area, patch tests a small area of skin to check for any potential sensitivities or reactions.

Remember, it is important to use essential oils safely and consult a qualified aromatherapist or healthcare professional if you have any concerns or specific health conditions.

When applying essential oils to your skin, be sure to follow safe dilution guidelines and best practices to ensure proper application and minimize the risk of skin irritation or sensitization. Here are some points to consider:

1. Dilution Guidelines: Essential oils are highly concentrated and should always be diluted before skin application. Diluting essential oils in a suitable carrier oil can help reduce the risk of adverse reactions. The recommended dilution ratio for general topical use in adults is 2 to 3%. This means using approximately 12 to 18 drops of essential oil per ounce (30 ml) of carrier oil.

2. Patch Test: Before applying a new essential oil or blend to a larger area of skin, it's important to conduct a patch test. Apply a small amount of diluted essential oil to a small area of skin, such as the inner forearm, and watch for any signs of irritation or allergic reaction within 24 hours. If any adverse reactions occur, discontinue use and seek medical advice if needed.

3. Targeted Application: When applying essential oils topically, consider your specific areas or concerns. For example, if you are using essential oils to treat muscle discomfort, you may choose to apply the mixture directly to the affected area. However, for general use or larger areas of skin, it is usually recommended to apply the diluted mixture to pulse points, the back of the neck, or the soles of the feet for optimal absorption.

4. Sensitivity and Skin Type: Everyone's skin is unique, and some people may have increased sensitivity to certain essential oils. If you have sensitive skin, starting with a lower dilution is recommended and gradually increasing if tolerated. Certain essential oils, such as citrus oils, may cause photosensitivity when applied to the skin, so avoiding exposure to sunlight for

at least 12 to 24 hours is important.

5. Duration of use: Short-term topical use of essential oils is generally recommended for a specific problem or as needed throughout the day. Long-term or overuse of certain essential oils may increase the risk of skin irritation. It's important to give your skin a " rest time " without constantly using essential oils.

6. Quality and Storage: To ensure the safety and effectiveness of essential oils, it is critical to select high-quality, pure, and selected organic oils from reputable sources. Storing essential oils properly in dark glass bottles away from direct sunlight and heat will help maintain their integrity and potency.

Remember, it is always a good idea to consult a qualified aromatherapist or healthcare professional, especially if you have any specific health concerns, are pregnant, nursing, or have a medical condition. They can provide personalized guidance and advice based on your circumstances.

By following these guidelines and the best application methods, you can safely and effectively enjoy the benefits of essential oils when applying them to your skin.

F. Pre-workout and Workout Support

Essential oils can be a great addition to your pre-workout routine to boost energy, focus, and stamina. Here are some essential oils known for their energizing and performance-enhancing properties:

1. Peppermint: Peppermint essential oil is refreshing and has a cooling effect. It can help increase alertness, improve concentration, and increase energy levels. Inhaling peppermint oil or applying it topically before a workout can provide a refreshing and stimulating effect.

2. Eucalyptus: Eucalyptus essential oil has a refreshing and revitalizing fragrance. It promotes deep breathing, clears airways, increases oxygen intake, and can enhance endurance during physical exercise. Consider diffusing eucalyptus oil in your workout space or applying it to your chest or pulse points before exercising.

3. Lemon: Lemon essential oil has a bright and uplifting aroma that

can help improve mood and increase energy levels. Its refreshing scent can provide a mental boost before a workout and promote a positive mindset. Consider diffusing lemon oil or inhaling lemon oil straight from the bottle for an instant energy boost.

4. Rosemary: Rosemary essential oil is known for its ability to improve focus, memory, and cognitive abilities. It can help stimulate the mind and improve mental clarity, which can be beneficial during exercises that require concentration. Consider diffusing rosemary oil before exercising or applying it topically.

5. Orange: Orange essential oil has a cheerful and uplifting scent that can help improve mood and increase motivation. It provides energizing results and increases enthusiasm for exercise. Consider diffusing orange oil or inhaling it straight from the bottle for a pre-workout energy boost.

6. Ginger: Ginger essential oil has warming and energizing properties. It can help energize the body, improve blood circulation, and provide a feeling of vitality. Consider applying diluted ginger oil to your muscles before exercising to support endurance and reduce muscle fatigue.

Remember to dilute essential oils appropriately in a carrier oil before applying them to your skin when using essential oils as a pre-workout aid. Perform a patch test to check for any skin sensitivities and follow the recommended dilution ratios and safety guidelines discussed previously.

It's important to note that individuals may react differently to essential oils, so it's best to experiment and find what works best for you. Listen to your body and adjust the amount and method used to suit your personal preferences and sensitivities.

If you have any underlying medical conditions or concerns, it is recommended that you consult a qualified aromatherapist or healthcare professional before incorporating essential oils into your pre-workout routine. They can provide personalized guidance based on your specific needs and circumstances.

Incorporating essential oils into your exercise routine is both enjoyable and beneficial for optimizing performance. Here are some practical ways to use essential oils during exercise:

1. Diffuse: Using an essential oil diffuser in your workout space can

create a stimulating and energizing environment. Diffuse energy oils like peppermint, eucalyptus, or citrus during your workout to enhance focus, increase alertness, and promote a positive mindset.

2. Pre-Workout Inhalation: Inhaling essential oils directly from the bottle or using a personal inhaler can provide a quick and convenient energy boost and focus before starting your workout. Just take a few deep breaths and inhale the aroma of an oil like peppermint, rosemary, or lemon to stimulate your senses and prepare you for your workout.

3. Topical Application: Dilute Energizing Essential Oil in a carrier oil and apply topically before exercising. You can apply the diluted mixture to your pulse points, such as your wrists, neck, or temples, to experience the scent throughout your workout. This can help promote mental clarity, increase stamina, and lift your mood. Some essential oils suitable for topical application include peppermint, eucalyptus, rosemary, or a personalized blend to suit your preference.

4. Cooling Spray: Create a refreshing cooling spray in a spray bottle by mixing peppermint or eucalyptus essential oil with water. Spraying this mixture on your face, neck, or body during exercise can provide a cooling sensation, stimulate your senses, and help regulate body temperature.

5. Post-workout massage: After a workout, consider combining a post-workout massage with essential oils to support muscle recovery and relaxation. Dilute an oil like lavender, eucalyptus, or peppermint in a carrier oil and gently massage the mixture into your muscles to relieve any discomfort and promote a calm and rejuvenated feeling.

6. DIY Workout Gear Freshener: Create a DIY workout gear freshener by adding a few drops of your favorite essential oil to a small spray bottle filled with water. Spray this mixture onto your gym bag, exercise mat, or equipment to freshen them up and add a pleasant scent to your workout space.

Remember to start with a low dilution and perform a patch test to ensure compatibility with your skin. Also, be aware of any specific sensitivities or allergies you may have when choosing and using essential oils.

It is important to note that essential oils should not replace a proper warm-up, stretching, or relaxation routine. They can supplement and enhance your workout experience, but they should not be relied upon as the sole means of achieving optimal performance or preventing injury.

Enjoy the invigorating and invigorating benefits of essential oils during your workout, and adjust your usage to your preference and comfort.

G. Aromatherapy for Mental Fatigue

Mental fatigue can significantly impact our energy levels, making it challenging to stay focused, motivated, and productive. It is important to address mental fatigue to maintain optimal energy levels. Here are some strategies to help combat mental fatigue:

1. Rest and sleep: Prioritize getting enough restful sleep every night. Aim for 7 to 9 hours of sleep to allow your brain to recover and recharge. Additionally, take breaks during the day to rest and refresh. Even a few minutes of deep breathing or meditation can help restore your mental energy.

2. Manage stress: Chronic stress can lead to mental fatigue. Identify the stressors in your life and find healthy ways to manage and reduce them. This may include practicing relaxation techniques such as deep breathing exercises and meditation or engaging in activities that bring you joy and relaxation.

3. Rest and exercise: Incorporate regular breaks into your day, especially during mentally demanding tasks. Taking short breaks to stretch, walk, or engage in light physical activity can help refresh your mind and prevent mental fatigue.

4. Prioritize tasks: Organize and prioritize your tasks based on importance and urgency. Breaking larger tasks into smaller, manageable steps can help prevent mental overwhelm and make it easier to focus on one thing at a time.

5. Mental stimulation: Engage in activities stimulating the mind and providing mental challenge. This might include reading, doing puzzles, learning a new skill, or engaging in a creative hobby. Mental stimulation helps keep the brain active and can reduce mental fatigue.

6. Healthy lifestyle: Healthy lifestyles can support mental and physical energy levels. This includes eating a balanced diet, staying hydrated, and engaging in regular physical activity. Proper nutrition and exercise contribute to overall health and help combat mental fatigue.

7. Essential oils for mental fatigue: Essential oils are also helpful in combating mental fatigue. Oils such as peppermint, rosemary, lemon, and lavender have uplifting and refreshing properties. Diffusing these oils or using them in an inhalation technique can help invigorate the mind and promote mental clarity.

Remember, if mental fatigue persists or interferes with your daily functioning, it is important to consult a healthcare professional for further evaluation and guidance.

By implementing these strategies and taking care of your mental health, you can effectively manage mental fatigue and maintain optimal energy levels throughout the day.

Essential oils and aromatherapy techniques can be powerful tools in combating mental exhaustion and promoting mental clarity. Here's how to introduce essential oils and aromatherapy into your daily routine:

1. Inhalation: Inhalation is one of the most common and effective ways to experience the mental fatigue benefits of essential oils. You can inhale the scent directly from the bottle, use a personal inhaler, or add a few drops to a tissue or cotton ball. Oils such as peppermint, rosemary, lemon, and eucalyptus are known for their uplifting and energizing properties. Inhaling these oils can help stimulate the mind, increase alertness, and promote mental clarity.

2. Diffuse: Using an essential oil diffuser is another popular way to enjoy the benefits of aromatherapy. Add a few drops of essential oil to a diffuser and let it disperse the scent throughout the space. Diffuse oils such as lemon, grapefruit, bergamot, or uplifting oil blends can create a fresh and energizing environment that can help combat mental exhaustion and enhance mental focus.

3. Topical application: The topical application of diluted essential oils provides a localized and sustained aroma experience. You can create a roll-on mixture by diluting essential oils with a carrier oil, such as jojoba or sweet almond, and applying it to your pulse points, temples, or the back of your neck. This allows you to enjoy the benefits of essential oils throughout the day and promotes mental clarity.

4. Aromatherapy bath: Adding a few drops of essential oils to your bath can create a relaxing and rejuvenating experience. Choose oils like lavender, frankincense, or chamomile to help calm the mind, reduce stress, and

promote mental clarity. Warm water and aroma can provide a soothing atmosphere and support mental health.

5. Mindfulness meditation: Incorporate essential oils into your mindfulness or meditation practice. Before you begin, apply a small amount of the diluted oil to your palms or wrists, rub them together, and inhale deeply. This can help create a sensory anchor and enhance your focus during meditation, promoting mental clarity and reducing mental exhaustion.

6. Personalized blends: Try creating your blend of essential oils to suit your specific needs and preferences. Mix oils with lifting and clarifying properties (such as peppermint, rosemary, lemon, and lavender) in proportions that resonate with you. You can create a roll-on blend, room spray, or inhalation blend based on your unique requirements.

When using essential oils topically, remember to follow proper dilution guidelines and safety precautions. Additionally, individuals may react differently to essential oils, so paying attention to your body's reactions and adjusting your use accordingly is important.

Incorporating essential oils and aromatherapy techniques into your daily life can combat mental exhaustion, promote mental clarity, and create a more balanced and energized state of mind.

H. Healthy Lifestyle Factors that Enhance Energy

Maintaining optimal energy levels involves more than just using essential oils and aromatherapy techniques. Lifestyle factors play a vital role in supporting your energy levels and overall health. Here are some important considerations:

1. Sleep: Prioritize getting enough restful sleep every night. Aim for 7 to 9 hours of uninterrupted sleep to recharge your body and mind. Establish a consistent sleep schedule, create a soothing bedtime routine, and create a sleep-friendly environment to promote quality sleep.

2. Nutrition: Provide energy to your body with a balanced diet that includes a variety of nutrient-dense foods. Focus on whole grains, lean proteins, fruits, vegetables, and healthy fats. Avoid excessive intake of processed foods, refined sugar, and caffeine, as they can cause energy crashes and affect sleep quality. Drink plenty of water throughout the day to stay hydrated.

3. Hydrate: Dehydration can lead to fatigue and a sluggish feeling. Make sure you drink enough water throughout the day to stay hydrated. Carry a reusable water bottle with you to remind you to drink water regularly.

4. Stress Management: Chronic stress can deplete your energy reserves. Find healthy ways to manage stress, such as practicing relaxation techniques, getting regular physical activity, spending time in nature, practicing mindfulness or meditation, and engaging in activities you enjoy. Prioritize self-care and make time for activities that promote relaxation and reduce stress.

5. Physical activity: Regular physical activity has many benefits, including improving energy levels. Engage in an activity you enjoy, whether it's walking, jogging, biking, dancing, or practicing yoga. Exercise helps increase circulation, releases endorphins, and enhances overall health.

6. Time management: Effective time management can prevent feelings of being overwhelmed and exhausted. Prioritize tasks, set realistic goals, and break them down into manageable steps. Practice delegation, eliminate unnecessary distractions, take regular breaks, and recharge.

7. Mindfulness and Relaxation: Incorporate mindfulness practices into your daily life. This can include deep breathing exercises, meditation, or engaging in activities that promote relaxation, such as listening to calming music or practicing gentle stretches.

Everyone's needs and circumstances are unique, so it's important to listen to your body and make adjustments that work best for you. Maintaining a balanced and healthy lifestyle, as well as incorporating essential oils and aromatherapy techniques, can help you maintain optimal energy levels and promote overall health.

Incorporating essential oils into a holistic energy-boosting approach can provide a synergistic effect. Here are some practical tips to help you get the most out of essential oils to boost your energy levels:

1. Create a daily ritual: Use essential oils to create a daily ritual to start your day. This might include diffusing an energy oil like peppermint, citrus, or rosemary as you get ready in the morning or applying a roll-on refreshing oil blend to your pulse points to start your day on a refreshing note.

2. Take your inhaler with you: Carry a personal inhaler or a small

bottle of essential oil with you throughout the day. Whenever you need a quick boost of energy, take a moment to inhale the scent directly from the bottle or use an inhaler to stimulate your senses. This is especially helpful during a mid-day slump or when you need a pick-me-up.

3. Vitality Workstation: Create an energizing environment in your workspace by diffusing stimulating essential oils. A blend of peppermint, lemon, or citrus oils can help improve focus, mental clarity, and productivity. Alternatively, you can keep a small plate of energy oil-infused cotton balls on your desk and inhale the scent when needed.

4. DIY Body and Massage Oils: Create your own energizing body or massage oil blend by combining carrier oil with invigorating essential oils. For example, mix a few drops of peppermint, rosemary, or eucalyptus essential oil with a carrier oil like sweet almond or jojoba. Apply the mixture to your wrists, temples, or the back of your neck for a boost of energy.

5. Refreshing Shower or Bath: Add a few drops of energizing essential oils to your shower or bath routine. Steam and warm water will help disperse the aroma, creating a refreshing and uplifting experience. You can use oils like eucalyptus, grapefruit, or citrus blends to awaken your senses and boost your energy.

6. Aromatherapy Blends for Exercise: Create a pre-workout or exercise blend using essential oils known for their invigorating properties. Mix oils like peppermint, orange, and ginger with a carrier oil and apply it to your pulse points before exercising. The uplifting aroma helps you feel energized and motivated during physical activities.

7. Relax before bed: While essential oils are often associated with energizing effects, they can also support a restful night's sleep. Establish a bedtime routine by diffusing a relaxing oil like lavender or chamomile in the evening to relax and promote quality sleep. Restful sleep plays a vital role in maintaining energy levels throughout the day.

Remember to follow proper dilution guidelines, perform a patch test, and consult resources for using essential oils safely. Additionally, listen to how your body responds to different oils and tailor your use to your preferences and needs.

Incorporating essential oils into your daily routine as part of a holistic energy-boosting approach can provide a natural and aromatic boost to support your overall health.

3.2 Support Muscle Recovery

This chapter'll explore how essential oils can support men's muscle recovery process. We delve into the soothing and rejuvenating properties of essential oils to guide you on using them safely and effectively to promote muscle recovery and relieve post-workout soreness.

A. Understanding Muscle Recovery

Muscle recovery is a critical process that occurs after strenuous physical activity or exercise. It involves several physiological mechanisms that help repair and rebuild muscle tissue, restore energy reserves, and reduce inflammation. Here's an overview of the muscle recovery process and the importance of proper rest and care:

1. Muscle damage: During exercise, especially high-intensity or resistance training, muscles experience microscopic damage at the cellular level. This damage triggers an inflammatory response and sets the stage for the recovery process.

2. Inflammation and repair: Inflammation occurs in response to muscle damage as a natural protective mechanism. It helps remove damaged cells and initiates the repair process. During this phase, the body releases various substances that promote tissue regeneration and healing.

3. Protein Synthesis: Protein synthesis is a key aspect of muscle recovery. It involves the production and incorporation of new proteins into muscle fibers, leading to muscle growth and repair. Adequate protein intake is essential to support this process.

4. Energy recovery: Intense exercise depletes energy stores in the form of glycogen. During the recovery phase, the body replenishes glycogen stores to ensure an adequate energy supply for future physical activity.

5. Rest and sleep: Rest is essential for muscle recovery. It allows the body to divert resources to repair and rebuild muscle tissue. Sleep plays a vital role in muscle recovery as it promotes hormone regulation, protein synthesis, and tissue repair.

6. Hydration: Proper hydration is important for muscle recovery because it helps maintain optimal cell function, nutrient delivery, and waste removal. Drink enough water and electrolyte-rich fluids to support the recovery process.

7. Nutrition: Providing the body with adequate nutrients is crucial for muscle recovery. A balanced diet that includes carbohydrates, protein, healthy fats, vitamins, and minerals supports tissue repair, energy replenishment, and overall recovery.

8. Active recovery: Mild, low-impact exercise or activities, called active recovery, can help muscles recover. Performing gentle movements, stretches, or low-impact exercises can help increase blood flow to your muscles, reduce muscle soreness, and promote healing.

9. Avoid overtraining: Overtraining can hinder muscle recovery and lead to chronic fatigue, decreased performance, and increased risk of injury. It is important to allow for adequate rest days and avoid excessive training volume or intensity.

10. Self-care practices: Incorporating self-care practices like massage, foam rolling, and heat or cold therapy can help relieve muscle soreness, improve circulation, and enhance the recovery process.

By prioritizing proper rest, nutrition, hydration, and self-care practices, you can optimize the muscle recovery process and promote overall muscle health and performance. Remember to listen to your body and adjust your training routine accordingly to allow for adequate recovery time.

Men face several common challenges with muscle recovery, including delayed onset muscle soreness (DOMS), inflammation, fatigue, and stress. Essential oils can provide potential benefits to address these challenges and support muscle recovery in the following ways:

1. Pain relief: Essential oils such as peppermint, lavender, and eucalyptus have analgesic properties that can help relieve muscle soreness and discomfort associated with DOMS. They can be used topically with a massage or added to bath water for a soothing effect.

2. Anti-inflammatory properties: Essential oils such as frankincense, turmeric, and ginger have anti-inflammatory properties that help reduce inflammation in muscles and joints. They can be applied topically or used in

aromatherapy to promote a calming effect.

3. Energy boost: Essential oils like citrus oils (such as lemon, grapefruit, and orange) and peppermint are known for their uplifting and energizing properties. Inhaling these oils or using them in a diffuser can provide a natural energy boost during exercise or help overcome fatigue.

4. Relieve stress: Stress and elevated cortisol levels can hinder muscle recovery. Essential oils like lavender, chamomile, and bergamot have calm and relaxing properties that can help reduce stress and promote restful sleep, which is essential for muscle repair.

5. Improves sleep: Essential oils like lavender, cedarwood, and vetiver are known for their sleep-inducing properties. Diffusing these oils or applying them topically before bed can promote better sleep quality for optimal muscle recovery.

6. Muscle relaxation: Essential oils such as marjoram, sage, and chamomile have muscle-relaxing properties that help relieve tension and promote muscle relaxation after an intense workout. They can be used in massage mixtures or added to bath salts.

7. Wound healing: Some essential oils, including helichrysum, tea tree, and lavender, have antibacterial and wound-healing properties. They can be applied topically to minor cuts, scrapes, or bruises that may occur during exercise, promoting faster healing and reducing the risk of infection.

It is important to note that while essential oils can provide potential benefits, they should be used safely and within proper dilution guidelines. Everyone may react differently to essential oils, so conducting a patch test and consulting a qualified aromatherapist or healthcare professional is recommended before incorporating essential oils into your muscle recovery routine.

B. Soothing Essential Oils Promote Muscle Recovery

Essential oils known for their calming and soothing properties include:

1. Lavender: Lavender oil is widely recognized for its relaxing and calming effects. It can help reduce stress, promote better sleep, and relieve muscle tension.

2. Chamomile: Chamomile oil, especially Roman chamomile, has mild sedative properties and is often used to promote relaxation, relieve anxiety, and support restful sleep.

3. Marjoram: Marjoram oil has soothing properties that can help calm the mind and relax the body. It may also help relieve muscle tension and promote a sense of tranquility.

4. Eucalyptus: While eucalyptus oil is best known for its respiratory benefits, it also helps calm the environment. Its uplifting and soothing aroma helps clear the mind and promotes a feeling of relaxation.

These essential oils can be used alone or in combination to create a calming and soothing blend. They can be diffused, inhaled, or used topically (diluted with a carrier oil) during relaxation practices, before bed, or when seeking tranquility and stress relief moments.

It's important to note that essential oils affect individuals differently, and personal preferences may vary. It is recommended to patch test and use essential oils following proper dilution guidelines and safety precautions.

The essential oils mentioned, such as lavender, chamomile, marjoram, and eucalyptus, can relieve muscle tension, reduce inflammation, and promote relaxation. Here's a closer look at how each oil promotes these effects:

1. Lavender: Lavender oil has calming properties that help relax the mind and body. It relieves muscle tension and promotes a feeling of relaxation. Lavender oil may also have mild analgesic properties, helping to relieve discomfort associated with muscle tension.

2. Chamomile: Chamomile oil is known for its calming and anti-inflammatory properties. It can help reduce muscle inflammation, relieve tension, and promote relaxation. Chamomile oil is especially beneficial for soothing sore muscles and aiding post-workout recovery.

3. Marjoram: Marjoram oil is known for its muscle-relaxing and anti-inflammatory properties. It can help relieve muscle tension, reduce inflammation, and promote a sense of calm. Marjoram oil may also help improve sleep quality, leading to better muscle recovery.

4. Eucalyptus: Eucalyptus oil has uplifting and soothing properties. It can help reduce muscle tension and promote relaxation through its cooling

and refreshing properties. Eucalyptus oil also has potential anti-inflammatory properties and can help reduce inflammation in muscles and joints.

When applied topically through massage or used in the bath, these essential oils can help release muscle tension, improve blood circulation, and provide a soothing sensation. Inhaling aromatic vapors through a diffuser or inhalation technique can also help with feelings of relaxation and calm.

It is important to note that essential oils should be used appropriately and diluted appropriately. They are generally safe for most people when used as directed, but individual sensitivities and allergies may vary. If you have any underlying health conditions or concerns, it is recommended that you consult a qualified aromatherapist or healthcare professional before using essential oils.

C. Topical Application for Muscle Recovery

When using essential oils topically for muscle recovery, be sure to follow these safe and effective application guidelines:

1. Dilution: Essential oils are highly concentrated and should be diluted before applying to the skin. Dilute essential oils in a carrier oil, such as sweet almond, coconut, or jojoba, to ensure proper absorption and reduce the risk of skin irritation. For most adults, a general guideline for dilution is 2 to 3 drops of essential oil per teaspoon (5 ml) of carrier oil.

2. Patch test: Conduct a patch test before applying the essential oil mixture to a larger area of the skin. Apply a small amount of diluted essential oil to a small area of skin, such as the inner forearm, and wait 24 hours to check for any adverse reactions or sensitivity.

3. Targeted application: Apply the diluted essential oil mixture directly to the affected area. Gently massage the oil into the skin using circular motions to promote absorption and circulation. If you have muscle soreness or tightness in multiple areas, you can also apply the oil blend to those specific areas.

4. Avoid sensitive areas: Keep essential oils away from sensitive areas such as eyes, ears, nose, and mucous membranes. If accidental contact occurs, flush the area with a carrier oil or water to dilute the oil and seek medical attention if necessary.

5. Start with a low concentration: When using essential oils for the

first time, start with a lower concentration and gradually increase if necessary. This allows you to assess your tolerance and sensitivity to the oil.

6. Use high-quality essential oils: Choose high-quality, pure essential oils from reputable sources. Look for oils that are labeled therapeutic grade or have been third-party tested for purity and quality.

7. Discontinue use if irritation occurs: If you experience any skin irritation or discomfort after using the essential oil blend, discontinue use immediately. Flush the area with a carrier oil and consult a health care professional if needed.

Please remember that essential oils are not a substitute for professional medical advice or treatment. If you have any underlying medical conditions, are pregnant or nursing, or are taking medications, please consult a qualified healthcare practitioner before using essential oils for muscle recovery.

By following these guidelines, you can safely and effectively incorporate essential oils into your muscle recovery routine to reap their potential benefits.

Proper dilution, carrier oil selection, and massage technique are critical to maximizing the benefits of essential oils during muscle recovery. Here's a breakdown of each aspect:

1. Dilution: Diluting essential oils in a carrier oil is critical to ensuring safe and effective application. For most adults, a general dilution guideline is 2 to 3 drops of essential oil per teaspoon (5ml) of carrier oil. For sensitive skin or when using the oil on children, a lower dilution is recommended. This dilution ratio helps prevent skin irritation and allows for better absorption of essential oils.

2. Carrier oil: Carrier oil is used to dilute essential oils and help them be absorbed into the skin. Some popular carrier oils for muscle recovery include sweet almond oil, coconut oil, jojoba oil, and grapeseed oil. These oils are gentle on the skin, provide nutrients, and enhance the benefits of essential oils. Choose a carrier oil based on your personal preference and skin type.

3. Massage techniques: Massage can further enhance the benefits of essential oils in the muscle recovery process. Here are some massage techniques to consider:

Soft touch: Use long, sweeping strokes and moderate pressure to warm muscles and evenly distribute the essential oil blend.

Kneading: Use kneading, rolling, and squeezing motions to gently engage muscles and release tension.

Rub: Use your fingertips or palms to rub in circular motions, targeting specific areas to allow the essential oil mixture to penetrate more deeply.

Tapping: A gentle tapping or tapping motion with cupped hands or fingertips to activate muscles and increase blood flow.

4. Massage direction: When applying the essential oil mixture, massage in the direction of the muscle fibers. This helps promote relaxation, reduces muscle tension, and supports the recovery process.

5. Allow time for absorption: After applying the essential oil mixture, allow some time for the skin to absorb the oil before covering the area or dressing. This ensures maximum absorption and effectiveness.

Remember that everyone's sensitivity to essential oils may vary, so pay attention to how your body reacts and adjust dilution ratios or carrier oil selection if needed. If you are unsure about the correct technique or have specific concerns, it is recommended that you consult a qualified aromatherapist or massage therapist for personalized guidance.

By following proper dilution techniques, choosing the right carrier oil, and using effective massage techniques, you can maximize the benefits of essential oils during muscle recovery and promote relaxation and relief in targeted areas.

D. Massage Mixture to Relieve Muscles

Here are some massage blend recipes to aid muscle recovery and relieve post-workout soreness:

1. Soothing Blend to Soothe Muscles

* 2 drops of peppermint essential oil
* 2 drops of lavender essential oil
* 2 drops of eucalyptus essential oil
* 2 tablespoons of sweet almond oil (carrier oil)

Combine all ingredients in a small glass bottle and mix well. After your workout, apply a small amount of the mixture to your target muscles. Massage gently in circular motions to promote relaxation and relief.

2. Deep Tissue Recovery Blend

* 4 drops of marjoram essential oil
* 3 drops of rosemary essential oil
* 2 drops of ginger essential oil
* 2 tablespoons of jojoba oil (carrier oil)

Mix essential oils with a carrier oil in a glass bottle. Shake and mix well. Apply the mixture to muscles in need of recovery and massage deeply using kneading and rolling motions to release tension and increase circulation.

3. Anti-Inflammatory Relaxing Blend

* 3 drops of chamomile essential oil
* 3 drops of frankincense essential oil
* 2 drops of geranium essential oil
* 2 tablespoons of coconut oil (carrier oil)

Combine the essential oils with the carrier oil in a small container and mix well. Apply the mixture to targeted muscles and massage gently to help reduce inflammation and induce relaxation.

Remember to patch-test any new mixture before using it on a larger area of skin. These blends are used for general muscle recovery, but individual reactions may vary. Adjust the number of essential oils or types of carrier oil based on personal preference and sensitivity.

Always consult a healthcare professional if you have any underlying medical conditions or concerns. These mixtures are not intended to replace professional medical advice or treatment.

Enjoy the soothing benefits of these massage blends as part of your muscle recovery routine.

Here are some essential oil combinations that can improve circulation, reduce inflammation, and relieve muscle discomfort:

1. Mixtures that Promote Circulation

* 3 drops of rosemary essential oil
* 3 drops of black pepper essential oil
* 2 drops of ginger essential oil
* 2 tablespoons of grapeseed oil (carrier oil)

This blend helps improve circulation and blood flow to support muscle recovery and reduce discomfort. Mix the essential oil with a carrier oil and massage the mixture into target areas with upward pressure.

2. Anti-Inflammatory Relief Blend

* 4 drops of lavender essential oil
* 3 drops of frankincense essential oil
* 2 drops of helichrysum essential oil
* 2 tablespoons of sweet almond oil (carrier oil)

This mixture can help reduce inflammation and relieve muscle discomfort. Mix the essential oil with a carrier oil and gently massage the mixture into the affected muscles in a circular motion.

3. Muscle Soothing Blend

* 3 drops of peppermint essential oil
* 3 drops of eucalyptus essential oil
* 2 drops of marjoram essential oil
* 2 tablespoons of coconut oil (carrier oil)

This mixture has a cooling and soothing effect on the skin, helping to relieve discomfort. Mix the essential oil with a carrier oil and apply the mixture to the muscles using gentle massage techniques.

Remember to patch-test these mixtures before applying them to larger areas of your skin. Adjust the number of essential oils or types of carrier oil based on personal preference and sensitivity. If you experience any adverse reactions, discontinue use and consult a health care professional.

These essential oil combinations can be used as part of a muscle discomfort management program. However, it is important to note that individual reactions may vary, and these mixtures are not intended to be a substitute for professional medical advice or treatment.

E. Bathing and Applying Muscle Recovery

Introducing essential oils into baths and compresses can be a great way to provide targeted muscle relief. Here's how to incorporate essential oils into these methods:

1. Bath and Soak

Fill the tub with warm water.

Add 5 to 10 drops of your chosen essential oil to a carrier substance such as Epsom salt, Himalayan salt, or a dispersing agent such as milk or natural liquid soap. This helps the essential oils disperse evenly throughout the bath water.

Swirl the water to ensure the oil is thoroughly mixed.

Soak yourself in the tub and soak for 15 to 20 minutes to let the oils work their magic on your muscles.

Breathe slowly and deeply to enjoy the benefits of aromatherapy fully.

Essential oils suitable for soaking include lavender, chamomile, eucalyptus, and rosemary. These oils can help promote relaxation, reduce muscle tension, and provide a soothing experience.

2. Apply

Fill a basin or large bowl with warm water.

Add 3 to 5 drops of your chosen essential oil to the water and mix gently.

Soak a clean cloth or towel in water so that it absorbs the essential oil-soaked water.

Wring out excess water and apply the heat directly to the target area of muscle discomfort.

Leave the dressing in place for 10 to 15 minutes, resoaking and re-wringing the cloth as needed to retain warmth and fragrance.

Relax and let the essential oils penetrate the muscles, relieving and relaxing.

The application is particularly effective for localized muscle discomfort or tension. Essential oils such as peppermint, ginger, and marjoram benefit this dressing because of their soothing and warming properties.

Remember, essential oils are highly concentrated, so be sure to dilute them before bathing or applying. If you have any allergies or sensitivities, do a patch test before using the oil. Additionally, if you have any underlying medical conditions or concerns, please consult a healthcare professional.

Enjoy the rejuvenating and relaxing benefits of essential oil soaks and wraps as part of a muscle relief routine.

Here are instructions for creating a bath mixture and using a compress to support muscle recovery:

Create a bath mix:

1. Muscle relaxing bath soak

Combine 1 cup Epsom salt and 5 drops of lavender essential oil in a small bowl.
Mix thoroughly so that the essential oils are evenly distributed.
Add the mixture to warm wash water and stir to dissolve.
Soak in the tub for 20 to 30 minutes to relax and soothe your muscles.

2. Refreshing muscle recovery bath soak

In a small bowl, combine 1 cup Himalayan salt, 5 drops of peppermint essential oil, and 3 drops of eucalyptus essential oil.
Stir the mixture well to incorporate the essential oils.
Add the mixture to warm wash water and swirl to dissolve.
Immerse yourself in the tub and enjoy the refreshing scent while the salts and oils support your muscle recovery.

Using patches for muscle recovery:

1. Hot compress

Fill a basin or sink with warm water.
Add 3 to 5 drops of your chosen essential oil to the water and mix gently.
Soak a clean cloth or towel in water so that it absorbs the essential oil-soaked water.
Wring out excess water and apply heat to targeted muscle areas.
Leave the dressing in place for 10 to 15 minutes to allow the warmth and essential oils to penetrate and relax your muscles.

2. Cold compress

Fill a basin or sink with cold water.

Add 3 to 5 drops of your chosen essential oil to the water and mix gently.

Soak a clean cloth or towel in water, making sure it absorbs the essential oil-soaked water.

Wring out excess water and apply a cold compress to the affected muscle area.

Leave the dressing in place for 10 to 15 minutes to help reduce inflammation and relieve symptoms.

Remember to adjust the amount of essential oil according to your preference and dilution guidelines. Always conduct a patch test before using the mixture on larger areas of skin, and consult a healthcare professional if you have any questions or underlying health conditions.

These soaking mixtures and dressing techniques provide relaxation and support muscle recovery. Incorporate them into your daily routine as needed, and enjoy the soothing benefits of essential oils for muscle relief.

F. Warm-up and Cool-down Rituals

Adding essential oils to your warm-up and cool-down routine can greatly enhance muscle recovery. Here's why it's important and how to do it:

1. Warm-up procedure:

Essential oils can help prepare your muscles for physical activity by increasing blood flow and promoting flexibility.

Apply the diluted essential oil mixture to the targeted muscles before beginning your warm-up exercise. Good choices include peppermint, eucalyptus, and rosemary, known for their uplifting and warming properties.

Gently massage the essential oil into your muscles to allow it to absorb and stimulate blood circulation.

As you begin your warm-up, breathe deeply to inhale aromatic molecules, which can help lift your mood and improve focus.

Incorporating essential oils into your warm-up routine can increase circulation, relax muscles, and mentally prepare for physical activity.

2. Cooling procedure:

Essential oils can aid the recovery process by reducing inflammation, soothing muscles, and promoting relaxation.

After completing your workout, apply the cooling essential oil blend to the targeted muscles. Consider oils like lavender, chamomile, or helichrysum, known for their calming and anti-inflammatory properties.

Gently massage the oil into the muscles to provide a cooling and soothing sensation.

Use this time to practice deep breathing exercises and inhale the aroma of essential oils, which can promote relaxation and help reduce stress.

Adding essential oils to your cooling routine can help relieve muscle soreness, reduce inflammation, and promote calm and relaxation.

Remember to dilute essential oils correctly before applying them to your skin, and do a patch test to make sure you don't have sensitivities. Additionally, please be aware of your body's specific needs and sensitivities and consult a healthcare professional if you have any concerns or underlying health conditions.

Incorporating essential oils into your warm-up and cool-down routine can enhance muscle recovery, promote relaxation, and support overall health during fitness.

Here are some specific essential oils and techniques that can prepare the body for exercise and promote post-workout relaxation:

1. Pre-workout essential oils and techniques:

* Peppermint: Peppermint essential oil is known for its uplifting properties that can help increase energy and mental focus. Apply the diluted solution to your temples, wrists, or chest before exercise for a refreshing effect.

* Eucalyptus: Eucalyptus essential oil has cooling and decongestant properties that can help clear the airways and enhance breathing. Diffuse it or apply a diluted solution to your chest or back before exercise to support respiratory function.

* Dynamic Stretching: Before a workout, incorporate dynamic stretching that involves active movement. Combine these stretches with deep inhales and exhales to energize your body and improve flexibility.

2. Post-Workout Essential Oils and Techniques:

* Lavender: Lavender essential oil is known for its calming and soothing properties, helping to promote relaxation and relieve muscle tension. Add a few drops to a warm bath or mix it with carrier oil for a relaxing post-workout massage.

* Chamomile: Chamomile essential oil is known for its calming effects on the mind and body. Diffuse it or use a diluted solution to promote relaxation and support restful sleep after exercise.

Static Stretching: After a workout, incorporate static stretching, including holding stretches for long periods. Combine these stretches with slow, deep breathing to help muscles recover and relax.

Additionally, you can combine different essential oils to create a personalized blend based on your preferences and desired effects. For example, combining lavender, peppermint, and eucalyptus can provide a refreshing and calming post-workout experience.

Remember to dilute essential oils correctly before applying them to your skin and perform a patch test to check for any sensitivities. If you have any underlying health conditions or concerns, please consult a healthcare professional before using essential oils.

Incorporating these specific essential oils and techniques into your pre- and post-workout routine can help prepare your body for your workout, enhance your workout experience, and promote relaxation and muscle recovery afterward.

G. Supports Joint Health and Flexibility

Here are some essential oils that are known for their potential to support joint health, reduce stiffness, and improve flexibility:

1. Frankincense: Frankincense essential oil has anti-inflammatory properties that may help reduce joint inflammation and discomfort. It can be applied topically to affected areas or diffused for its soothing aroma.

2. Ginger: Ginger essential oil is known for its warming and anti-inflammatory properties. It can help relieve joint stiffness and promote better flexibility. Dilute with a carrier oil and massage into joints, or add a few drops to a warm compress for topical relief.

3. Wintergreen: Wintergreen essential oil contains a compound called methyl salicylate, which has analgesic and anti-inflammatory properties. It can be applied topically to support joint health and relieve discomfort. However, it is important to use wintergreen oil with caution and in diluted form, as it is effective.

4. Cypress: Cypress essential oil has astringent properties that may help improve circulation and reduce fluid retention around joints. It can be mixed with carrier oil and massaged into affected areas to support joint health.

5. Helichrysum: Helichrysum essential oil is known for its anti-inflammatory properties and may help reduce inflammation and promote joint comfort. It can be diluted and applied topically to the affected joint.

6. Turmeric: Although not an essential oil, turmeric essential oil contains the active compound curcumin, which is known for its powerful anti-inflammatory effects. It can be used topically by diluting it with a carrier oil and applying it to the affected area.

Remember to dilute essential oils correctly before applying them to your skin, and do a patch test to check for any sensitivities. Everyone may react differently to essential oils, so it's important to find the oil and dilution ratio that works best for you. If you have any underlying health conditions or concerns, please consult a healthcare professional before using essential oils.

Incorporating these essential oils into your wellness routine, along with proper joint care and exercise, can support joint health, reduce stiffness, and improve flexibility.

Here are some guidelines for incorporating essential oils known for promoting joint mobility and comfort into your daily routine:

1. Local application:

Dilute 2 to 3 drops of essential oil, such as sweet almond or coconut oil, with a carrier oil to create a topical mixture.
Massage the mixture into the affected and surrounding areas using gentle circular motions.
Apply the mixture morning and evening or as needed throughout the day to support joint health and mobility.

2. Hot compress:

Add a few drops of essential oil to a bowl of warm water.

Soak a clean cloth or towel in water, wring out the excess, and apply it to the affected joint.

Leave the compress on for 10 to 15 minutes to allow the warmth and essential oil vapor to penetrate the joints and provide relief.

3. Aromatherapy:

Use an essential oil diffuser or aromatherapy necklace to diffuse essential oils in your living space.

Choose essential oils like frankincense, ginger, or cypress to create a soothing and supportive environment for joint health.

Inhale aromatic molecules throughout the day and experience their benefits.

4. Bath and soak:

Add a few drops of essential oil to a warm bath.

Stir the water to disperse the oil.

Soak in the bathtub for 15 to 20 minutes to relax muscles and promote joint comfort.

5. Mix:

Try creating your blends using the essential oils listed above, or try premade blends designed for joint support.

Mix different oils in a roller bottle for easy and targeted application.

Personalize the proportions and scent to your preferences and needs.

Remember to follow proper dilution guidelines and perform a patch test before applying essential oils to your skin. It's crucial to listen to your body and adjust the frequency and amount of essential oil use based on your comfort and response.

Incorporating these essential oils into your daily routine can help promote overall joint mobility and comfort. However, it is important to note that essential oils should not be used as a substitute for professional medical advice. If you have chronic or severe joint problems, it is recommended that you consult a healthcare professional for a comprehensive approach to joint health.

H. Lifestyle Factors for Optimal Muscle Recovery

Proper nutrition, hydration, sleep, and stress management play important roles in supporting muscle recovery. Here's why each of these factors is important:

1. Nutrition:

Eat a balanced diet with enough protein, carbohydrates, and healthy fats to provide the necessary nutrients for muscle repair and growth.

Protein is particularly important because it provides the amino acids needed for muscle tissue repair. Include lean protein sources such as chicken, fish, beans, and tofu in your meals.

Carbohydrates provide energy for exercise and replenish glycogen stores in muscles. Choose complex carbohydrates such as whole grains, fruits, and vegetables.

Healthy fats, like those found in avocados, nuts, and olive oil, help reduce inflammation and support overall health.

2. Hydration:

Staying hydrated is crucial for muscle recovery. Water helps transport nutrients to muscles and remove waste products.
Aim to drink enough water throughout the day, especially during and after exercise. The exact amount varies based on factors such as weight, activity level, and climate.

3. Sleep:

Quality sleep is essential for muscle recovery and growth. during sleep, The body repairs damaged tissue and release growth hormones.

Aim for 7 to 9 hours of uninterrupted sleep every night. Establish a consistent sleep schedule and create a relaxing bedtime routine to promote better sleep.

4. Stress management:

Chronic stress can interfere with muscle recovery. High levels of stress hormones, such as cortisol, can negatively impact muscle growth and repair.

Engage in stress-reducing activities such as meditation, deep breathing exercises, yoga, or a hobby you enjoy.

Prioritize relaxation and self-care to support your overall health and enhance muscle recovery.

By focusing on these aspects of your lifestyle, you can create an environment that supports optimal muscle recovery and growth. Remember, it's important to listen to your body and give yourself enough rest and recovery time between workouts. Additionally, please consult a healthcare professional or registered dietitian for personalized advice based on your specific needs and goals.

Essential oils can complement lifestyle and enhance the recovery process. Here's how to integrate them to optimize muscle recovery:

1 Massage and topical application:

Essential oils can be diluted with a carrier oil and used to massage sore muscles. Gentle massage helps improve blood circulation and relax muscles.

Popular essential oils used for muscle recovery include lavender, peppermint, eucalyptus, and rosemary. These oils have soothing, cooling, and anti-inflammatory properties.

Apply a diluted essential oil mixture to affected areas after exercise or before bed to promote relaxation and aid muscle recovery.

2. Aromatherapy:

in a recovery space, using them in your bath can create a relaxing and rejuvenating atmosphere.

Lavender, chamomile, and frankincense are known for their calming and stress-relieving properties. They can help promote relaxation and quality sleep, which is essential for muscle recovery.

Peppermint and eucalyptus oils are energizing and cooling. Inhaling these oils during or after a workout can provide a refreshing feeling and relieve muscle fatigue.

3. Epsom Salt Bath Soak:

Add a few drops of essential oils to your Epsom salt bath to further enhance the relaxation and recovery process. Epsom salt baths help soothe sore muscles and provide minerals like magnesium to aid muscle recovery. Consider using essential oils like lavender, chamomile, or eucalyptus to create a therapeutic bath experience.

4. Inhalation technique:

Inhaling essential oils directly or through an inhalation device can produce an energizing or calming effect, depending on the essential oil used. For example, inhaling citrus oils like lemon or orange can provide refreshing and uplifting effects that can help combat mental fatigue and improve mood.

It is important to note that essential oils should be used with caution, and individual reactions may vary. Always dilute essential oils correctly and perform a patch test before applying them to your skin. If you have any underlying health conditions or concerns, please consult a healthcare professional before using essential oils.

Incorporating essential oils into your recovery routine can enhance relaxation, promote muscle recovery, and create a more enjoyable and rejuvenating experience. Experiment with different oils to find the best scent and method for you.

3.3 Relieve Joint and Muscle Discomfort

This section will explore how essential oils can relieve joint and muscle discomfort. We discuss the soothing properties of essential oils and provide practical guidance on their safe and effective use to relieve pain, reduce inflammation, and promote overall comfort.

A. Understanding Joint and Muscle Discomfort

Men may experience joint and muscle discomfort due to various factors. Here are some common causes and types of discomfort:

1. Physical overexertion: Engaging in strenuous physical activities or repetitive movements can lead to muscle strain, fatigue, and discomfort. It can occur during exercise, lifting weights, or even everyday activities that involve

lifting weights or repetitive movements.

2. Joint conditions: Men may experience joint discomfort due to diseases such as osteoarthritis, rheumatoid arthritis, gout, or tendonitis. These conditions can lead to joint inflammation, stiffness, and joint pain.

3. Injuries: Accidents, falls, or sports-related injuries can cause joint and muscle discomfort. Sprains, strains, dislocations, and fractures can cause acute pain and require appropriate medical care.

4. Posture and Ergonomics: Poor posture, improper lifting technique, and sitting or standing in incorrect postures for long periods can strain muscles and joints, causing discomfort over time.

5. Age-related factors: As men age, they may experience joint and muscle discomfort due to the natural wear and tear of the body. Conditions such as degenerative disc disease, spinal stenosis, or age-related joint degeneration can cause discomfort.

6. Inflammation: Inflammatory conditions such as bursitis, tendinitis, or fibromyalgia can cause ongoing joint and muscle discomfort. Inflammation in the body can cause pain and reduced mobility.

It is important for men who experience joint and muscle discomfort to consult a healthcare professional for proper diagnosis and treatment. Understanding the underlying cause of discomfort is critical to developing an appropriate management plan.

NOTE: This information is for educational purposes only and should not replace professional medical advice. If you are experiencing severe or persistent joint and muscle discomfort, seek medical care for an accurate diagnosis and personalized treatment.

Addressing joint and muscle discomfort is critical to improving mobility and overall quality of life. Here are some key points to highlight:

1. Increased mobility: Joint and muscle discomfort can severely limit mobility, making it challenging to perform daily activities or perform physical exercise. By addressing discomfort, individuals can regain mobility and enjoy a more active lifestyle.

2. Improved function: Joint and muscle discomfort can affect the

function of the affected area, making it difficult to perform tasks that require strength, flexibility, or coordination. By addressing discomfort, individuals can regain function and perform daily activities more easily.

3. Pain management: Joint and muscle discomfort can lead to ongoing pain that affects a person's ability to concentrate, work, and enjoy daily life. Effectively managing discomfort can reduce pain levels, improve comfort, and enhance overall well-being.

4. Prevent further complications: Ignoring joint and muscle discomfort may lead to further complications over time. Discomfort must be addressed promptly to prevent the worsening of the underlying condition and potential long-term consequences.

5. Improves quality of life: Ongoing joint and muscle discomfort can significantly impact a person's overall quality of life, leading to depression, reduced productivity, and emotional distress. By effectively managing and resolving discomfort, individuals can experience a better quality of life and enjoy the activities they enjoy.

It is important to note that appropriate management of joint and muscle discomfort may involve a combination of approaches, including lifestyle changes, physical therapy, medications, and natural remedies such as essential oils. Consulting a healthcare professional or specialist in this area can provide tailored guidance and support to address discomfort and improve mobility.

B. Anti-inflammatory Essential Oils

Certain essential oils are known for their anti-inflammatory properties when it comes to addressing joint and muscle discomfort. Here are some examples:

1. Ginger essential oil: Ginger contains compounds with anti-inflammatory properties, such as gingerol and curcumin. It can help reduce inflammation and relieve joint and muscle discomfort.

2. Frankincense Essential Oil: Frankincense has been traditionally used for its anti-inflammatory effects. It may help reduce inflammation in joints and muscles and promote relief.

3. Turmeric essential Oil: Turmeric contains a compound called cur-

cumin, which has powerful anti-inflammatory properties. It can help relieve joint and muscle discomfort and support overall joint health.

4. Helichrysum essential oil: Helichrysum oil is known for its anti-inflammatory and analgesic properties. It can help reduce inflammation and relieve joint and muscle discomfort.

These essential oils can be used alone or in combination with each other to create a personalized blend to address joint and muscle discomfort. It is important to note that essential oils should be diluted and used correctly according to safety guidelines. Additionally, people who have certain health conditions or are taking medications should consult a healthcare professional before using essential oils.

Ginger, frankincense, turmeric, and helichrysum essential oils have potential benefits in reducing inflammation, swelling, and pain associated with joint and muscle discomfort. Let's take a closer look at their specific properties:

1. Ginger essential oil: Ginger contains gingerol, whose anti-inflammatory effects have been studied. It may help reduce inflammation, swelling, and pain in joints and muscles. Ginger essential oil can be used topically through massage or added to a warm compress.

2. Frankincense essential oil: Frankincense has anti-inflammatory and analgesic properties. It may help relieve inflammation and reduce pain associated with joint and muscle discomfort. It can be applied topically to affected areas or used in aromatherapy because of its calming effects.

3. Turmeric essential oil: Turmeric contains curcumin, a potent anti-inflammatory compound. Turmeric essential oil can help reduce inflammation, swelling, and pain associated with joint and muscle discomfort. It can be used topically or added to a carrier oil for massage.

4. Helichrysum essential oil: Helichrysum oil has anti-inflammatory and analgesic properties, helping to reduce inflammation, swelling, and pain. It can be applied topically to affected areas or used in a massage mixture for targeted relief.

These essential oils can be used individually or in combination, depending on personal preference and needs. They can be diluted in a carrier oil, such as jojoba or coconut oil, and applied to the skin. It is important to perform a patch test and follow proper dilution guidelines to ensure safety and effectiveness.

While essential oils can provide relief, a healthcare professional must be consulted for a proper diagnosis and treatment plan, especially for chronic or severe joint and muscle discomfort.

C. Topical Application for Targeted Relief

When using essential oils topically to treat joint and muscle discomfort, be sure to follow these guidelines for safe and effective use:

1. Dilute essential oils: Essential oils are highly concentrated and should be diluted before applying to the skin. Dilute them with carrier oil, such as coconut oil, sweet almond oil, or jojoba oil. A general guideline is to use a 2 5 dilution, which means adding 10 to 15 drops of essential oil per 1 ounce (30ml) of carrier oil.

2. Conduct a patch test: Before applying any essential oil mixture to a larger area, conduct a patch test. Apply a small amount of the diluted oil to a small area of skin, such as the inside of your forearm. Wait 24 hours and watch for any adverse reactions, such as redness, itching, or irritation.

3. Gentle massage: When applying essential oil, use gentle massage techniques to help the essential oil penetrate the skin and promote absorption. Massage in a circular motion or along the affected area, applying light to moderate pressure.

4. Targeted application: Apply a diluted essential oil mixture directly to affected joints or muscles. You can also apply the mixture to nearby areas for broader coverage. Avoid applying essential oils to broken or irritated skin.

5. Start with a low concentration: If you are new to using essential oils, start with a lower concentration and gradually increase as needed. This allows you to gauge your sensitivity and ensure a comfortable experience.

6. Avoid sensitive areas: Keep essential oils away from sensitive areas such as eyes, ears, nose, and mucous membranes. If accidental contact occurs, rinse with carrier oil or milk and seek medical advice if necessary.

7. Avoid sun exposure: Some essential oils, especially citrus oils, can

cause photosensitivity, making the skin more sensitive to sunlight. Stay out of the sun or use sun protection on areas where you are applying essential oils.

8. Listen to your body: Pay attention to how your body reacts to essential oils. If you experience any discomfort, irritation, or adverse reactions, discontinue use and seek medical advice if necessary.

Remember, it's important to consult a healthcare professional or aromatherapist before using essential oils, especially if you have any underlying health conditions or are taking medications. They can provide personalized guidance based on your specific needs and ensure safe and effective use.

Proper dilution, carrier oil selection, and massage application methods play a vital role in maximizing the effects of essential oils on joint and muscle discomfort. Here are some guidelines to follow:

1. Dilution: Essential oils should be diluted before applying to the skin to avoid skin irritation or sensitization. A common dilution ratio is 2 ~5%, which means adding 10 to 15 drops of essential oil per 1 ounce (30 ml) of carrier oil. Adjust the dilution based on your sensitivity and the specific essential oil you are using.

2. Carrier oil: Carrier oil is used to dilute essential oils and promote their safe application to the skin. Choose a carrier oil that is nourishing and easy to absorb, such as coconut oil, sweet almond oil, jojoba oil, or grapeseed oil. Each carrier oil has unique properties, so choose one that suits your skin type and preferences.

3. Massage techniques: Massage helps enhance the absorption and efficacy of essential oils. Apply the oil mixture to the affected area using gentle circular motions or long, sweeping strokes. Apply light to moderate pressure depending on your comfort and discomfort level.

4. Focus on the affected area: Directly message and apply it to the specific joint or muscle where you are feeling discomfort. Spend extra time in these areas, applying the oil blend in a targeted manner for maximum stress relief.

5. Heat: Consider using a heat compress alongside your essential oils for added comfort and relaxation. Soak a clean cloth in warm water, wring out the excess, and place it over the affected area. This can help relax muscles and enhance the absorption of essential oils.

6. Take your time: Allow enough time for the essential oils to be absorbed and work their magic. Take a moment to relax and enjoy the soothing effects of the massage and the aromatic properties of the essential oils.

Remember to listen to your body and adjust the pressure and intensity of the massage to your comfort level. If you experience any adverse reactions or discomfort, discontinue use and consult a health care professional.

It is important to note that these guidelines are general recommendations, and personal preferences and sensitivities may vary. Always consider your specific needs and consult a qualified aromatherapist or healthcare professional for personalized advice and guidance.

D. Pain Relief Mixtures and Formulations

Here are some blends and formulas that provide targeted pain relief for joint and muscle discomfort:

1. Joint Soothing Blend:

* 5 drops of peppermint essential oil
* 5 drops of lavender essential oil
* 4 drops of eucalyptus essential oil
* 3 drops of ginger essential oil
* 2 tablespoons of carrier oil (such as sweet almond or jojoba)

Mix essential oils with a carrier oil in a dark glass bottle. Shake well before each use. Apply a small amount of the mixture to the affected joint and massage gently.

2. Muscle Relaxation Blend:

* 6 drops of marjoram essential oil
* 4 drops of lavender essential oil
* 3 drops of rosemary essential oil
* 2 drops of frankincense essential oil
* 2 tablespoons of carrier oil (such as coconut oil or grapeseed oil)

Mix essential oils with a carrier oil in a dark glass bottle. Shake well before use. Apply the mixture to the affected muscles and massage gently.

3. Anti-Inflammatory Blend:

* 4 drops of helichrysum essential oil
* 4 drops of turmeric essential oil
* 4 drops of chamomile essential oil
* 3 drops of peppermint essential oil
* 2 tablespoons of carrier oil (such as jojoba or avocado oil)

Mix essential oils with a carrier oil in a dark glass bottle. Shake well before each use. Apply a small amount of the mixture to the affected area and massage gently into the skin.

Remember to do a patch test before using these mixtures on larger areas of the body. Everyone's sensitivity to essential oils may vary, so it's important to adjust the dilution or choose a different essential oil if needed. If you have any existing medical conditions or are taking medications, please consult a healthcare professional before using these mixtures.

These mixtures are for topical use only. If you experience persistent or worsening discomfort, please consult a healthcare professional for further evaluation and guidance.

Here are some combinations of essential oils that can help increase circulation, relax muscles, and relieve pain and inflammation:

1. Circulation Boosting Blend:

* 5 drops of rosemary essential oil
* 4 drops of peppermint essential oil
* 3 drops of ginger essential oil
* 2 drops of cypress essential oil
* 2 tablespoons of carrier oil (such as sweet almond or coconut oil)

Mix essential oils with a carrier oil in a dark glass bottle. Shake well before each use. Apply a small amount of the mixture to the desired area and massage gently to promote blood circulation.

2. Muscle Relaxation Blend:

* 6 drops of lavender essential oil
* 4 drops of marjoram essential oil

* 3 drops of chamomile essential oil
* 2 drops of sage essential oil
* 2 tablespoons of carrier oil (such as jojoba or grapeseed oil)

Mix essential oils with a carrier oil in a dark glass bottle. Shake well before use. Apply the mixture to tense or sore muscles and massage gently to promote relaxation.

3. Pain Relief and Inflammation Blend:

* 4 drops of eucalyptus essential oil
* 4 drops of peppermint essential oil
* 3 drops of helichrysum essential oil
* 2 drops of frankincense essential oil
* 2 tablespoons of carrier oil (such as coconut oil or olive oil)

Mix essential oils with a carrier oil in a dark glass bottle. Shake well before use. Apply the mixture to the affected area and massage gently to help reduce pain and inflammation.

Remember to do a patch test before using these mixtures on larger body areas. Adjust the dilution or choose a different oil if you have sensitivities or allergies. These mixtures are for topical use only, and if you have any underlying health conditions or are taking medications, it is recommended that you consult a healthcare professional before use.

Always listen to your body and discontinue use if any adverse reactions occur. If your symptoms persist or worsen, please seek medical advice for further evaluation and treatment options.

E. Hot Compresses and Soothing Baths

Warm compresses and soothing baths are effective ways to relieve joint and muscle discomfort. Here's how to incorporate essential oils into these practices:

Hot compress:

1. Fill the basin with warm water.
2. Add a few drops of essential oil to the water. Suitable options for joint and muscle discomfort include lavender, eucalyptus, ginger, or chamo-

mile.

3. Gently stir the water to disperse the essential oils.

4. Soak a clean cloth or towel in water and wring out the excess.

5. Apply a hot compress to the affected area and leave it for 10 to 15 minutes.

6. Repeat the process as needed for relief.

Soothing bath:

1. Fill the bathtub with warm water.

2. Add 8 to 10 drops of essential oil of your choice to the water. You can use a single oil or create a blend of complementary oils.

3. Swirl the water to disperse the essential oils.

4. Soak yourself in the bathtub and soak for 15 to 20 minutes to let the essential oils work their magic.

5. Relax and enjoy the soothing effects.

6. Rinse with clean water after bathing.

For hot compresses and baths, it is essential to use high-quality, pure essential oils. Be sure to dilute essential oils in a carrier oil or emulsifier before adding them to water, as essential oils do not mix well with water on their own.

Remember, if you have any pre-existing medical conditions or are taking medications, consult a healthcare professional before using essential oils. Additionally, if you experience any adverse reactions, discontinue use and avoid using essential oils on broken or irritated skin.

Enjoy the therapeutic benefits of essential oils in hot compresses and baths and relieve joint and muscle discomfort.

Here are instructions for creating a hot compress mixture and adding essential oils to your bathing ritual to relieve symptoms:

Hot compress mixture:

1. Fill the basin with warm water.

2. Add 2 cups of warm water to the bowl.

3. Add 3 to 5 drops of essential oil of your choice to warm water. Suitable options for joint and muscle discomfort include lavender, eucalyptus, ginger, or chamomile.

4. Gently stir the water to disperse the essential oils.

5. Soak a clean cloth or towel in water and wring out the excess.

6. Apply a hot compress to the affected area and leave it for 10 to 15 minutes.

7. Repeat the process as needed for relief.

Bathing ritual:

1. Fill the bathtub with warm water.

2. Add 8 to 10 drops of essential oil of your choice to the water. You can use a single oil or create a blend of complementary oils.

3. To ensure proper dispersion, dilute essential oils in a carrier oil or emulsifier before adding them to your bath water. You can mix the essential oil with 1 tablespoon of carrier oil (such as sweet almond or jojoba) or unscented liquid soap.

4. Gently swirl the water to disperse the essential oil mixture.

5. Soak yourself in the bathtub and soak for 15 to 20 minutes to let the essential oils work their magic.

6. Relax, take a deep breath, and enjoy the soothing effects.

7. Rinse with clean water after bathing.

Remember to use high-quality, pure essential oils and perform a patch test before using the mixture on larger areas of the body. If you have sensitivities or allergies, adjust the dilution or choose a different oil. If adverse reactions occur, please stop using it.

Please note that heat and bathing are supportive measures and should not replace professional medical advice. If you have persistent or severe joint and muscle discomfort, please consult a healthcare professional for appropriate evaluation and treatment options.

Enjoy the therapeutic and comforting benefits of essential oils in hot compresses and baths and relieve your joint and muscle discomfort.

F. Support Joint Health and Flexibility

Here are some essential oils known for their potential to support joint health, improve flexibility, and reduce stiffness:

1. Frankincense: Frankincense essential oil is known for its anti-inflammatory properties, which can help reduce inflammation and support joint health. It can also promote relaxation and relieve muscle tension.

2. Peppermint: Peppermint essential oil has a cooling effect and can help soothe and relax muscles. It can also temporarily relieve joint discomfort and stiffness.

3. Ginger: Ginger essential oil has warming properties and is often used to support joint health and relieve muscle discomfort. It may help improve flexibility and mobility.

4. Rosemary: Rosemary essential oil is known for its stimulating and uplifting properties. It may help reduce muscle tension, support circulation, and promote joint flexibility.

5. Marjoram: Marjoram essential oil is often used to soothe tired and overworked muscles. It may help relieve muscle stiffness and promote relaxation.

6. Lavender: Lavender essential oil is known for its calming and soothing effects. It may help reduce muscle tension, relieve joint discomfort, and promote a feeling of relaxation.

7. Helichrysum: Helichrysum essential oil has anti-inflammatory properties and is often used to support joint health. It may help reduce swelling, relieve stiffness, and improve flexibility.

When using essential oils to promote joint health and flexibility, it's important to dilute them appropriately in a carrier oil, such as coconut oil or sweet almond oil, before applying them topically. You can massage the diluted mixture into the affected area or use it for gentle stretching.

It is important to note that essential oils should be used as complementary and not replace professional medical advice. If you have chronic or severe joint problems, it is recommended that you consult a healthcare professional for appropriate evaluation and treatment options.

Experiment with these essential oils to find the one that works best for you to support joint health, increase flexibility, and reduce stiffness.

Here are some ways to incorporate essential oils into your daily life to promote overall joint comfort and mobility:

1. Topical application: Dilute the essential oil of your choice in a carrier oil and apply the mixture to the affected joints. Gently massage the oil into

the skin to promote absorption. You can do this in the morning and evening or throughout the day as needed.

2. Hot compress: Create a hot compress by soaking a cloth in warm water and infusing it with a few drops of essential oil of your choice. Leave the dressing on the joint for 10 to 15 minutes to help soothe and relax the muscles and joints.

3. Bath and soak: Add a few drops of essential oil to warm water and soak for 15 to 20 minutes. Warm water and essential oils can help relax muscles, reduce tension, and support joint comfort.

4. Aromatherapy diffuser: Use an essential oil diffuser to disperse the aroma of essential oils into the air. Inhaling essential oils can be calming and soothing, promoting overall relaxation and joint comfort.

5. Gentle stretching and massage: Perform gentle stretching exercises on your joints before or after physical activity. Apply a diluted essential oil mixture to the skin before stretching or use it during a massage to promote relaxation and movement.

6. Personal care products: Look for natural personal care products like lotions, creams, or balms that contain essential oils known for their joint-supporting properties. Apply these products to your joints as part of your daily skincare routine.

7. Custom blends: Try creating your custom blend by combining different essential oils known for their joint-supporting properties. You can mix and match oils to suit your preferences and needs.

Remember to start with a low dilution and do a patch test before applying the oil to larger areas of the body. Listen to your body and adjust the frequency of use based on your comfort and personal response.

Incorporating these methods into your daily life can help support joint comfort, promote mobility, and enhance overall health. However, it is important to note that essential oils should complement, not replace, professional medical advice. If you have any underlying joint conditions or concerns, it is best to consult a healthcare professional for appropriate guidance.

G. Managing Uncomfortable Lifestyle Factors

Maintaining a healthy lifestyle is crucial to managing joint and muscle discomfort. Here are some key factors to consider:

1. Proper nutrition: A balanced diet that contains a variety of nutrients is essential to support joint and muscle health. Focus on eating foods rich in omega-3 fatty acids (such as fatty fish and walnuts), antioxidants (found in fruits and vegetables), and foods rich in vitamin D and calcium (such as dairy products and green leafy vegetables).

2. Exercise regularly: Regular physical activity helps strengthen the muscles around your joints, improves flexibility, and supports overall joint health. Choose low-impact and gentle exercises on your joints, such as swimming, walking, or biking. Prioritize stretching and strengthening exercises to maintain joint mobility and stability.

3. Weight management: Maintaining a healthy weight is essential for joint health. Being overweight can stress your joints, leading to increased discomfort. Focus on achieving and maintaining a healthy weight through a combination of a balanced diet and regular exercise.

4. Stress management: Chronic stress can exacerbate joint and muscle discomfort. Find healthy ways to manage stress, such as practicing relaxation techniques (such as deep breathing or meditation), taking up hobbies, spending time in nature, or seeking support from a therapist or counselor.

5. Proper posture and body mechanics: Pay attention to your posture and body mechanics during daily activities. Maintaining good posture and using proper body mechanics can help reduce stress on your joints and minimize discomfort.

6. Rest and recovery: Make sure you give your body adequate rest and recovery time between physical activities. Allow adequate sleep and incorporate relaxation techniques into your daily routine to support overall muscle and joint recovery.

By combining these lifestyle factors, along with the use of essential oils and other supplements, you can create a holistic approach to managing joint and muscle discomfort. It is important to consult with a healthcare professional to receive personalized advice and guidance based on your specific needs and conditions.

Essential oils can complement lifestyles and support long-term joint and muscle comfort in a variety of ways:

1. Topical application: Essential oils can be applied topically to the affected area to provide local relief. Dilute the essential oil in a carrier oil and massage it into the skin. This helps increase circulation, reduces inflammation, and promotes relaxation. Popular essential oils for joint and muscle comfort include lavender, eucalyptus, peppermint, and rosemary.

2. Bath: Adding essential oils to your bath can create a soothing and therapeutic experience. Fill the tub with warm water and add a few drops of essential oil. Soak in the bathtub for 15 to 20 minutes to allow the oil to penetrate the skin and provide relief. Lavender, chamomile, and frankincense are commonly used for their calming and anti-inflammatory properties.

3. Dressings: Using hot or cold compresses infused with essential oils can provide targeted relief for sore joints and muscles. Soak a clean cloth in warm or cold water, mix a few drops of essential oil, and apply it to the affected area. This can help reduce inflammation, relieve pain, and promote relaxation.

4. Aromatherapy: Diffusing essential oils into the air via a diffuser or inhaler can create a relaxing and supportive environment. Inhaling essential oils directly impacts the nervous system, promoting relaxation and reducing discomfort. Diffuse oils like lavender, peppermint, or chamomile throughout your living space or workplace to create a soothing atmosphere.

5. Mind-body techniques: Combining the use of essential oils with mind-body techniques such as meditation, deep breathing exercises, or gentle yoga can provide additional benefits. The aroma of essential oils can enhance relaxation and promote a sense of calm, indirectly supporting joint and muscle comfort by reducing stress and tension.

Remember to choose high-quality essential oils from reputable sources and follow proper dilution guidelines and safety precautions. Also, be sure to consult a healthcare professional if you have any underlying medical conditions or are taking medications that may interact with essential oils. Incorporating essential oils into your lifestyle can create a comprehensive approach to support long-term joint and muscle comfort. It's important to listen to your body, stay consistent with your practice, and adjust as needed to find the best combination.

Chapter 4

Men's Grooming and Skin Care

Essential Oils

Chapter 4 will discuss the use of essential oils in men's grooming and skin care routines. Topics covered include shaving and aftershave care, beard maintenance, and addressing skin problems and irritations.

4.1 Shaving and After-shave Care

This section will explore how essential oils can enhance your shaving experience and provide soothing care to your skin during your aftershave session. We discuss the benefits of using essential oils for shaving, preventing razor burns, and promoting overall skin health.

A. Understand the Shaving Process

Shaving is a regular part of many men's grooming routines. Understanding the shaving process is essential to maintaining a clean, smooth look or managing facial hair growth. Let's take a deeper look at the steps involved in a typical shaving routine and some common challenges men may encounter along the way.

Steps involved in a typical shaving routine:

1. Preparation before shaving: This is a critical step that is often overlooked but can significantly improve your shaving experience. It involves cleansing and moisturizing the skin. Start by washing your face with warm water and a mild cleanser to remove dirt and oil. This step softens the hair and opens the pores for a smoother shave.

2. Application of shaving cream or gel: Apply a generous amount of shaving cream or gel to your face. The purpose of this is to create a barrier between the skin and the razor, reducing friction and providing extra hydration to the hair, making it easier to cut.

3. Shaving: Using a sharp, clean razor, start shaving in the direction of hair growth (also called "against the grain"). This technique can help reduce the likelihood of irritation and razor bumps.

4. Rinse and dry: After shaving, rinse your face with cold water to close pores and soothe your skin. Then, gently pat your skin dry with a clean towel.

5. Aftershave: Use an alcohol-free aftershave or moisturizer to hydrate and soothe your skin. This step helps prevent irritation and dryness after shaving.

Common challenges men face when shaving:

Although shaving is routine, some challenges may arise during the process. These include:

1. Razor burn: These are usually caused by shaving too close to the skin, using a dull blade, or shaving against the grain. Razor burn appears as red, irritated skin, sometimes accompanied by a burning sensation.

2. Irritation: Skin irritation can occur due to various factors, such as using irritating shaving products, not properly preparing the skin before shaving, or not moisturizing after shaving.

3. Ingrown hairs: This occurs when cut hair curls back into the skin instead of growing outward. This can lead to red, itchy bumps and, in more severe cases, painful, pus-filled ulcers.

4. Scratches and cuts: These are common, especially for those who are new to shaving or who use dull or dirty blades. Small cuts can be treated with a styptic pencil or alum block to stop bleeding and aid healing.

Understanding these challenges is the first step in learning how to prevent and treat them. Incorporating quality shaving products and maintaining a healthy skincare routine can greatly enhance your shaving experience. The next section will explore how essential oils can help address these challenges and improve your overall shaving routine.

B. Shaving Preparation Essential Oils

Essential oils offer a wide range of benefits for men's grooming routines, especially when it comes to shaving. They have properties that clean the skin, soften facial hair, and create a lubrication barrier for the razor, helping to provide a smoother, more comfortable shave. Let's explore some essential oils known for these properties – tea tree, eucalyptus, and lavender.

Tea tree oil:

Tea tree oil is known for its powerful antibacterial and anti-inflammatory properties and can be a helpful addition to your shaving routine.

Cleansing the skin: Tea tree oil is very effective in clearing the skin. Its antibacterial properties fight bacteria and other microorganisms on the skin, reducing the risk of infection and breakouts.
Softens facial hair: While not directly helping to soften hair, the overall cleansing and hydration tea tree oil provides can indirectly help soften facial hair by keeping the skin underneath healthy.
Lubricating barrier: When mixed with a carrier oil or included in shaving cream or gel, tea tree oil can help provide a lubricating barrier between the skin and the razor, reducing friction that can lead to irritation and razor burn.

Eucalyptus essential oil:

Eucalyptus oil is widely recognized for its uplifting aroma and ability to promote clear skin and respiratory health.

Cleans skin: Its antiseptic properties make it an excellent choice for cleansing skin before shaving, helping to reduce bacteria that can cause skin irritation.

Softens facial hair: Eucalyptus oil can be mixed with carrier oil to create a pre-shave oil that moisturizes and softens facial hair, making it easier to cut and reducing the risk of razor pull.

Lubricating barrier: Like tea tree oil, eucalyptus oil, when used in shaving cream or gel, provides a lubricating barrier to help the razor glide smoothly over the skin.

Lavender essential oil:

Lavender oil is known for its calming fragrance and numerous skin benefits, making it an excellent addition to any shaving routine.

Cleansing the skin: The antibacterial properties of lavender oil can help cleanse the skin and reduce bacteria that can cause irritation or infection.

Softens Facial Hair: While lavender oil does not directly soften facial hair, its soothing and moisturizing properties can help keep skin and hair hydrated, indirectly helping to make facial hair softer and more manageable.

Lubricant barrier: Lavender oil can be added to shaving cream or gel to provide a smoother, more comfortable shave. Its calming aroma also adds a soothing element to your shaving routine.

Incorporating these essential oils into your shaving routine can enhance the experience and help solve common shaving challenges. However, essential oils should always be used with caution. They are effective and should be diluted with a carrier oil before being used directly on the skin. A patch test is also recommended to check the skin's sensitivity to these oils. Finally, it's always a good idea to consult a professional or aromatherapist for advice on using essential oils.

C. Create Pre-Shave Mixtures and Solutions

Essential oils can be blended with a variety of carrier oils, astringents, and other ingredients to customize a pre-shave solution based on your skin type and personal preferences. Here are some suggestions:

Tea Tree, Eucalyptus, and Lavender Pre-Shave Oil:

This pre-shave oil blend is designed to cleanse, soothe, and prepare skin for a smooth, comfortable shave.

* Element:
* 2 tablespoons of jojoba oil (carrier oil)
* 4 drops of tea tree essence
* 4 drops of eucalyptus essential oil
* 4 drops of lavender essential oil

* Guide:
* Mix the essential oil with jojoba oil (carrier oil) in a small dark glass bottle.
* Before shaving, apply a small amount of essential oil to damp skin and massage gently.
* Wait a minute for the skin and beard to absorb the essential oil, then continue shaving as usual.

Refreshing Pre-Shave Astringent Witch Hazel and Peppermint:

This refreshing pre-shave astringent cleanses and tightens skin, providing a tight, smooth surface for shaving.

* Element:
* 1/2 cup of witch hazel (astringent)
* 10 drops of peppermint essential oil

* Guide:
* Mix peppermint essential oil with witch hazel in a small, dark glass bottle.
* Shake well to mix.
* After washing your face, use a cotton pad to apply the astringent to your skin, avoiding the eye area.
* Wait until dry before applying shaving cream or gel.

Nourishing Pre-shave Scrub with Coconut Oil and Lemon Essential Oil:

This scrub can help exfoliate your skin, remove dead skin cells, and lift facial hair for a closer shave.

* Element:
* 1/2 cup of coconut oil (carrier oil)
* 1/2 cup of granulated sugar (exfoliating)
* 10 drops of lemon essential oil

* Guide:
* Combine the coconut oil and sugar in a small bowl.
* Add lemon essential oil and stir until well mixed.
* Before shaving, apply the scrub to your face in circular motions, avoiding the eye area.
* Rinse off the scrub with warm water and continue with your shaving routine.

Remember, when using a new essential oil or blend, always do a patch test to make sure there are no adverse reactions. It's also important to remember that essential oils are potent and should never be applied directly to the skin unless diluted in a carrier oil or other suitable medium. As always, when in doubt, consult a professional or aromatherapist.

D. Aftershave Soothing and Healing

Essential oils have been used for centuries for their healing and soothing properties. Regarding aftershave care, certain oils can help soothe skin irritation, reduce redness, and even prevent infection. Let's look at some essential oils that are great for after-shave care:

Chamomile essential oil:

Chamomile essential oil, especially Roman chamomile, is known for its calming and soothing properties. It's rich in azure, a compound that reduces inflammation and promotes skin healing. Chamomile essential oil can help soothe razor burn and reduce post-shave redness. Its mild, calming fragrance also adds to feelings of relaxation and well-being.

Cedarwood essential oil:

Cedarwood essential oil is an effective antiseptic that can help prevent post-shave infections and breakouts. Its soothing properties help relieve irritation and reduce redness, while its woody, masculine scent makes it a great aftershave option for men.

Sandalwood oil:

Sandalwood essential oil is highly valued for its anti-inflammatory and antiseptic properties. It is often used in aftershave products because of its ability to soothe and heal the skin. Its rich, woody scent is also appreciated in men's grooming products.

How to use these oils in your after-shave care:

After Shave Balm with Chamomile, Cedarwood, and Sandalwood:

This aftershave balm is designed to soothe skin, reduce redness, and prevent infection while delivering a refreshing, masculine scent.

* Element:
* 1/4 cup of shea butter (carrier base)
* 1 tablespoon of jojoba oil (carrier oil)
* 4 drops of chamomile essential oil
* 4 drops of cedarwood essential oil
* 4 drops of sandalwood essential oil

* Guide:
* Melt the shea butter in a double boiler and remove from the heat.
* Add jojoba oil and essential oils and stir.
* Pour the mixture into a small dark glass jar and allow it to cool and set.
* After shaving, apply a small amount of balm on your face and massage gently into the skin.

Remember, when using a new essential oil or blend, always do a patch test to make sure there are no adverse reactions. Essential oils are potent and should not be applied directly to the skin without being diluted. When in doubt, always seek professional advice.

E. DIY After-shave Balm and Lotion

After shaving, the skin often feels dry, irritated, or even damaged due to the friction caused by the razor. Therefore, using a nourishing aftershave balm or lotion that promotes skin healing and hydration is essential. With the right ingredients, you can make your aftershave balms and lotions at home that are not only effective but also free of harsh chemicals. Here are some recipes that incorporate the benefits of essential oils:

Aloe Vera and Tea Tree Oil Aftershave Lotion:

This lotion harnesses the soothing properties of aloe vera and the antiseptic benefits of tea tree oil to create a cooling, healing aftershave.

* Element:
* 1/2 cup of aloe vera gel
* 1/4 cup of witch hazel
* 2 tablespoons of jojoba oil
* 10 drops of tea tree essential oil
* 10 drops of peppermint essential oil

* Guide:
* Combine all ingredients in a bowl and stir until well combined.
* Pour mixture into a small dark glass bottle for storage.
* After shaving, shake the bottle well, then apply a small amount of lotion to the shaved area and massage gently into the skin.

Coconut Oil and Lavender After-Shave Balm:

This balm harnesses coconut oil's hydrating power and lavender's calming properties to create a soothing, hydrating aftershave.

* Element:
* 1/4 cup of coconut oil
* 1 tablespoon of shea butter
* 10 drops of lavender essential oil
* 5 drops of chamomile essential oil

* Guide:
* Melt coconut oil and shea butter in a double boiler and remove from heat.
* Add essential oil and stir.
* Pour the mixture into a small dark glass jar and allow it to cool and set.
* After shaving, apply a small amount of balm on your face and massage gently into the skin.

Remember, homemade aftershave should be stored in a cool, dark place to maintain its potency and shelf life. Also, do a patch test to make sure there are no adverse reactions before applying it to a large area of the skin. Not only does making your aftershave help you maintain healthy skin, but it also gives you the freedom to experiment with different essential oils to create a personalized skin care regimen.

F. Addressing Ingrown Hairs and Razor Bumps

Ingrown hairs and razor bumps can be painful and frustrating side effects of shaving. They occur when hair grows back into the skin instead of rising out of it, causing inflammation and bumps. Fortunately, essential oils have powerful properties that can relieve or even prevent these skin irritations.

Here are some beneficial essential oils that can help manage ingrown hairs and razor bumps:

Tea tree oil: Known for its powerful antiseptic properties, tea tree oil can help cleanse the skin, reduce inflammation, and prevent infection, making it great for treating razor bumps and ingrown hairs.

Lavender oil: Lavender oil is highly regarded for its anti-inflammatory and soothing properties. Applying this oil can help reduce the redness, inflammation, and irritation associated with ingrown hairs.

Frankincense oil: This oil is known for its anti-inflammatory and antibacterial properties. It can help reduce inflammation and protect the skin from potential infection.

Here are some tips and techniques for incorporating these essential oils into your aftershave routine for smoother, healthier skin:

1. Aftershave oil mixture: In a small glass bottle, mix 1 tablespoon of jojoba oil (or other carrier oil) with 2 to 3 drops each of tea tree oil, lavender oil, and frankincense oil. After shaving, apply a few drops of this mixture to the affected area and gently massage the skin. This will help soothe irritation, reduce inflammation, and prevent the development of razor bumps and ingrown hairs.

2. Cold compress: Add a few drops of lavender oil and tea tree oil to a bowl of cold water. Soak a clean washcloth in this mixture, wring it out, and apply a cold compress to the irritated skin area. This provides instant relief from razor burn and helps prevent ingrown hairs.

3. Essential oil exfoliating scrub: Exfoliation can help prevent ingrown hairs by removing dead skin cells that can clog hair follicles. Mix 1/2 cup sugar, 1/4 cup jojoba oil (or other carrier oil), and 10 drops each of tea tree oil and lavender oil. Use this scrub once or twice a week to exfoliate and keep your skin healthy.

Remember, essential oils are potent and should always be diluted with a carrier oil before applying directly to the skin. Do a patch test to ensure you have no adverse reactions to the oil. Incorporating these essential oils into your daily routine can promote smoother, healthier skin and enhance your overall shaving experience.

G. Natural Antiseptic and Antibacterial Properties

Due to their diverse properties, essential oils can play an important role in enhancing your shaving experience and promoting skin health. Certain essential oils' antiseptic and antibacterial properties can protect the skin from potential infections that may result from minor cuts or razor burns. Here, we will explore some of these essential oils:

1. Tea tree oil: This oil is known for its powerful antiseptic and anti-inflammatory properties. It cleans the skin, prevents cuts from becoming infected, and soothes any inflammation or redness. Using tea tree oil as part of your pre- or post-shave routine can help ensure your skin remains healthy and irritation-free.

2. Lavender oil: Lavender oil has antiseptic and anti-inflammatory properties that can prevent infection and reduce inflammation. Its soothing effect is perfect for calming skin after shaving and promoting healing in the case of minor nicks or cuts.

3. Lemon oil: Lemon oil is an excellent natural preservative. It can help cleanse the skin from microorganisms that can cause infection. Its refreshing and invigorating scent can make it a pleasant addition to your shaving routine.

How to incorporate these essential oils into your shaving routine:

1. Pre-shave cleanser: Add a few drops of lemon oil and tea tree oil to a carrier oil like coconut or jojoba oil. Apply this mixture to your face before shaving to clean your skin and prepare it for shaving.

2. Aftershave soothing solution: Combine lavender oil and tea tree oil with carrier oil in a small glass bottle. After shaving, gently massage a few drops into your skin. This will not only relieve any irritation but also prevent potential infection.

3. Cut healing roll-on: Mix lavender oil with carrier oil in a roll-on bottle. Apply it to any cuts or nicks as needed. Lavender oil will help speed healing and prevent any infection.

It's important to note that due to their potency, essential oils should always be diluted with a carrier oil before applying to the skin. Additionally, some people may be allergic or sensitive to certain oils, so doing a patch test before full use is always a good idea. Incorporating these oils into your shaving routine ensures a smoother, more comfortable shave while keeping your skin healthy and vibrant.

H. Aromatherapy Benefits During Shaving

Shaving is more than just a daily grooming task; It can be an opportunity for self-care and relaxation. With the right essential oils, shaving can be transformed into an aromatherapy experience. Here are some essential oils that can enhance mood, reduce stress, and promote relaxation during your shaving routine:

1. Bergamot oil: Known for its uplifting and calming properties, Bergamot Oil is great for reducing stress and promoting positive emotions. Its citrusy and spicy aroma can also stimulate your senses, leaving you feeling refreshed and energized.

2. Lavender oil: One of the most popular essential oils in aromatherapy, lavender oil is prized for its calming and soothing properties. Its sweet and floral scent can help reduce anxiety and promote relaxation.

3. Sandalwood oil: This oil has a rich, warm, woody aroma and promotes mental clarity and relaxation. Sandalwood oil can help create a calming and peaceful atmosphere during your shaving routine.

4. Peppermint oil: Peppermint oil has a cool, uplifting, and refreshing scent that helps boost energy and reduce fatigue, making it perfect for morning shaving.

5. Rosemary oil: Rosemary's fresh, herbal scent reduces stress and increases alertness, helping to stimulate the senses and improve concentration.

Adding these oils to your shaving routine can elevate the experience from mundane to relaxing. Here are a few ways to do this:

1. Aromatherapy shaving cream: Add a few drops of essential oil of your choice to your shaving cream. As you apply the cream, the heat from your skin will help release the aroma of the essential oils, creating a soothing atmosphere.

2. Pre-shave oil: Add a few drops of essential oil to pre-shave oil. Massage it into your skin. Take a moment to take a deep breath and enjoy the scent.

3. Scented hot towels: Add a few drops of essential oils to a damp towel to create a hot towel experience at home. Warm the towel in the microwave for a few seconds. Heat activates the aroma of essential oils. Placing a warm washcloth on your face for a few minutes before shaving helps open pores and soften your beard, while the scent of the oil can boost your mood.

Remember to always dilute essential oils in a carrier oil before applying them to your skin to avoid irritation. Also, do a patch test first to make sure you're not allergic or sensitive to the oil. With these essential oils, your shaving routine can become a peaceful and enjoyable ritual that refreshes and prepares you for the day ahead.

4.2 Beard Care and Maintenance

In this chapter, we'll explore how essential oils can enhance beard care and maintenance for men. We discuss the benefits of using essential oils to promote beard health, address common beard problems, and provide nutrients to your beard hair and underlying skin.

A. Learn about Beard Care

Understanding the importance of proper beard care and maintenance is crucial for anyone who wishes to grow and maintain a healthy, attractive beard. This includes regular cleaning, moisturizing, trimming, and shaping your beard, all of which work together to prevent common beard-related issues like dryness, itchiness, and dandruff.

Dry beards can occur due to several factors, such as exposure to harsh weather conditions, use of harsh soaps or shampoos, and not adequately moisturizing your beard. This can lead to itchy beards and beard dandruff, also known as beard dandruff. If not treated properly, these problems can cause discomfort and negatively impact the appearance of your beard.

Essential oils can play an important role in solving these common beard problems. For example, oils like argan and jojoba have high moisturizing properties and can help relieve dryness, thereby reducing itching. They closely resemble your skin's natural oils and help effectively moisturize your beard and skin underneath.

Tea tree oil is known for its antifungal and antibacterial properties and can help with beard dandruff. Its application can help maintain the skin's health beneath your beard, preventing the build-up of oil and dead skin cells known to cause dandruff.

Lavender and chamomile are known for their soothing properties and can help relieve itchiness, while peppermint oil provides a cooling effect for immediate relief from irritation.

By incorporating these essential oils into your beard care routine, men can not only address common beard problems but also enhance the health and appearance of their beard. However, it's important to remember that essential oils are potent and should always be diluted in a carrier oil before use. A patch test is also recommended to ensure there are no adverse skin reactions.

B. Beard Health Essential Oil

Essential oils have long been appreciated for their beneficial properties that promote a healthy beard. Let's take a deeper look at some of these oils and their benefits:

1. Cedarwood: Cedarwood oil is popular in many beard oil recipes for its woody scent and potential benefits for beard health. It is known to have antiseptic and anti-inflammatory properties that can help keep the skin under your beard healthy and free from irritation. Additionally, some research suggests that cedarwood oil may help stimulate hair growth, although more research is needed to confirm these effects.

2. Sandalwood: Another oil with a pleasant masculine scent, sandalwood is believed to have anti-inflammatory and antiseptic properties. It is also known to be a great moisturizer, helping prevent beard dryness and the result-

ing itchiness.

3. Jojoba oil: Technically a wax ester rather than an oil, jojoba oil is prized for its similarity to sebum (the natural oil produced by the human skin). This makes it great for moisturizing beards and the skin underneath, reducing dryness and associated itchiness. Jojoba oil is also non-comedogenic, which means it won't clog pores, which helps prevent acne and inflammation.

4. Bergamot: This citrus oil provides a refreshing scent and is known for its antiseptic properties, which can help keep the skin under your beard clean and infection-free. It is also thought to stimulate blood flow to hair follicles, potentially promoting beard growth.

By incorporating these oils into your beard care routine, you can provide your beard with nutrients, prevent dryness, and possibly even support beard growth and thickness. However, remember that essential oils are highly concentrated and should always be diluted or mixed with a carrier oil like jojoba or coconut oil. It is also important to perform a patch test to ensure no adverse skin reactions.

C. Beard Oil Blend

Beard oil is a simple yet effective addition to your beard care routine. Creating your blend allows you to customize your beard oil to suit your specific needs and preferences. Here are some recipes and tips to get you started:

1. Basic Beard Oil Blend

* 1 oz jojoba oil (carrier oil)
* 5 drops of cedarwood essential oil
* 5 drops of sandalwood essential oil

Combine the essential oils in a small glass container with the jojoba oil. Place a few drops of the mixture on your hands, rub them together, and massage the oil into your beard, making sure to reach the skin underneath.

2. Refreshing Citrus Beard Oil Blend

* 1-ounce sweet almond oil (carrier oil)
* 4 drops of bergamot essential oil
* 3 drops of lemon essential oil

* 3 drops of cedarwood essential oil

Combine all the oils in a small glass bottle. The application is similar to the above, focusing on moisturizing the beard and skin underneath.

3. Growth Support Beard Oil Blend

* 1 oz argan oil (carrier oil)
* 4 drops of rosemary essential oil
* 4 drops of peppermint essential oil
* 2 drops of lavender essential oil

As in the previous recipe, mix the oils in a glass bottle. Apply to the beard as part of your grooming routine.

Tips for effective application:

* The best time to apply beard oil is after showering when your hair follicles and pores are open and can easily absorb the oil.
* Always start with a small amount of oil. You can add more if necessary, but remember, a little goes a long way.
* Make sure to massage the oil into your skin, not just your beard. This ensures that the skin underneath your beard remains moisturized and healthy, thus promoting better beard growth.

Remember to patch test when using new essential oils to avoid adverse skin reactions. These are just a few example blends; feel free to experiment with your favorite essential oils to create the perfect blend for your beard.

D. Solve Beard Itching and Dandruff

Essential oils with soothing and anti-inflammatory properties are very beneficial in relieving beard itch and tackling dandruff. Here are some oils commonly used for this purpose:

Tea tree oil: Known for its powerful antiseptic properties, tea tree oil can help relieve itching and irritation. It also has antifungal properties that can help manage dandruff.

Lavender oil: Lavender is known for its soothing and anti-inflammatory properties. It helps relieve irritation and aids skin healing.

Peppermint oil: Peppermint provides a cooling sensation that can relieve itching. It also has antiseptic properties that can help keep skin clean.

Here are some ways to incorporate these oils into your beard care routine:

Beard Oil: Add a few drops of these oils to your beard oil mixture. For example, you can add 2 to 3 drops each of tea tree oil, lavender oil, and peppermint oil to one ounce of carrier oil of your choice. Apply this mixture to your beard, ensuring it reaches the skin underneath.

Beard Shampoo / Conditioner: Add a few drops of these oils to a mild, unscented shampoo or conditioner. Use it to wash your beard regularly.

DIY Beard Rinse: Rinse your beard by adding 5 to 10 drops of lavender and peppermint oil to a cup of distilled water. After washing your beard, pour a rinse solution over it and rinse it with cold water.

Skill:

* While these oils may be beneficial, they are potent and should be used with caution. Always dilute essential oils in a carrier oil or other product before use.
* It's important to do a patch test before using any new oil to make sure you don't have adverse reactions.
* If your symptoms persist or worsen, you may want to consult a dermatologist or healthcare provider.

E. Beard Grooming and Styling

Essential oils play an important role in beard grooming and styling, not only in enhancing the health and appearance of your beard but also in contributing to an overall enjoyable grooming experience.

Here are a few ways essential oils can be used to groom and style your beard:

Shine and health: Certain essential oils, such as argan, jojoba, and castor oil, are known to give beards a healthy shine. They deeply nourish the hair and can help your beard look smooth and neat.

Hold and style: While essential oils won't provide much hold on their own, they can complement other natural ingredients in beard balms and waxes, like beeswax or shea butter. Essential oils help nourish and protect hair while adding a pleasant fragrance.

Fragrance: Essential oils are often used to provide natural and pleasant scents to beard care products. Some popular choices include sandalwood for its warm, woody scent, peppermint for its refreshing, uplifting scent, and lavender for its calming, soothing scent.

To make homemade beard balm, for example, you can melt together 1 part beeswax, 1 part shea butter, and 2 parts carrier oil (such as jojoba or argan oil). Once the ingredients are melted and mixed, you can add a few drops of the essential oil of your choice for a scent. Once the mixture has cooled and set, it can be applied to your beard for styling and hold.

Remember, less is more when using essential oils in your beard care routine. A few drops can provide fragrance and extra benefits to your beauty routine. Always remember to do a patch test to make sure you are not having an allergic reaction to the essential oils you choose to use.

F. Beard Cleaning and Conditioning

Maintaining a clean and well-groomed beard is vital to its health and appearance; just like the hair on your head, beard hair benefits from regular cleaning and conditioning. Not only does this help keep your beard clean and debris-free, but it also ensures your hair stays soft, manageable, and hydrated. This is especially important because beard hair tends to be coarser and more prone to dryness than scalp hair.

Clean:

Essential oils can provide a variety of benefits when it comes to cleaning. Certain essential oils, such as tea tree, peppermint, and eucalyptus, are known for their antibacterial properties. This means they can help cleanse your beard and skin underneath, keeping them free of bacteria and promoting overall skin health.

To make a homemade beard cleanser, you can mix a mild natural soap with a few drops of an essential oil of your choice. Alternatively, many pre-made beard washes also contain essential oils.

Adjust:

Conditioning your beard is equally important. This helps keep your beard soft and manageable, reducing problems like itching and dandruff. Essential oils can play a key role here, too. Oils like argan, jojoba, and coconut oil are rich in fatty acids and other nutrients that nourish and moisturize hair, making it softer and more manageable.

To condition your beard, you might consider making a beard oil or balm containing one or more essential oils. You can also look for a commercial beard conditioner that contains essential oils in its ingredients.

Whether cleansing or conditioning, it's important to ensure you're using the correct number of essential oils. These potent plant extracts are very concentrated, so a little goes a long way. Always dilute them in a carrier oil or other product before applying them to your skin or hair. Remember to do a patch test first to make sure you won't have an allergic reaction to the oil.

G. Promote Beard Growth and Thickness

Essential oils do more than make your beard smell good; some of them may also help promote beard growth and thickness. Here are some examples:

Rosemary essential oil: Rosemary oil is known for its potential to stimulate hair growth. When used topically, it is thought to enhance blood circulation, which may help nourish hair follicles and promote healthier, thicker hair. A 2015 study published in the journal Skinmed compared rosemary oil to minoxidil, a conventional treatment for hair loss, and found that both were equally effective, although rosemary had fewer side effects.

Cedarwood essential oil: Cedarwood oil is another essential oil known for its potential to stimulate hair growth. It is thought to work by balancing the oil-producing glands in the skin and promoting circulation to the hair follicles. While more research is needed, a study published in the Archives of Dermatology found that a blend of essential oils, including cedarwood, improved hair growth in 44 percent of people with alopecia areata.

Peppermint essential oil: Peppermint oil is another potentially useful oil for promoting hair growth. A study published in Toxicological Research found that it promotes hair growth by increasing dermal thickness, hair follicle number, and hair follicle depth.

When using these essential oils in your beard care routine, it is crucial to dilute them in a carrier oil first. Never apply essential oils directly to the skin, as they can irritate. For beard care, good carrier oils include jojoba, argan, or coconut oil, which are all non-comedogenic (meaning they won't clog pores) and have health benefits for your hair. A typical dilution might be 2 to 3 drops of essential oil per teaspoon of carrier oil.

To use these blends, apply a few drops to your palms, rub your hands together, and massage the oil into your beard and skin underneath. It's best to apply these oils after a shower when your beard is clean and your pores are open.

Remember to do a patch test with any new oil to make sure you don't have an adverse reaction. Everyone's skin is different, and what works for one person may not work for another. If you are unsure about how to use these oils safely, be sure to consult a healthcare provider or a trained aromatherapist.

H. Aromatherapy Benefits of Beard Care

Aromatherapy, the therapeutic use of plant-derived aromatic essential oils, can significantly improve your beard care routine. When used correctly, essential oils not only improve your beard's health and appearance but also engage the senses and positively impact your mood and overall health.

Here are some essential oils known for their aromatherapy properties that may be beneficial in your beard care routine:

Lavender essential oil: Lavender essential oil is known for its calming and relaxing properties. Inhaling the scent of lavender can help reduce stress and anxiety and promote good sleep. Beard care is good for nourishing the skin and may promote hair growth.

Peppermint essential oil: Peppermint oil is refreshing and uplifting. It stimulates the mind, enhances concentration, and provides a cooling sensation to the skin, which is especially soothing for itchy beards.

Cedarwood essential oil: Cedarwood oil has a warm, woody scent that promotes comfort and grounding. It is also known for its potential to stimulate hair growth and balance skin oil production.

Bergamot essential oil: Bergamot Oil has a fresh and citrus scent that improves mood, relieves stress, and promotes a sense of freshness and vitality. It is also beneficial for oily and acne-prone skin.

Sandalwood essential oil: Sandalwood oil has a rich, sweet aroma that promotes relaxation and mental clarity. It's also great for moisturizing dry skin and hair.

You can create a custom beard oil blend using your favorite essential oils diluted in a carrier oil like jojoba or argan oil to reap these benefits. A typical dilution might be 2 to 3 drops of essential oil per teaspoon of carrier oil. Then, as part of your beard care routine, massage a few drops of the mixture into your beard and underlying skin.

As always, do a patch test with any new oil to ensure you don't have an adverse reaction. If you're unsure how to use these oils safely, talk to a healthcare provider or a trained aromatherapist.

4.3 Solve Skin Problems and Irritations

In this chapter, we'll look at how you can use essential oils to address a variety of skin problems and irritations common to men. We discuss essential oils' soothing and healing properties and guide on using them safely and effectively to promote skin health and relieve discomfort.

A. Understand Common Skin Problems

Men often experience a variety of skin issues that can affect their overall skin health and well-being. Here are some common skin problems among men and why it's important to address them:

1. Acne: Acne can occur due to hormonal changes, excess oil production, bacteria, or clogged pores. It can cause blemishes, inflammation, and discomfort. Treating acne is important not only for aesthetics but also to prevent long-term scarring and promote skin health.

2. Drying: Dry skin is characterized by rough, flaky, and sometimes

itchy patches. Factors such as harsh weather conditions, over-washing, or using harsh skin care products can cause dryness. Proper hydration and moisturization are essential to maintaining healthy and comfortable skin.

3. Redness and Irritation: Redness and irritation can be caused by a variety of reasons, including shaving, environmental factors, or skin sensitivity. It can lead to discomfort, sensitivity to certain products, and overall dissatisfaction with the appearance of your skin. Addresses redness and irritation to help maintain a calm and balanced complexion.

4. Sensitive: Some men have naturally sensitive skin, which external factors may cause. Sensitivity can manifest as redness, itching, burning, or stinging. It's important to be aware of potential irritants and choose gentle skin care products that won't exacerbate sensitivity.

Addressing these skin concerns is vital to overall skin health and well-being. It promotes skin comfort, reduces the risk of infection or inflammation, and enhances the appearance and texture of the skin. By incorporating a proper skincare routine and using the right products, including essential oils, men can effectively manage these skin concerns and maintain healthy, nourished skin.

It's important to note that individuals may react differently to skin care products, and what works for one person may not work for another. If you have ongoing or severe skin concerns, it is recommended that you consult a dermatologist or skin care specialist for personalized advice and treatment.

B. Soothing and Healing Essential Oils

Certain essential oils are known for their soothing and healing properties, making them valuable for addressing skin concerns and promoting overall skin health. Here are some essential oils that have the potential to reduce inflammation, promote skin regeneration, and relieve irritation:

Tea tree essential oil: Tea tree oil has antibacterial and anti-inflammatory properties that are beneficial for acne-prone skin. It can help reduce inflammation, fight bacteria, and soothe skin irritations. Tea tree oil is often used in skincare products for its purifying and calming effects.

Lavender essential oil: Lavender essential oil is known for its calming and soothing properties. It can help reduce inflammation, relieve itching, and promote skin healing. Lavender oil is mild and well tolerated by most skin types, making it suitable for a variety of skin concerns.

Chamomile essential oil: Chamomile oil has anti-inflammatory and skin-soothing properties. It can help calm redness, irritation, and sensitivity. Chamomile oil is often used in skin care products because of its gentle and soothing effect on the skin.

Frankincense essential oil: Frankincense oil has anti-inflammatory and skin-regenerating properties. It can help reduce inflammation, promote cell regeneration, and improve the appearance of scars and blemishes. Frankincense oil is often used in skin care formulas to support overall skin health and rejuvenation.

When using these essential oils for soothing and healing purposes, it is important to dilute them appropriately before applying them to the skin. Dilute essential oils in a carrier oil such as jojoba or almond at a safe concentration, depending on the specific oil and your skin sensitivity.

To incorporate these essential oils into your skincare routine, you can create a custom blend by mixing a few drops of your chosen essential oil with a carrier oil. Gently massage the mixture into affected areas or use it as part of an overall skincare routine. Always do a patch test before applying any new oil to a larger area of skin.

While these essential oils show potential benefits, it's important to note that personal experience may vary. Some people may be sensitive or allergic to certain oils. If you experience any adverse reactions, discontinue use and seek medical advice.

C. Topical Application for Skin Problems

When using essential oils topically to address skin concerns, be sure to follow guidelines for safe and effective use. Here are some tips for using essential oils safely and effectively:

1. Proper dilution: Essential oils are highly concentrated and should be diluted before applying to the skin. Dilution helps reduce the risk of skin irritation and sensitization. A safe dilution ratio for most adults is usually 2 to 3 parts essential oil to carrier oil. This means adding approximately 6 to 12 drops of essential oil per ounce (30 ml) of carrier oil. For sensitive skin

or when using the oil on the face or children, a lower dilution (1% or less) is recommended.

2. Carrier oil: Carrier oils are used to dilute essential oils and help spread them evenly on the skin. Some popular carrier oils include jojoba oil, sweet almond oil, coconut oil, and grapeseed oil. Choose a carrier oil that suits your skin type and personal preferences. It is best to use a cold-pressed organic carrier oil for the best quality.

3. Patch test: A patch test is necessary before applying any new essential oil blend to a larger skin area. Apply a small amount of the diluted oil to a small area of skin (such as the inner forearm) and wait 24 hours. The mixture should be safe for wider use if no adverse reactions occur.

4. Spot treatment: You can apply the dilute essential oil mixture directly to the affected area using clean fingertips or a cotton swab for targeted relief. Spot treatments are especially useful for addressing specific skin concerns, such as acne, blemishes, or irritation.

5. General application: When applying essential oil mixtures to larger areas of the body, such as for general skin care or massage, it is recommended to use gentle, sweeping motions to distribute the oils evenly. Avoid applying essential oils to broken or injured skin.

6. Consistency: Maintaining a consistent skincare routine is important for ongoing skin care concerns. Consistent use of essential oil blends can help achieve the desired results over time. However, discontinue use and seek professional advice if any adverse reactions occur or your condition worsens.

7. Personal Sensitivities: Everyone's skin is unique, and individuals may have specific sensitivities or allergies to certain essential oils. Pay attention to skin reactions and discontinue use if any adverse reactions occur.

Following these guidelines, you can safely and effectively use essential oils topically to address various skin concerns. It's always a good idea to consult a healthcare professional or qualified aromatherapist for personalized guidance, especially if you have any underlying health conditions or concerns.

D. DIY Skincare Products

Here are some homemade skin care recipes using essential oils that can help with specific skin concerns:

1. Soothing Facial Toner for Sensitive Skin:

* Element:
* 1/2 cup of rose water
* 2 tablespoons witch hazel
* 5 drops of lavender essential oil
* 3 drops of chamomile essential oil

* Guide:
* In a small glass bottle, combine rose water and witch hazel.
* Add lavender and chamomile essential oils.
* Shake well to combine all ingredients.
* Apply toner on a cotton pad and gently wipe onto the face after cleansing. Avoid eye area.

2. Nourishing Dry Skin Essence:

* Element:
* 1 tablespoon jojoba oil
* 1 tablespoon rosehip oil
* 4 drops of frankincense essential oil
* 3 drops of geranium essential oil

* Guide:
* In a small glass dropper bottle, combine jojoba oil and rosehip oil.
* Add frankincense and geranium essential oils.
* Gently shake the bottle to mix all ingredients.
* After cleansing and toning, apply a few drops of essence on your fingertips and massage gently on the face and neck.

3. Purifying Mask for Acne-prone Skin:

* Element:
* 2 tablespoons bentonite clay
* 1 tablespoon apple cider vinegar
* 2 drops of tea tree essential oil
* 2 drops of lavender essential oil

* Guide:
* In a small bowl, combine bentonite clay and apple cider vinegar

until you reach a smooth paste.
* Add tea tree and lavender essential oils and stir evenly.
* Apply the mask evenly on a clean face, avoiding the eye area.
* Keep it on for about 10 ~ 15 minutes or until it starts to dry.
* Rinse with warm water and apply moisturizer.

Remember to do a patch test before using any new skincare product on a larger area of skin, especially if you have sensitive skin or are allergic to specific ingredients. It's important to choose high-quality, pure essential oils from reputable sources.

Feel free to modify these recipes to suit your personal preferences and needs. You can also explore different combinations of essential oils and natural ingredients to create customized skin care products to address your specific skin concerns.

E. Calming and Soothing Mask

Here are some homemade face mask recipes using essential oils that can help calm and soothe irritated skin while providing nutrition and hydration:

1. Calming Honey and Lavender Mask:

* Element:
* 1 tablespoon raw honey
* 1 teaspoon aloe vera gel
* 3 drops of lavender essential oil

* Guide:
* In a small bowl, combine raw honey and aloe vera gel.
* Add lavender essential oil and stir evenly.
* Apply the mask to a clean face, avoiding the eye area.
* Keep it on for 15 to 20 minutes.
* Rinse with warm water and pat the skin dry.

2. Soothing Oatmeal and Chamomile Mask:

* Element:
* 2 tablespoons oat flour (or oatmeal powder)
* 1 tablespoon chamomile tea (cooled)

* 2 drops of chamomile essential oil

* Guide:
* In a small bowl, combine oat flour and chamomile tea to form a paste.
* Add chamomile essential oil and stir evenly.
* Apply the mask to a clean face, avoiding the eye area.
* Keep it on for 15 to 20 minutes.
* Use wet fingertips to massage the face to exfoliate gently, then rinse with warm water.

3. Hydrating Avocado and Rose Mask:

* Element:
* 1/2 ripe avocado
* 1 tablespoon rose water
* 1 teaspoon jojoba oil
* 2 drops of rose essential oil
* Guide:
* Place avocado in a small bowl and mash until smooth.
* Add rose water, jojoba oil, and rose essential oil.
* Mix well to form a creamy paste.
* Apply the mask on a clean face, avoiding the eye area.
* Keep it on for 15 to 20 minutes.
* Rinse with warm water and pat the skin dry.

Before using any new mask on your face, remember to do a patch test, especially if you have sensitive skin or are allergic to specific ingredients. Adjust the amounts of ingredients as needed to achieve your desired consistency.

When applying the mask, gently massage the skin in circular motions to promote blood circulation and enhance absorption. Relax and let the mask work its magic before rinsing it off.

These masks can be used once or twice weekly depending on your skin's needs. Enjoy the soothing and nourishing benefits of these homemade face masks with essential oils!

F. Support skin regeneration

Here's a discussion of essential oils known for their potential to support skin regeneration and repair, as well as ways to incorporate them into your daily skincare routine:

1. Helichrysum essential oil: Helichrysum oil is known for its skin-rejuvenating properties. It can help promote skin cell regeneration, reduce the appearance of scars and blemishes, and soothe skin irritations. You can incorporate helichrysum essential oil into your daily skincare routine in the following ways:
 * Add a few drops of helichrysum oil to your favorite moisturizer or facial oil and apply to the face and neck.
 * Mix a carrier oil like rosehip seed oil with a few drops of helichrysum oil for a targeted serum. Apply serum to areas with scars, blemishes, or signs of aging.

2. Rosehip seed oil: Rosehip Seed Oil is rich in vitamins, antioxidants, and essential fatty acids, making it great for skin regeneration and repair. It can help improve skin texture, reduce the appearance of scars, and improve overall skin radiance. Here's how to incorporate rosehip seed oil into your daily skincare routine:
 * Take a few drops of rosehip seed oil and apply it directly to your face, then massage gently after cleansing and toning.
 * Mix a few drops of rosehip seed oil with your favorite moisturizer to enhance its nourishing properties.
 * Mix rosehip seed oil with other skin-loving oils like jojoba, argan, or evening primrose to create a revitalizing facial oil.

3. Geranium essential oil: Geranium oil is known for its balancing and regenerating properties, making it beneficial for various skin types. It can help improve skin elasticity, promote a youthful appearance, and soothe skin irritations. Here's how to incorporate geranium essential oil into your daily skincare routine:
 * Add a few drops of geranium oil to your facial cleanser or toner for enhanced results.
 * Mix distilled water with a few drops of geranium oil to create a DIY facial mist. Spray on your face throughout the day for refreshed and balanced skin.
 * Add geranium oil to your facial massage routine, dilute a few drops with carrier oil, and massage gently into your face and neck.

When using essential oils for skin rejuvenation and repair, it's important to start with a small amount and see how your skin reacts. Everyone's skin is unique, so it's important to listen to your skin's needs and adjust the concentration or frequency of application as needed.

Remember to choose high-quality, pure essential oils and carrier oils from reputable sources. If you have any underlying skin conditions or concerns, it is recommended that you consult a dermatologist or qualified aromatherapist for personalized guidance.

By incorporating these essential oils into your daily skincare routine, you can support skin regeneration, improve texture and appearance, and enjoy their rejuvenating benefits.

G. Reduce Acne and Breakouts.

Here are some essential oils with antibacterial and anti-inflammatory properties that can help reduce acne and breakouts, along with tips for incorporating them into your skincare routine:

1. Tea tree oil: Tea tree oil is known for its powerful antibacterial properties. It can help kill acne-causing bacteria, reduce inflammation, and promote clearer skin. Here's how to incorporate tea tree oil into your skincare routine:
* Add a few drops of tea tree oil to your facial cleanser, or mix a few drops with a mild, unscented cleanser to create a DIY facial cleanser.
* Add a few drops of tea tree oil to witch hazel or rose water to create a DIY toner. After cleansing, use a cotton pad to apply toner to your face.
* For spot treatment, dilute tea tree oil with a carrier oil (such as jojoba or grapeseed oil) and apply directly to blemishes with a cotton swab.

2. Lavender essential oil: Lavender essential oil has soothing and antibacterial properties that help reduce inflammation and promote healing. It can also help calm irritated skin. Here's how to incorporate lavender oil into your skincare routine:
* Add a few drops of lavender oil to your facial moisturizer or make a DIY moisturizer by mixing a carrier oil (such as jojoba or almond oil) with a few drops of lavender oil.
* Mix distilled water with a few drops of lavender oil to create a DIY facial mist. Spray onto the face throughout the day to refresh and soothe the skin.
* Dilute lavender oil with a carrier oil and apply to the skin after cleansing as a calming and spot-care solution.

3. Chamomile essential oil: Chamomile oil has anti-inflammatory and

calming properties that help reduce redness and soothe irritated skin. Here's how to incorporate chamomile oil into your skincare routine:
* Add a few drops of chamomile oil to a gentle cleanser or mix it with chamomile tea to create a DIY chamomile-infused facial cleanser.
* Soak chamomile in hot water, let it cool, then apply it on your face with a cotton pad; use the chamomile-soaked water as a facial toner.
* Dilute chamomile oil with a carrier oil and apply it to the skin as a calming spot treatment or soothing facial massage oil.

When using essential oils on acne-prone skin, it's important to start with low concentrations and see how your skin reacts. Some people may be more sensitive to certain oils, so doing a patch test before applying them to your face is crucial.

Remember to dilute essential oils correctly in a carrier oil before applying them to your skin, as undiluted essential oils can cause skin irritation. Additionally, consistency is key when using essential oils to treat acne, so incorporate them into your skincare routine regularly for the best results.

If you have severe acne or an underlying skin condition, it is recommended that you consult a dermatologist for personalized advice and treatment options.

Incorporating these essential oils into your skincare routine can harness their antibacterial and anti-inflammatory properties to help reduce acne and breakouts, promote clearer skin, and enjoy a healthier complexion.

H. Moisturizing and Moisturizing Solutions

Below is a discussion of essential oils and ingredients known for their moisturizing and moisturizing properties, as well as guidance on incorporating them into your skincare routine:

1. Jojoba oil: Jojoba oil is a well-known moisturizer that is very similar to the natural oils produced by our skin. It's easily absorbed, helps balance oil production, and provides long-lasting hydration. Here's how to incorporate jojoba oil into your skincare routine:
* Use jojoba oil as a stand-alone moisturizer, apply a few drops to the face, and massage gently after cleansing and toning.
* Mix jojoba oil with your favorite moisturizer or facial oil to enhance its moisturizing properties.

* Mix jojoba oil with a few drops of other nourishing oils, such as rosehip seed oil or argan oil, to create a DIY facial serum.

2. Rose water: Rose water is a natural moisturizing ingredient that helps soothe and refresh the skin. It has moisturizing properties and can help maintain the skin's pH balance. Here's how to incorporate rose water into your skincare routine:

* After cleansing, use a cotton pad to apply rose water on your face as a toner. It will help moisturize and prepare your skin for subsequent products.

* Mix rose water with distilled water and a few drops of your favorite essential oil to create a DIY facial mist. Spray on your face throughout the day for quick hydration and a refreshing experience.

3. Neroli essential oil: Neroli oil comes from the flowers of the bitter orange tree and is known for its moisturizing and regenerative properties. It helps maintain moisture balance, promotes smoothness, and improves skin elasticity. Here's how to incorporate neroli essential oil into your skincare routine:

* Add a few drops of Neroli oil to your facial moisturizer or make a DIY moisturizer by mixing a carrier oil like jojoba or almond oil with a few drops of Neroli oil.

* Mix distilled water with a few drops of Neroli oil to create a rejuvenating facial mist. Spray onto the face throughout the day to moisturize and revitalize the skin.

When using essential oils and ingredients for moisturizing and moisturizing purposes, it's important to choose high-quality, pure oils and ingredients from reputable sources. Do a patch test before applying them to your face to check for any potential sensitivities.

Also, remember to adjust the concentration according to your skin's needs and sensitivity. If you have oily or combination skin, you may prefer a lighter oil and use it less frequently. If your skin is dry, you may choose a richer oil and use it more frequently.

Incorporating these essential oils and ingredients into your skincare routine provides your skin with the necessary moisture and moisture to keep it nourished, soft, and healthy.

Chapter 5

Essential Oils for Stress Management

and Mental Health

Stress management and mental health are crucial to men's overall health. This chapter will explore relaxation techniques and calming blends, enhance focus, and promote restful sleep.

5.1 Relaxation Techniques and Calming Blends

In this chapter, we'll explore how essential oils can be used as relaxation techniques and calming blends to promote a sense of tranquility and reduce stress in men. We discuss the therapeutic properties of essential oils and provide guidance on calming blends for various relaxation practices.

A. Understand the Importance of Relaxation

Below is a discussion of the benefits of relaxation for overall health and stress management, as well as the role of essential oils in enhancing relaxation practices:

1. Benefits of Relaxation:

Relaxation plays a vital role in maintaining overall health and managing stress. When we practice relaxation, our body and mind enter a state of rest and rejuvenation, allowing us to release tension, reduce anxiety, and restore balance. Some of the key benefits of relaxation include:

a. Stress reduction is a key benefit of relaxation techniques. When we engage in relaxation exercises, our bodies activate the relaxation response, which counteracts stress's physiological and psychological effects. Here's a more in-depth explanation of how relaxation techniques can help reduce stress: 1. Relaxation response: The relaxation response is the body's natural counterpart to the stress response (also known as the " fight or flight " response). When we encounter a physical or psychological stressor, our bodies release stress hormones like cortisol and adrenaline to prepare us for action. This response may be helpful in some situations, but chronic activation of the stress response can lead to various health problems. Relaxation techniques, on the other hand, trigger the relaxation response, also known as the "rest and digest" response. When we engage in activities like deep breathing, meditation, progressive muscle relaxation, or other relaxation exercises, our bodies release neurotransmitters and hormones that promote relaxation, reduce stress hormones, and induce feelings of calm and well-being. 2. Reduce stress hormones: During relaxation, the body's production of stress hormones, such as cortisol and adrenaline, decreases. These hormones are associated with physiological changes that prepare us to deal with stressors. Still, over time, elevated levels can lead to a variety of health problems, including anxiety, insomnia, and digestive problems. By triggering the relaxation response, relaxation techniques help reduce stress hormone levels and promote a state of calm and relaxation. 3. Relieve Muscle Tension: Muscle tension is a common physical manifestation of stress. When we are stressed, our muscles tend to contract and tighten, causing discomfort and even pain. Relaxation exercises such as progressive muscle relaxation and stretching help release muscle tension and allow our bodies to experience physical relaxation and comfort. 4. Promotes emotional health: Chronic stress can take a toll on our emotional health, causing anxiety, irritability, and mood swings. Engaging in relaxation techniques can help calm the mind, reduce anxiety, and promote a more positive emotional state. Practices like meditation and deep breathing have been shown to positively impact emotional health and increase feelings of peace and happiness. 5. Improve sleep quality: Stress and anxiety can disrupt sleep patterns, making it difficult to fall asleep and stay asleep. By promoting relaxation, relaxation techniques can improve sleep quality and duration. When we relax, our bodies can enter a restful sleep state, allowing for better physical and mental recovery at night. Overall, relaxation techniques play a vital role in managing stress and promoting overall health. By incorporating practices like deep breathing, meditation, yoga, or mindfulness into your daily life, you can activate your relaxation response, reduce stress hormones, relieve muscle tension, and experience a greater sense of calm and balance in your life.

b. Mental clarity and focus are important aspects of relaxation and can greatly benefit our cognitive abilities and overall health. Here's how relaxation exercises can help with mental clarity and improve focus: 1. Reduce mental clutter: When we feel stressed or overwhelmed, our minds can become cluttered with thoughts, worries, and distractions. Engaging in relaxation techniques can help calm mental chatter and bring a sense of calm and clarity to the mind. This reduction in mental clutter allows us to think more clearly and make decisions more easily. 2. Enhanced focus: Stress and anxiety can negatively impact our ability to stay focused on a task or focus on a specific activity. By triggering the relaxation response, relaxation techniques promote a state of relaxation and concentration, allowing us to better focus on our work, studies, or any other activity that requires sustained attention. 3. Improve problem-solving skills: When we are relaxed and clear-minded, we can better approach problems from a new perspective. Relaxation exercises develop mental flexibility and creativity, allowing us to think outside the box and develop innovative solutions to challenges we may encounter. 4. Stress reduction and cognitive function: Chronic stress can impair cognitive function and affect memory, learning, and information processing. By reducing stress through relaxation techniques, we can help protect our cognitive abilities and maintain optimal brain function. 5. Mindfulness and present-moment awareness: Many relaxation techniques, such as mindfulness meditation, emphasize being fully present. This heightened awareness and mindfulness allow us to focus on the task at hand, resulting in increased focus and productivity. 6. Enhanced learning: When our minds are relaxed and stress-free, we are better able to absorb and retain information. This is especially beneficial for students or anyone engaged in learning new skills or knowledge. 7. Reduce stress and mental fatigue: Chronic stress can lead to mental fatigue and burnout. By practicing relaxation exercises, we can relieve mental fatigue, recharge our cognitive resources, and increase our overall mental stamina.

c. Emotional health is an important aspect of our overall health, and relaxation exercises play an important role in promoting positive emotions and reducing feelings of anxiety and feeling overwhelmed. Here's how relaxation techniques can boost emotional health: 1. Reduce stress: Chronic stress can take a toll on our emotional health, causing feelings of anxiety, irritability, and tension. By triggering the relaxation response, relaxation exercises help reduce the production of stress hormones and promote feelings of calm and relaxation.

This stress reduction contributes to a more balanced emotional state. 2. Relieve Anxiety: Relaxation techniques, such as deep breathing and meditation, have been shown to reduce symptoms of anxiety and panic. These practices help activate the parasympathetic nervous system, which counteracts the " fight or flight " response associated with anxiety. As a result, individuals experience feelings of ease and relaxation, reducing the impact of anxious thoughts and feelings. 3. Mood Enhancement: Practicing relaxation exercises can have a positive impact on mood and emotional health. Practices such as mindfulness meditation can promote present-moment awareness, helping individuals break away from negative thought patterns and develop a more positive outlook on life. 4. Emotional resilience: Regular relaxation practices can enhance emotional resilience, which refers to our ability to adapt to stressors and bounce back from challenging situations. By reducing the impact of stress on our emotional health, relaxation techniques enable us to cope more effectively with life's ups and downs. 5. Increase self-awareness: Many relaxation exercises encourage self-reflection and self-awareness. This heightened level of self-awareness enables individuals to identify and acknowledge their emotions without judgment, resulting in a greater sense of emotional acceptance and well-being. 6. Improve sleep and rest: Quality sleep is essential for emotional health. By promoting relaxation and reducing stress, relaxation exercises help improve sleep quality, which in turn supports emotional well-being. 7. Positive coping strategies: Engaging in relaxation exercises provides individuals with healthy coping strategies for managing stress and emotional challenges. Rather than turning to unhealthy coping mechanisms, such as excessive substance use or emotional eating, individuals can turn to relaxation techniques for comfort and relief. 8. Strengthen the mind-body connection: Many relaxation practices, such as yoga and tai chi, involve mind-body exercises to promote a deeper connection between mind and body. Combining mind and body can lead to increased emotional awareness and a greater sense of inner peace.

d. Chronic stress significantly impacts our physical health, and relaxation exercises play a vital role in promoting overall health and reducing the negative effects of stress on the body. Here's how relaxation techniques can help improve physical health: 1. Lower blood pressure: High levels of stress can lead to increased blood pressure, a risk factor for cardiovascular disease. Relaxation exercises, such as deep breathing and meditation, have been shown to help lower blood pressure and promote cardiovascular health. 2. Improve sleep quality: Chronic stress can disrupt sleep patterns and lead to insomnia. Relaxation exercises, such as progressive muscle relaxation and guided imagery, promote relaxation and stress reduction, resulting in improved sleep quality and better overall rest. 3. Enhance immune function: Chronic stress can weaken the immune system, making individuals more susceptible to infection and disease. By reducing stress through relaxation practices, the immune system is better able to fight off pathogens and maintain optimal health. 4. Relieves Stress-Related Illnesses: Many physical conditions, such as tension headaches, migraines, digestive disorders, and chronic pain, can be exacerbated by stress. Relaxation techniques help relieve these symptoms by reducing stress and promoting physical relaxation. 5. Enhance respiratory function: Deep breathing exercises are a common relaxation technique that can improve respiratory function by enhancing lung capacity and increasing oxygen intake. This is especially beneficial for people with respiratory conditions such as asthma. 6. Muscle Relaxation: Chronic stress can cause muscle tension and discomfort. Progressive muscle relaxation and other relaxation exercises help release muscle tension, reduce the risk of musculoskeletal problems, and promote better mobility and flexibility. 7. Manage Chronic Pain: For people with chronic pain conditions, relaxation exercises can serve as an effective complementary therapy to reduce pain intensity and improve overall pain management. 8. Supports digestive health: Stress can disrupt digestive function and lead to irritable bowel syndrome (IBS) and Gastrointestinal problems. Relaxation exercises help calm the nervous system and promote better digestive function. 9. Hormone balance: Chronic stress disrupts the production and regulation of hormones, causing imbalances in cortisol, adrenaline, and other hormones. Reducing stress through relaxation exercises can restore hormonal balance. 10. Overall health: When the body is relaxed and has reduced stress, it functions optimally, allowing individuals to experience a greater overall sense of well-being and a higher quality of life.

2. Essential oils and relaxation:

Essential oils can enhance relaxation habits by creating an aromatherapy environment that promotes a sense of calm, tranquility, and well-being. Inhaling certain essential oils stimulates the olfactory system, which is closely related to the brain's limbic system, which is responsible for mood and relaxation. Here's how essential oils can enhance relaxation habits:

Essential oils like lavender, chamomile, and bergamot are known for their calming and soothing effects on the mind and body. These oils contain compounds that interact with our olfactory system, affecting our mood and promoting feelings of relaxation. Here's how these essential oils contribute to a calming and soothing experience: 1. Lavender Essential Oil: Lavender is one of the most popular essential oils for relaxation and stress relief. It contains linalool and linalyl acetate, which have sedative properties. When inhaled, lavender's sweet and floral aroma can help reduce anxiety, soothe nervous tension, and induce a state of relaxation, making it ideal for promoting better sleep and reducing stress. 2. Chamomile essential oil: Chamomile has a mild and soothing fragrance, and its essential oil is often used for its calming effects. Chamomile contains compounds such as alpha* bisabol and chamazulene, which have anti-inflammatory and sedative properties. In aromatherapy, chamomile oil is often used to relieve anxiety, reduce irritability, and promote a sense of inner calm. 3. Bergamot Essential Oil: Bergamot's citrusy and refreshing scent makes it uplift and calming at the same time. It contains the compound linalool, which contributes to its soothing properties. Bergamot essential oil is often used to improve mood, reduce feelings of stress and depression, and create a more relaxing atmosphere. 4. Ylang-ylang essential oil: Ylang-ylang has a strong floral fragrance that is both relaxing and uplifting. This essential oil contains compounds such as linalool and geranyl acetate, which have calming and mood-enhancing effects. Ylang-ylang is often used in aromatherapy to reduce stress, promote relaxation, and improve emotional well-being.

When these essential oils are diffused, inhaled, or applied topically, they create a calming environment that helps relieve stress and tension. The aroma of these oils interacts with the limbic system in the brain, which is responsible for mood and memory, causing the release of neurotransmitters like serotonin and endorphins. This release contributes to a positive and relaxed emotional state.

To incorporate these essential oils into your relaxation practice, consider the following:

1. Aromatherapy Diffuser: Use an aromatherapy diffuser to spread the calming aroma of these essential oils throughout the room to create a peaceful and peaceful atmosphere.

2. Inhalation: Add a few drops of your choice of essential oil to a tissue or inhaler stick and inhale the scent deeply for instant calming effects.

3. Topical Application: Dilute the essential oil with a suitable carrier oil and apply it to pulse points or the back of the neck for a calming and grounding experience.

4. Bath: Add a few drops of essential oil to a warm bath to create a relaxing and soothing experience that calms the mind and body.

Essential oils like ylang-ylang, sage, and frankincense are known for their stress-relieving properties, making them valuable allies in relaxation practices. Here's how these essential oils can help relieve stress and promote a more relaxed state: 1. Ylang-Ylang Essential Oil: Ylang-ylang has a pleasant floral aroma that is not only calming but is also known for its ability to reduce stress and anxiety. Inhaling the sweet taste of ylang-ylang can help reduce cortisol levels and stress hormones and promote tranquility and emotional balance. 2. Sage Essential Oil: Sage has an earthy and herbal scent that is deeply relaxing and uplifting. This essential oil contains compounds such as linalyl acetate and linalool, which help it relieve stress. Inhaling sage oil can help relieve nervous tension, reduce anxiety, and cultivate a peaceful mind. 3. Frankincense Essential Oil: Frankincense has a woody and resinous aroma and is often used in spiritual and relaxation practices. It contains compounds such as alpha* pinene and limonene, which have calming properties. Inhaling frankincense essential oil can help calm the mind, reduce stress, and create a peaceful atmosphere.

Incorporating these stress-relieving essential oils into your relaxation practice can enhance the overall experience and provide effective support in managing stress. Here are some ways to use these oils during relaxation:

1. Aromatherapy Diffuser: Use an aromatherapy diffuser to disperse the calming scent of ylang-ylang, sage, or frankincense into the air to create a peaceful atmosphere that helps reduce stress.

2. Massage or Topical Application: Dilute the essential oil with a carrier oil and apply it to the skin during massage or self-massage. The calming aroma and gentle touch can help soothe the mind and body.

3. Meditation and Breathing Exercises: Inhale the aroma of these stress-relieving essential oils directly from the bottle or through an inhaler stick as you practice meditation or deep breathing exercises. Scent can support relaxation and promote a focused state of mind.

4. Bath Ritual: Add a few drops of these essential oils to a warm bath for a calming and stress-relieving soak. Warm water combined with aromatherapy can provide a rejuvenating experience.

Essential oils like lemon, rosemary, and peppermint are excellent choices for enhancing mindfulness practices, improving focus, and improving mental clarity during relaxation exercises. Here's how these essential oils can contribute to a more focused and focused experience: 1. Lemon Essential Oil: Lemon has a bright and uplifting citrus aroma that stimulates the senses and promotes mental alertness. Inhaling lemon essential oil during a mindfulness practice can help clear mental fog, improve focus, and create a sense of freshness and positivity. 2. Rosemary Essential Oil: Rosemary has an herbal and stimulating aroma and is known for its cognitive-enhancing properties. Inhaling rosemary oil can help improve memory, increase focus, improve mental clarity, and facilitate mindfulness and meditation practices. 3. Peppermint Essential Oil: Peppermint has a refreshing and energizing fragrance that can provide a natural pick-me-up during relaxing exercise. Inhaling peppermint oil can increase mental alertness, promote clear thinking, increase motivation, and enhance the overall mindfulness experience.

Here are some ways to incorporate these mindfulness-enhancing essential oils into your relaxation practice:

1. Inhalation: Inhale the scent of these essential oils directly from the bottle or through a personal inhaler before and during mindfulness practice. The uplifting aroma promotes mental clarity and creates a more focused and present state of mind.

2. Aromatherapy Diffuser: Use an aromatherapy diffuser to disperse the uplifting scent of lemon, rosemary, or peppermint into the air. Diffusing these essential oils can create an inspiring and focused atmosphere for mindfulness practice.

3. Blend to create: Use lemon, rosemary, and peppermint to create a custom essential oil blend diluted with an appropriate carrier oil. Before a meditation or mindfulness session, apply the mixture to your pulse points or chest to experience its clarifying effects.

4. Scented Environment: Spray a diluted mixture of these essential oils into water to create a refreshing and purifying room spray. Spraying the mixture into your environment before a relaxation practice can help set the mood for mindful awareness.

Aromatherapy diffusers are a great way to create a soothing, aromatic atmosphere to enhance relaxation practices. Essential oils like lavender, bergamot, or a special relaxation blend can help create a calming environment that supports relaxation and promotes a sense of tranquility. Here's how these essential oils help create a peaceful atmosphere during aromatherapy diffusion: 1. Lavender Essential Oil: Lavender is one of the most popular and well-known essential oils for relaxation. Its sweet floral scent has calming and sedative properties that can help reduce stress and anxiety and promote feelings of relaxation. Diffusing lavender oil before or during relaxation exercises can create a calming atmosphere and create a peaceful space for mindfulness and meditation. 2. Bergamot essential oil: Bergamot has a refreshing and up-lifting citrus scent and has a calming effect on the nervous system. Diffusing bergamot oil can help relieve feelings of tension and anxiety, promoting relax-ation and a positive mindset during relaxation exercises. 3. Relaxation Blends: Many essential oil companies offer premade relaxation blends designed to induce feelings of calm and relaxation. These blends often combine sooth-ing oils such as lavender, chamomile, and ylang-ylang. Diffusing relaxation blends quickly creates a comfortable and stress-relieving environment, perfect for relaxation exercises.

Use aromatherapy (diffuse) to relax:

1. Choose a high-quality diffuser: Choose an ultrasonic or atomizing diffuser because it can effectively disperse essential oils into the air without using heat, which can change the oil's therapeutic properties.

2. Dilute the essential oil: If your diffuser requires water, add the ap-propriate amount of essential oil directly to the water. Use undiluted essential oils directly in the diffuser chamber for a mist diffuser.

3. Start with a few drops: Start with a small amount (usually 3 to 5 drops) of your chosen essential oil or relaxation blend. You can always adjust the number of drops to suit your preference and the size of your room.

4. Diffuse carefully: Open the diffuser and let it disperse the aroma into the air. Enjoy the calm and comforting atmosphere created by essential oils during your relaxation exercises.

5. Safe use: Follow the manufacturer's instructions for your specific diffuser and avoid diffusing essential oils for extended periods. A typical dif-fusion process usually lasts from 30 minutes to an hour.

Diffusing aromatherapy can enhance relaxation practices, create a soothing environment, and cultivate a greater sense of calm and tranquility during mindfulness practices. It is crucial to choose high-quality essential oils and diffusers and practice safe and careful use to experience the benefits of aromatherapy during your relaxation routine.

Adding essential oils to massages and baths can further enhance the relaxing experience and provide deep, soothing, and therapeutic benefits. Es-sential oils like lavender, chamomile, and sandalwood are great choices for massage and bath rituals because of their calming and relaxing properties.

Here's how to use essential oils for massage and bathing:

1. Essential oil massage:

    a. Choose a carrier oil: Choose a carrier oil, such as sweet almond oil, jojoba oil, or coconut oil, and dilute the essential oil for massage. A carrier oil helps spread the essential oil onto the skin and provides nutrients to the skin.
    b. Dilution ratio: For massage, use a safe and effective dilution ratio, about 2 to 3 drops of essential oil per tablespoon of carrier oil. This ensures proper dilution and minimizes the risk of skin sensitivity.
    c. Relaxation Blend: Create a relaxing massage blend by combining essential oils such as lavender, chamomile, and sandalwood. This blend can help relieve tension, reduce stress, and promote relaxation during massage.
    d. Massage Technique: Apply the dilute essential oil mixture to the skin and use gentle massage techniques to promote relaxation. Focus on muscle tension or stress areas and let the oil's calming aroma enhance your massage experience.

2. Essential oil aromatic bath:

    a. Choose bath salts or carrier oil: For bathing, you can add essential oils to bath salts or dilute them in carrier oil before adding them to the bath water. Mixing essential oils with bath salts or carrier oil helps disperse the oil in the water and prevents direct contact with the skin.
    b. Safe dilution: For a complete bath, use approximately 4 to 6 drops of essential oil, premixed with bath salts or carrier oil, dispersed in warm bath water. Swirl the water to ensure even distribution.
    c. Relaxing Soak: Choose essential oils known for their calming properties, such as lavender, chamomile, or sandalwood, to create a soothing, aromatic bath experience. Warm water combined with aromatic oils helps release tension and promote relaxation.

3. Relaxing bath salt recipe:

    * 1 cup Epsom salt
    * 1/4 cup baking soda
    * 10 drops of lavender essential oil
    * 5 drops of chamomile essential oil
    * 5 drops of sandalwood essential oil

    Mix Epsom salt and baking soda in a bowl. Add essential oils and mix thoroughly. Store bath salts in an airtight container. Add a tablespoon (about

1/2 cup) to warm bath water and enjoy a relaxing soak.

4. Bath oil formula:

* 2 tablespoons carrier oil (such as sweet almond or jojoba)
* 6 drops of lavender essential oil
* 4 drops of chamomile essential oil
* 2 drops of sandalwood essential oil

Combine the carrier oil and essential oil in a small bowl or bottle. Add the mixture to warm bath water, swirling the water to disperse the oil before entering the tub. The carrier oil will help create a luxurious and hydrating experience during bath time.

Please note that when using essential oils in the bath, always ensure the oil is properly diluted and fully dispersed in the water. Avoid using undiluted essential oils directly on the skin or adding them directly to bath water without dilution, as this can cause skin irritation. Additionally, essential oils are not soluble in water, so combining them with bath salts or carrier oil is crucial for safe and effective use in the bath.

Using essential oils during massage and bathing can enhance relaxation, promote serenity, and create a calm atmosphere, making the overall relaxation experience more enjoyable and beneficial to your health.

When using essential oils for relaxation, it's important to consider personal preferences and sensitivities. Start with a low concentration and, if applying topically, dilute the essential oil in a suitable carrier oil. Use in moderation and avoid overuse to prevent sensitization or adverse reactions.

B. Calm Essential Oils

Essential oils are known for their various therapeutic properties, and some are known for their calming and soothing effects. The following are essential oils known for their calming and soothing properties:

1. Lavender: Lavender essential oil is one of the most popular and versatile oils, prized for its calming and relaxing effects. It has a sweet floral scent that promotes tranquility, reduces stress, and helps improve sleep quality.

2. Chamomile: Chamomile essential oil is known for its calming and

soothing properties. Its mild apple aroma can help reduce anxiety, soothe nerves, and promote relaxation.

3. Bergamot: Bergamot essential oil has a citrusy, sweet aroma and calming qualities. It enhances mood, relieves tension, and supports emotional well-being.

4. Ylang-ylang: Ylang-ylang essential oil has a rich floral fragrance that makes people feel deeply relaxed and comfortable. It can help reduce stress, promote relaxation, and improve mood.

5. Frankincense: Frankincense essential oil has a warm, woody aroma that is grounding and calming. It can help relieve stress and anxiety and promote a sense of peace.

6. Vetiver: Vetiver essential oil has an earthy, smoky aroma that is deeply grounding and calming. It can help reduce tension and promote relaxation.

7. Neroli: Neroli essential oil has a sweet floral aroma and is known for its calming and uplifting effects. It can help reduce anxiety, improve mood, and promote relaxation.

8. Marjoram: Marjoram essential oil has a warm herbal aroma that is soothing and comforting. It can help relieve tension, calm the mind, and promote relaxation.

9. Geranium: Geranium essential oil has a floral, rosy scent that can help balance emotions, reduce stress, and create a calm atmosphere.

These essential oils can be used individually or blended to create a custom calming and soothing aromatherapy blend. Whether used in aromatherapy diffusers, massage oils, bath products, or personal inhalers, these essential oils promote relaxation, reduce stress, and provide a sense of peace and well-being.

Remember to use high-quality, pure essential oils and consider personal preferences and sensitivities when using these oils. Essential oils can be powerful, so always dilute them correctly and follow recommended safe and effective use guidelines.

These essential oils have specific properties that can help reduce anxiety, promote relaxation, and improve sleep quality:

1. Lavender: Lavender is widely recognized for its calming and relaxing properties. It can help reduce feelings of anxiety and promote a sense of tranquility. Lavender is often used to support better sleep by soothing the mind and promoting relaxation before bed.

2. Chamomile: Chamomile is known for its mild and soothing effects. It can help reduce feelings of stress and anxiety, making it conducive to relaxation and promoting a peaceful mind. Chamomile is also popular for supporting restful sleep.

3. Bergamot: Bergamot has a refreshing citrus aroma with a subtle calming quality. It can help lift your mood and relieve stress and anxiety, making it an excellent choice for relaxation exercises and promoting emotional balance.

4. Ylang-ylang: Ylang-ylang has a rich, sweet floral fragrance that is deeply relaxing. It can help reduce stress and nervous tension, create a soothing atmosphere of relaxation, and promote a sense of well-being.

5. Frankincense: Frankincense is known for its grounding and meditative properties. It can help relieve anxiety and promote inner peace and tranquility, making it suitable for relaxation exercises and mindfulness practices.

6. Vetiver: Vetiver has a deep, earthy aroma and has calming and stabilizing effects. It can help reduce restlessness and promote relaxation during times of stress or anxiety. Vetiver is also known for supporting restful sleep.

7. Orange Blossom: Orange blossom has a sweet, uplifting, calming floral fragrance. It can help relieve anxiety and promote relaxation, helping to create a soothing environment.

8. Marjoram: Marjoram has a warm, herbal fragrance and a comforting quality. It can help reduce nervous tension and stress, supporting relaxation and emotional well-being.

9. Geranium: Geranium has a balancing and uplifting aroma. It can help relieve anxiety and promote relaxation, creating a harmonious atmosphere for relaxation exercises.

These essential oils can be used individually or blended to create a personalized aromatherapy experience that promotes relaxation and reduces anxiety. They can be diffused, used topically in appropriate dilutions, or used in massage oils, bath mixes, or personal inhalers to create a calming environment and support emotional well-being.

To improve sleep quality, consider incorporating these oils into your bedtime routine. Apply the relaxing blend to your bedroom before bed, add a few drops to a warm bath, or apply diluted essential oil to your wrists or chest before bed to help create a peaceful atmosphere and promote a restful night's sleep.

As with any essential oil use, it is crucial to use high-quality, pure essential oils and consider personal sensitivities. If you have specific health concerns or are pregnant or breastfeeding, it is best to consult a qualified aromatherapist or healthcare professional before using essential oils for anxiety or sleep support.

C. Relaxing Aromatherapy Techniques

Aromatherapy offers a variety of relaxation techniques, each providing a unique and enjoyable experience. Here are some popular aromatherapy techniques to promote relaxation:

1. Aromatherapy diffuser: Using an aromatherapy diffuser is one of the most common and convenient ways to enjoy the benefits of essential oils. Diffusers disperse aromatic molecules into the air, creating a calming and aromatic atmosphere in any room. Diffusing essential oils like lavender, chamomile, or bergamot can help reduce stress, promote relaxation, and create a soothing environment.

2. Inhalation: Inhalation is a simple and straightforward way to relax using essential oils. You can add a few drops of your favorite calming oil, such as ylang-ylang or frankincense, to a tissue or inhaler stick. Take a deep breath from a tissue or inhaler to experience the benefits of aromatherapy on the go, at work, or in stressful situations.

3. Aromatherapy massage: Aromatherapy massage combines the therapeutic benefits of essential oils with the relaxing touch of massage. Diluted essential oils are applied to the skin with gentle massage, allowing the oils to be absorbed into the body while promoting relaxation and emotional well-being. Lavender, chamomile, and geranium are popular choices for aromathera-

py massages due to their calming properties.

4. Aromatherapy bath: Aromatherapy bath provides a luxurious and relaxing experience. Add a few drops of essential oil, such as vetiver or marjoram, to warm water and enjoy a soothing soak. The steam and aromatic molecules released from the oil create a peaceful atmosphere, helping to relieve tension and promote relaxation.

5. Personal inhaler: A personal inhaler or aromatherapy inhaler stick is a convenient tool for relaxation on the go. Create a calming blend of essential oils like bergamot and lavender in an inhaler stick and breathe deeply when you need a moment of peace and stress relief.

6. Pillow spray: Spray a mixture of water and a few drops of soothing essential oil (such as neroli or ylang-ylang) onto your pillow before bed. The relaxing aroma will help you relax, improve sleep quality, and promote a sense of calm.

7. Steam inhalation: Steam inhalation is good for breathing and relaxation. Add a few drops of essential oil, such as eucalyptus or peppermint, to hot water, cover your head with a towel, and inhale the steam deeply. Aromatic steam can help clear your mind, relieve tension, and soothe your senses.

8. Aromatherapy roll-on: Create a custom roll-on blend using essential oils like bergamot, chamomile, and frankincense. Dilute the oil in a carrier oil and apply the mixture to pulse points for a quick and calming aromatherapy experience throughout the day.

Each aromatherapy technique offers a unique way to incorporate essential oils into your relaxation practice. Remember to use high-quality, pure essential oils and follow proper dilution guidelines to ensure safe and effective use. Whether you're diffusing essential oils at home, enjoying a soothing massage, or using a personal inhaler on the go, aromatherapy can be a powerful tool to promote relaxation, reduce stress, and enhance overall well-being.

Each aromatherapy technique has its own unique benefits and best practices for maximizing the calming effects of essential oils. Let's explore the benefits and best practices of each technique to help you get the most out of your relaxation experience:

1. Aromatherapy diffuser:

Benefits: Diffusing essential oils creates a calming atmosphere and disperses aromatic molecules throughout the room. This method promotes relaxation, reduces stress, and creates a soothing environment in your home or office.

Best practices:

Use a high-quality ultrasonic or nebulizer diffuser to ensure proper dispersion of essential oils.

Add 3 to 5 drops of essential oil per 100 ml of water in the diffuser.

Diffuse the oil for 30 minutes to an hour at a time, taking breaks in between to prevent olfactory fatigue.

Adjust the number of drops based on the size of the room and personal preference.

2. Inhalation:

Benefits: Inhalation provides direct and immediate access to the aromatic benefits of essential oils. This technique is great for quick stress relief, relaxation, and emotional support.

Best practices:

Use a personal inhaler or tissue for discreet and portable inhalation.

3 to 5 drops of essential oil to a personal inhaler or tissue.

Breathe deeply 3 to 5 times or as needed to experience the desired calming effect.

Choose calming oils to inhale, like lavender, chamomile, or bergamot.

3. Aromatherapy massage:

Benefits: Aromatherapy massage combines the relaxing benefits of touch with the therapeutic properties of essential oils to promote deep relaxation and emotional well-being.

Best practices:

Dilute the essential oil in a carrier oil such as sweet almond, jojoba, or coconut oil before applying it to the skin.

Use 10 to 20 drops of essential oil per 30 ml of carrier oil as a massage mixture.

Enjoy a full body or targeted massage with slow, gentle strokes to relax muscles and calm the mind.

Choose essential oils like lavender, chamomile, or geranium for a calming massage experience.

4. Aromatherapy bath:

Benefits: Aromatherapy baths provide a luxurious and immersive relaxation experience, making them ideal for relaxing after a long day and promoting restful sleep.

Best practices:

Before adding it to warm wash water, add 5 to 10 drops of essential oil to a tablespoon of carrier oil, bath salts, or unscented liquid soap.

Stir the water to disperse the oil evenly.

Soak in the aromatic bath for at least 15 to 20 minutes to fully enjoy the calming effect.

Choose essential oils like vetiver, marjoram, or ylang-ylang for a peaceful bathing experience.

5. Personal inhaler:

Benefits: Personal inhalers provide a discreet and convenient way to enjoy essential oils on the go, quickly relieving stress and promoting relaxation during busy times.

Best practices:

Get a custom blend of calming oils like bergamot, lavender, or frankincense in a personal inhaler.

Use the inhaler as needed throughout the day, take deep breaths in the aroma, and experience relaxation.

Replace the wick in your inhaler every few weeks to ensure freshness and potency.

6. Pillow spray:

Benefits: Pillow spray helps create a restful sleep environment, promoting relaxation and better sleep quality.

Best practices:

Add 10 to 15 drops of essential oil to 30 ml of water in a spray bottle.

Shake well before each use and gently massage pillows and bedding before bed.

Choose soothing essential oils like neroli, ylang-ylang, or lavender to help you drift off to sleep.

7. Steam inhalation:

Benefits: Steam inhalation is great for breathing and relaxation, helping clear the mind and relieve tension.

Best practices:

3 to 5 drops of essential oil to a bowl of hot water.

Cover your head with a towel to form a steam tent, and inhale deeply for 5 to 10 minutes.

Choose an invigorating oil like eucalyptus, peppermint, or rosemary to inhale the refreshing steam.

8. Aromatherapy roller balls:

Pros: Aromatherapy roll-ons allow for easy targeted application and can be carried in your purse or pocket for quick relaxation throughout the day.

Best practices:

Dilute 5 to 10 drops of calming oil in a 10 ml roller bottle with a carrier oil such as jojoba or sweet almond oil.

Apply the rollerball to pulse points such as wrists, temples, and behind ears when you need to relax and unwind.

By following these best practices, you can enhance the calming effects of essential oils in your relaxation practice and experience their full potential in reducing stress, promoting relaxation, and improving overall well-being. Always use pure and high-quality essential oils and consider personal preferences and sensitivities when choosing blends.

D. Create a Calming Mixture

Creating custom calming blends using essential oils allows you to tailor your aromatherapy experience to your personal preferences and needs. Here are some guidelines to help you create your personalized calming blend:

1. Choose your base oil: Start by choosing a base oil, as it forms the base of your blend and provides a long-lasting scent. Common base oils used in calming blends include:

Sandalwood is A woody and grounding scent that promotes relaxation and mental clarity.

Vetiver: An earthy and deep scent known for its calming and balancing properties.

Patchouli: A warm, musky scent that helps relieve tension and anxiety.

2. Add a mid-note oil: A mid-note oil adds complexity to the mix and acts as a mediator between the base and top notes. Some popular mid-note oils used in calming blends are:

Lavender: A versatile soothing oil known for its calming effects on the mind and body.

Roman Chamomile: A mild, comforting scent that promotes relaxation and restful sleep.

Geranium: A floral and balancing oil that helps relieve nervous tension and lift mood.

3. Include top note oil: Top note oil provides freshness and initial fragrance to your blend. They are often light and uplifting. Consider adding these top-note oils for a calming and refreshing touch:

Bergamot: A citrusy and bright oil that helps reduce stress and promote positive emotions.

Sweet orange: A cheerful, sweet scent that induces relaxation and happiness.

Ylang-Ylang: A rich floral scent known for its calming and aphrodisiac properties.

4. Experiment with proportions: Essential oil mixtures have no one-size-fits-all ratio. Start with equal parts of the oil of your choice and adjust the proportions based on your scent preference. For example, you could use a 2 to 3%: 2 ratios (2 drops of base notes, 3 drops of midrange, and 2 drops of top notes) as a starting point and modify it from there.

5. Dilute and Carrier Oil: Since essential oils are highly concentrated, dilute the calming mixture in carrier oil before use. Common carrier oils include sweet almond oil, jojoba oil, coconut oil, or grapeseed oil. A 2 to 3% dilution rate is generally safe for most adults. For example, use 6 to 9 drops of essential oil blend per 10 ml carrier oil.

6. Safety precautions: Some essential oils, especially citrus oils, can cause skin sensitivity when exposed to sunlight. If you plan to use the calming mixture on your skin, avoid direct sunlight or UV rays for at least 12 hours after application.

7. Document: As you try different essential oil combinations, document the blends you create and their impact on your mood and relaxation. This will help you identify your favorite combinations for future use.

Here are examples of custom calming blends:

*3 drops of sandalwood (base note)
*4 drops of lavender (middle note)
*2 drops of bergamot (top note)

Dilute the mixture in 10ml of carrier oil (such as jojoba oil) and use it in an aromatherapy diffuser, massage, or as a calming roll-on.

Aromatherapy is a personal experience, so feel free to adjust the mixture to suit your preferences. Be aware of any allergies or sensitivities and perform a patch test before applying the mixture to larger areas of the body. Enjoy the calming benefits of a custom essential oil blend and embrace the tranquility it brings to your daily life.

Proper mixing ratios, complementary scents, and application methods play a vital role in maximizing the calming effects of essential oils for a variety of relaxation purposes. Here are some guidelines for different relaxation options:

1. Aromatherapy diffuser:

5 to 10 drops of essential oil in the diffuser. You can adjust the number of drops depending on the size of your diffuser and the intensity of your preferred scent.

Complementary scents: Blending 2 to 3 essential oils belonging to different aroma categories (base, middle, and top notes) together to create a balanced and complex blend. For example, you could mix 2 drops of sandalwood (base note), 3 drops of lavender (middle note), and 1 drop of bergamot (top note).

How to use: Add the essential oil blend to your diffuser according to the manufacturer's instructions and enjoy the calming aroma as it fills the room.

2. Relaxing massage combination:

Mixing ratio: For massage mixes, use a 2 to 3% dilution rate. Mix 6 to 9 drops of essential oil with 10 ml of carrier oil (such as sweet almond or jojoba oil).

Complementary scents: Choose essential oils with soothing properties, such as lavender, chamomile, and ylang-ylang. You can also add a touch of grounding oil like vetiver or a floral scent like geranium.

How to use: Apply the massage mixture to your skin and enjoy relaxation as you gently massage into your muscles.

3. Relaxation bath:

Mixing ratio: For a relaxing bath, use 8 to 10 drops of essential oil mixed with a dispersing agent like Epsom salt or a carrier oil before adding it to the bath water.

Complement your scent: Consider essential oils like lavender, chamomile, and bergamot for a relaxing bath experience. You can also add a few drops of citrus oil, such as sweet orange, for a refreshing flavor.

How to use: Mix the essential oil mixture with a dispersant or carrier oil and add it to warm water. Relax and soak in the calming aroma.

4. Calming ball:

Mixing ratio: For rolling mixes, use a dilution rate of 2 to 3%. Mix 6 to 9 drops of essential oil with 10 ml of carrier oil (such as fractionated coconut oil).

Complementary Fragrance: Blend soothingly with essential oils like lavender, chamomile, and frankincense. Add a little cedar wood for a grounding effect.

Directions: Roll the mixture onto your pulse points, such as wrists, temples, and neck. Carry the roller balls with you for instant relaxation throughout the day.

5. Pillow spray before bed:

Mixing ratio: For pillow spray, use 20 to 30 drops of essential oil mixed with water and a solubilizer (a dispersing agent that helps essential oils mix with water).

Complement your scent: Choose calming oils like lavender, chamomile, and ylang-ylang. Add a touch of vetiver or cedar wood to create a cozy sleeping environment.

How to use: Gently spray the mixture on your pillow before bed to promote restful and restful sleep.

Remember, essential oils are potent and should be used with caution. Always do a patch test before applying the mixture to larger areas of the body. Customize your blend to your personal preferences and needs and enjoy the relaxation and tranquility that essential oils bring to your relaxation practice.

E. Sleep Support

Exploring essential oils known for their sleep-enhancing properties can be beneficial for those looking to improve their sleep quality and experience a more restful night. Here are some essential oils known for their calming and sleep-promoting effects:

1. Lavender: Lavender is one of the most popular essential oils for promoting relaxation and sleep. Its soothing aroma has been shown to reduce stress and anxiety, helping individuals achieve a calmer state before bed.

2. Vetiver: Vetiver has a deep, earthy scent that is grounding and comforting. It is often used to calm a restless mind and promote a sense of tranquility, perfect for those who struggle with racing thoughts before bed.

3. Cedar: Cedar has a warm, woody aroma that can create a peaceful atmosphere. Its calming properties make it useful for those seeking peaceful and undisturbed sleep.

4. Marjoram: Marjoram has a sweet and herbal fragrance and is known for its relaxing and calming effects. It can help relieve nervous tension, promote relaxation, and prepare the mind and body for a restful sleep.

These essential oils can be used alone or blended to create a synergistic sleep-enhancing blend. Here is a simple bedtime blend recipe using these essential oils:

Calming Sleep Blend:

*4 drops of lavender essential oil
*3 drops of vetiver essential oil
*3 drops of cedar essential oil
*2 drops of marjoram essential oil

Dilute this mixture in 10 ml of carrier oil (such as fractionated coconut oil) for topical application or add it to an aromatherapy diffuser to create a relaxing atmosphere in the bedroom. You can also make a bedtime pillow spray by combining this mixture with water and a solubilizer.

It's crucial to establish a relaxing bedtime routine to signal your body that it's time to wind down. Incorporate these essential oils into your bedtime ritual, such as diffusing them at night, applying a diluted mixture to your pulse points, or using them in a soothing bedtime bath.

As with any essential oil use, individual reactions may vary. If you have any known allergies or sensitivities, perform a patch test before applying the mixture to larger areas of the skin. Creating a calming and sleep-promoting environment with these essential oils can be a powerful addition to your sleep hygiene routine.

Incorporating essential oils into your nighttime routine can significantly improve sleep quality and promote a more restful night. Here are some tips and tricks for using sleep-enhancing essential oils effectively:

1. Diffuse: Use an aromatherapy diffuser in the bedroom to disperse sleep-promoting essential oils into the air. Start diffusing about 30 minutes before bed to create a calming atmosphere. Consider using the calming sleep blend mentioned earlier, or try different combinations to find one that works best for you.

2. Topical application: Dilute the essential oil of your choice in a carrier oil, such as coconut oil or jojoba oil, and apply the mixture to your pulse points, temples, neck, or soles of your feet. Gently massage the essential oil into the skin to help it absorb and enhance the relaxing experience.

3. Bath before bed: Add a few drops of your favorite sleep-enhancing essential oil to your bath water. Warm water will help release the scent of the oil, and the soothing experience can prepare your mind and body for sleep.

4. Pillow spray: Create a calming pillow spray by mixing essential oils with water and a solubilizer (a substance that helps oil and water mix). Lightly spray your pillows and bedding before bed, and enjoy the relaxing scent as you fall asleep.

5. Relaxation techniques: Incorporate relaxation techniques such as deep breathing, meditation, or gentle stretching before bed. Combine these practices with the use of essential oils to enhance their calming effects and reduce stress and anxiety.

6. Consistency: Make using essential oils a part of your nightly routine. Consistency is key to reaping the full benefits of its sleep-enhancing properties. As you create a bedtime ritual using essential oils, your body will begin to associate the scents with relaxation and sleep.

7. Limit screen time: Reduce screen time (phone, computer, TV) at least an hour before bed. The blue light emitted by screens can interfere with melatonin production and disrupt your sleep-wake cycle.

8. Create a soothing environment: Make your bedroom a sleep haven

by keeping it cool, dark, and quiet. Consider using blackout curtains, earplugs, or a white noise machine to minimize distractions.

9. Relaxing activities: Carry out calming activities before going to bed, such as reading, listening to soft music, and taking a hot bath. Avoid stimulating or stressful activities that may interfere with relaxation.

Keep in mind that essential oils can complement healthy sleep habits, but individual reactions may vary. If you experience any adverse reactions or have a pre-existing medical condition, consult a healthcare professional before using essential oils to support sleep. By incorporating these tips and tricks into your nighttime routine, you can harness the calming and soothing power of essential oils to improve the quality of your sleep and wake up feeling refreshed and rejuvenated.

F. Relaxation Rituals and Practices

Incorporating essential oils into relaxation rituals and practices can deepen the calming and soothing effects. Here are some ideas for using essential oils in meditation, yoga, and bath rituals:

1. Meditation:

Diffuse your meditation space with calming essential oils like lavender, chamomile, or frankincense to create a peaceful atmosphere.

Place a drop of the oil of your choice on the palms of your hands, rub them together, and take a deep breath to center and calm the mind before starting your meditation session.

Mix a few drops of essential oil with a carrier oil and apply it to your pulse points before meditation to help you stay present and focused.

If you use a meditation cushion or eye pillow, add a drop of essential oil to it to enhance relaxation during your practice.

2. Yoga:

Enhance your yoga practice by diffusing grounding essential oils like vetiver, cedarwood, or patchouli in your yoga space to promote a sense of stability and connection.

Before starting a yoga class, apply a mixture of essential and carrier oils to your wrists, neck, or heart center to encourage mindfulness and intention.

DIY yoga mat spray using essential oils, water, and a little witch hazel or white vinegar. Spray your mat before practice for an uplifting and uplifting experience.

3. Bathing ritual:

Add a few drops of your favorite essential oil to a carrier oil, Epsom salt, or body wash before adding it to your bath water. Immerse yourself in the calming aroma and relax.

For a luxurious and skin-nourishing experience, create a bath oil by blending essential oils like lavender, geranium, and ylang-ylang with a carrier oil like jojoba or sweet almond oil.

Consider using essential oil-infused bath bombs for an indulgent and aromatic bathing ritual.

4. Aromatherapy massage:

If you do a self-massage or receive a massage from a partner or professional, add essential oils for a soothing and sensual experience.

Create a massage oil blend using essential oils known for their relaxing properties, such as chamomile, sage, and bergamot, combined with a carrier oil like coconut or almond oil.

5. Breathing techniques:

Practice deep breathing exercises while inhaling the calming scent of essential oils from the palm of your hand or a diffuser. The combination of breathwork and aromatherapy can amplify the relaxation response.

6. Personal inhaler:

Use a personal inhaler stick infused with your favorite essential oil blend. Carry it with you throughout the day, and enjoy calming aromatherapy when you need a moment to relax.

When using essential oils, remember to follow proper dilution guidelines topically and consult a qualified aromatherapist or healthcare professional if you have any concerns or medical conditions. By incorporating essential oils into your relaxation rituals and practices, you can create a more immersive and transformative experience that nourishes the body, mind, and spirit.

Incorporating essential oils into your relaxation practice can enhance the overall experience and provide additional relaxation benefits. Here are guidelines on how to use essential oils in specific practices:

1. Meditation:

Diffuse: Use an aromatherapy diffuser to diffuse calming essential oils like lavender, chamomile, or frankincense in your meditation space.

Personal Inhalation: Inhale the aroma directly from the bottle or apply a drop of essential oil to your palms, rub them together, then cover your nose with your hands and breathe deeply.

Topical application: Apply a dilute blend of essential oils to your pulse points or heart center before meditation to promote feelings of calm and focus.

2. Yoga:

Diffuse: Choose to ground essential oils like vetiver, cedarwood, or patchouli to diffuse in your yoga space to enhance a sense of stability and connection during your practice.

Topical Application: Before starting a yoga class, apply a diluted essential oil blend to your wrists, neck, or temples to support mindfulness and intention.

3. Bathing ritual:

Bath oil: Make a bath oil blend by mixing a few drops of essential oil (such as lavender, geranium, or ylang-ylang) with a carrier oil like jojoba or sweet almond oil. Add this mixture to your bath water for a relaxing and aromatic experience.

Bath salts: Combine Epsom salts with your favorite essential oils for a soothing and muscle-relaxing bath. Add a few drops to the bath water when filling the tub.

4. Aromatherapy massage:

Massage oil: Make a massage oil blend using calming essential oils like chamomile, sage, and bergamot mixed with a carrier oil like coconut or almond oil. Use this mixture for self-massage or massage with a partner or professional.

5. Breathing techniques:

Inhalation: Inhale the calming scent of essential oils while practicing deep breathing exercises. You can use a diffuser, a personal inhaler wand, or inhale directly from the bottle.

6. Personal inhaler:

DIY Inhaler: Create a personal inhaler stick by adding a few drops of your favorite essential oil blend to the inhaler tube. Carry it with you throughout the day and relax anytime, anywhere.

7. DIY products:

Customize your relaxation experience by using essential oils to create DIY products, such as pillow spray, room spray, or massage oil, to promote relaxation and calmness.

Always follow proper dilution guidelines and safety precautions when using essential oils in these relaxation exercises. If you are new to essential oils or have specific health concerns, consider consulting with a certified aromatherapist or healthcare professional for personalized guidance.

Remember, relaxation exercises vary from person to person, so feel free to experiment with different oils and techniques to find the one that resonates best with you. By incorporating essential oils into your relaxation ritual, you can create a more immersive and peaceful experience that supports overall health and reduces stress.

G. Stress Management and Mood Enhancement

Essential oils have long been valued for their stress-relieving and mood-enhancing properties. Here are some essential oils known for their positive effects on stress and mood:

1. Citrus oils: Citrus essential oils, such as sweet orange, lemon, grapefruit, and bergamot, are known for their uplifting and uplifting scents. They are rich in compounds such as limonene, which promotes positive emotions, reduces stress, and increases feelings of well-being and relaxation. Diffusing these oils or using them in a personal inhaler can provide a quick and effective mood boost.

2. Sage: Sage essential oil is known for its calming and soothing effects on the nervous system. It contains linalyl acetate and linalool, which

contribute to its stress-relieving properties. This oil can help relieve tension, reduce anxiety, and create a sense of tranquility during relaxation exercises.

3. Frankincense: Frankincense essential oil has been used for centuries in spiritual and meditative practices. It is thought to promote feelings of grounding and deep relaxation. The woody and resinous aroma of frankincense can help calm the mind and reduce feelings of stress and anxiety.

4. Lavender: Lavender essential oil is a well-known favorite for relaxing and relieving stress. Its floral and soothing fragrance can help calm the mind, promote better sleep, and reduce nervous tension. Lavender is often used in diffusers, bath salts, and massage oils to create a relaxing atmosphere.

5. Vetiver: Vetiver essential oil has a rich, earthy aroma that is deeply grounding and calming. It's great for promoting relaxation and relieving feelings of restlessness and stress. Vetiver can be diffused or used topically in dilute form for calming and focusing effects.

6. Rose: Rose essential oil has a beautiful and uplifting fragrance and is known for its mood-enhancing properties. It can help reduce feelings of sadness, anxiety, and stress. The luxurious scent of rose oil can be enjoyed by inhalation, diffusion, or topical application.

When using essential oils to relieve stress and lift your mood, consider these tips:

Diffusing is one of the most popular and effective ways to use essential oils to create a calming and uplifting environment. Here's how to use an aromatherapy diffuser for best results:

1. Choose a high-quality diffuser: Choose a high-quality ultrasonic diffuser or atomizer that does not use heat-dispersing oils. Heat can change the chemical composition of essential oils and reduce their therapeutic effectiveness.

2. Add water: Fill the diffuser with clean room temperature water until it reaches the marked level as directed by the manufacturer. Make sure not to exceed the maximum fill line.

3. Add essential oils: Add 3 to 10 drops of your chosen essential oil or blend with the water in your diffuser. The number of drops will depend on the size of the room, the intensity of the desired scent, and the specific essential

oil used.

4. Customize your blend: Create your custom blend by combining different essential oils known for their stress-relieving and mood-enhancing properties. For example, a blend of lavender, bergamot, and sage can create a calming and uplifting atmosphere.

5. Turn on the diffuser: After adding the essential oils to the water, follow the manufacturer's instructions to turn on the diffuser. Diffusers disperse a fine mist into the air, carrying the aromatic molecules of essential oils throughout the room.

6. Set the duration: Some diffusers have settings that control the duration of the diffuser. You can choose to diffuse the oil continuously or set it to intermittent mode, depending on your preference.

7. Enjoy the aroma: Relax and enjoy the calming and uplifting aroma of the essential oils dispersed into the air. The scent will create a soothing atmosphere, helping to reduce stress, promote relaxation and improve mood.

8. Clean your diffuser: Remember to clean your diffuser according to the manufacturer's instructions after each use to prevent essential oil residue buildup and maintain your diffuser's effectiveness.

When diffusing essential oils, make sure the room is well-ventilated and never leave the diffuser unattended. If you have pets in your home, be aware that some essential oils can be harmful to animals, so research pet-safe oils or place your diffuser in a pet-free area.

Diffusing essential oils is a simple and enjoyable way to incorporate aromatherapy into your daily life. Whether you're winding down in the evening or starting your day on a positive note, using an aromatherapy diffuser can help create a calming and uplifting environment that supports relaxation and relieves stress.

Inhalation is a quick and easy way to experience the stress-relieving and mood-enhancing effects of essential oils. Here's how to use inhalation techniques to relieve the stress of moving:

1. Direct inhalation: Open the essential oil bottle of your choice and hold it close to your nose. Take a deep breath through your nose and inhale the aroma directly from the bottle. Repeat this process a few times, focusing on the

scent and letting it calm your senses.

2. Personal Inhaler Sticks: Personal inhalers are portable devices that allow you to take your favorite essential oils with you wherever you go. To use a personal inhaler wand, follow these steps:

a. Remove the cap from the inhaler and remove the absorbent wick.
b. Add 5 to 10 drops of your favorite essential oil or mixture on the cotton wick.
c. Place the wick back into the inhaler and secure the cap.
d. Hold the inhaler in one nostril while closing the other nostril with your finger.
e. Take a deep breath through your nose and inhale the aroma of the inhaler.
f. If necessary, repeat the process on the other nostril.

3. Pocket tissue or handkerchief: If you don't have a personal inhaler, you can also add a few drops of essential oil to a tissue or handkerchief. Hold the scented tissue close to your nose, take a deep breath, and experience the scent.

4. Hand rubbing technique: Add a few drops of essential oil to your palms, rub them together, and then cover your nose and mouth with your hands. Take a deep breath and inhale the aromatic vapor.

5. Steam inhalation: For a more intense inhalation experience, add a few drops of essential oil to a bowl of steaming water. Lean against the bowl, drape a towel over your head to create a steam tent, and inhale deeply.

When using the inhalation technique, be sure to choose essential oils known for their stress-relieving and mood-enhancing properties, such as lavender, bergamot, sage, or frankincense. These oils can quickly help you relax, reduce anxiety, and promote a sense of well-being.

Remember, essential oils go a long way, so start with a few drops and adjust as needed. Additionally, if you have any respiratory conditions or sensitivities, please consult a healthcare professional before using essential oil inhalation techniques. With the convenience of the inhalation method, you can easily incorporate essential oils into your daily routine for stress relief and relaxation.

Topical application is another effective way to enjoy the stress-relieving and mood-enhancing benefits of essential oils. When using essential oils topically, they must be diluted in an appropriate carrier oil to ensure safe and comfortable use. Here's how to use essential oils topically to relieve stress:

1. Choose a carrier oil: Choose a carrier oil that suits your skin type and preferences. Some popular carrier oils include sweet almond oil, jojoba oil, coconut oil, and grapeseed oil. A carrier oil helps dilute the essential oil and bring its properties to the skin without irritating it.

2. Determine the dilution ratio: The appropriate dilution ratio depends on the individual's age, skin sensitivity, and the specific essential oil being used. As a general guideline for adults, use a 1~2% dilution, which means adding 1 to 2 drops of essential oil per teaspoon (5 ml) of carrier oil. For children or those with sensitive skin, use a lower dilution.

3. Conduct a patch test: Before using a new essential oil or blend, a patch test must be performed on a small area of skin. This will help you check for any potential allergic reactions or sensitivities to the oil.

4. Apply to pulse points: Pulse points are areas where blood vessels are close to the surface of the skin, allowing the aroma of essential oils to be released more easily. Common pulse points include the wrists, temples, behind the ears, and inside the elbows.

5. Back of neck: Applying an essential oil blend to the back of the neck can promote relaxation and relieve tension, especially when experiencing stress-related headaches.

6. Hand massage: Mix a few drops of essential oil with your favorite unscented hand lotion or carrier oil. Rub your hands together to warm the oil, then gently massage your temples and forehead for a calming experience.

7. Self-massage: If you have some time to relax, consider giving yourself a brief neck and shoulder massage with an essential oil blend. Use gentle circular motions to massage the oil into the skin and release tension.

8. Aromatherapy bath: Spice up your bath time by adding a few drops of your chosen essential oil blend to warm water. The steam generated by the bath will dissipate the aroma, creating a soothing aromatic experience.

Always remember to store essential oils safely, away from direct sunlight and out of the reach of children and pets. If you experience any skin irritation or discomfort, discontinue use immediately and wash the affected area with carrier oil.

By using topical applications, you can integrate the stress-relieving and mood-enhancing properties of essential oils into your self-care routine and enjoy their calming effects throughout the day.

Bathing is a great way to incorporate stress-relieving essential oils into your relaxation routine. By adding a few drops of stress-relieving essential oils to your bath water, you can create a soothing and aromatic soak that helps melt away stress and tension. Here's how to use essential oils in your bath:

1. Choose a relaxing essential oil: Choose a stress-relieving essential oil that you find calming and pleasurable. Lavender, chamomile, ylang-ylang, bergamot, and sage are great choices for promoting relaxation and reducing stress.

2. Dilute essential oils: Essential oils are highly concentrated, so it's important to dilute them before adding them to your bath water. Mix the essential oils with the dispersant, making sure they are thoroughly mixed with the water. Some options for dispersants include Epsom salts, bath oil, or a small amount of unscented liquid soap.

3. Make the bath mixture: In a small bowl, mix a few drops of the stress-relieving essential oil of your choice with the dispersant. Stir the mixture well to ensure an even distribution of essential oils.

4. Add to bath water: Fill the tub with warm water and add the bath mixture you created. Swirl the water with your hands to disperse the essential oils throughout the tub.

5. Relax and enjoy: Step into the tub, take a deep breath, and inhale the calming aroma of the essential oils. Allow yourself to relax and let go of any stress or tension. You can stay in the bathtub for 15 to 30 minutes to fully enjoy the benefits of essential oils.

6. NOTE: Be careful when adding essential oils to the bath, as they can make the bath slippery. Use a bathmat or towel to prevent slipping and ensure your safety.

7. Combine with Epsom Salts: If you have sore muscles or want to enhance your relaxation experience, consider adding Epsom salts to your bath-

tub. Epsom salt can help relax muscles and provide additional therapeutic benefits.

8. Personalize your bath: Feel free to try different combinations of stress-reducing essential oils to create a bath blend that suits your preferences and needs. You can also add dried flowers or herbs to enhance the visual and aromatic experience.

Remember, before using any new essential oil in the bath, be sure to dilute it correctly and perform a patch test to avoid any skin irritation or sensitivity. Bathing with stress-relieving essential oils is a pleasant and effective way to relax, relieve stress, and enjoy a moment of relaxation and tranquility.

Massage is a great way to incorporate stress-relieving essential oils into your relaxation routine. The combination of soothing touch and aromatic essential oils creates a deeply calming and therapeutic experience. Here's how to use essential oils in massage to enhance relaxation:

1. Choose relaxing essential oils: Choose stress-relieving essential oils to complement the massage experience and promote relaxation. Lavender, chamomile, ylang-ylang, bergamot, sage, and frankincense are some popular choices for their calming properties.

2. Dilute essential oils: Essential oils are potent and should be diluted before applying to the skin. Mix the essential oil with a carrier oil (such as sweet almond, jojoba, or coconut oil) at the appropriate dilution ratio. A common dilution ratio for massage is 2 to 3 drops of essential oil per tablespoon of carrier oil.

3. Create the massage mixture: In a small bowl or bottle, combine the selected stress-relieving essential oil with the carrier oil. Mix thoroughly to ensure the essential oil is evenly dispersed in the carrier oil.

4. Perform a patch test: Before massaging, perform a patch test on a small area of the skin to check for any sensitivity or allergic reactions.

5. Massage technique: Begin your massage by heating a small amount of the massage mixture in your hands. Apply the oil to the recipient's skin using gentle, smooth stroking and kneading motions. Focus on areas of tension or stress, such as your neck, shoulders, back, and feet.

6. Aromatherapy benefits: When you massage the mixture into your

skin, the calming aroma of the essential oils is released, enhancing the relaxing experience. Recipients are encouraged to breathe deeply to inhale the soothing scent, promoting relaxation and reducing stress.

7. Custom blend: Feel free to customize your massage blend to the recipient's preferences and needs. You can adjust essential oil combinations and dilutions to create a personalized experience.

8. Relaxing environment: Create a relaxing atmosphere for your massage by dimming the lights, playing soft music, and using an aromatherapy diffuser to diffuse the scent of your chosen essential oil.

9. Communicate: During the massage, communicate with the recipient to ensure their comfort and adjust pressure or focus areas as needed.

10. Relax after the massage: After the massage, encourage the recipient to take a moment to rest and relax to enjoy the stress-reducing effects of the essential oils fully.

Massage with stress-relieving essential oils can provide physical and emotional benefits, helping to reduce muscle tension, relieve stress, and promote a sense of tranquility and well-being. Massage must be performed with care and sensitivity to create a comfortable and nourishing experience for the recipient.

Remember that individuals may react differently to essential oils, so it's important to find the scent that resonates most with you. Also, consider any potential sensitivities or allergies and perform a patch test before using a new essential oil. Incorporating these essential oils into your daily life and relaxation practices can promote positive emotions, reduce stress, and enhance your overall well-being.

Using essential oils to manage stress and lift mood throughout the day involves a variety of techniques that are quick and easy to use. Here are some ways to incorporate stress-relieving and mood-enhancing essential oils into your daily life:

1. Aromatherapy diffuser: Use an aromatherapy diffuser in your home or office to disperse stress-relieving essential oils into the air. Diffusing oils like lavender, bergamot, or sage can create a calming and uplifting vibe throughout the day.

2. Personal inhalation stick: Carry a personal inhalation stick filled with stress-relieving essential oils to relieve stress on the go. Breathe directly from your inhaler when you need a quick mood boost or a moment of calm.

3. Roll-on blend: Create a roll-on blend in a roller bottle by diluting stress-relieving essential oils with carrier oil. Apply the mixture to your pulse points, temples, or the back of your neck whenever you feel stressed or need a mood boost.

4. Aromatherapy jewelry: Wearing diffuser jewelry, such as a necklace or bracelet, allows you to apply essential oils directly to the porous surface of the jewelry. This way, you can enjoy the benefits of aromatherapy throughout the day.

5. Desk diffuser: Place a small bowl of cotton balls or a clay diffuser on your desk. Add a few drops of stress-relieving essential oil and let the scent gently diffuse while you work.

6. Decompression bath: Add a few drops of decompression essential oil to warm bath water to take a decompression bath. Soak in and inhale the soothing scent to relax and unwind after a long day.

7. Aromatherapy inhalation: Inhale the stress-relieving essential oil directly from the bottle, a few inches away from your nose, and take a deep breath.

8. Hand sanitizer spray: Make a homemade hand sanitizer spray with stress-relieving essential oils. Take it with you and use it throughout the day for a refreshing and mood-enhancing spray.

9. Mood-lifting room spray: Make a mood-lifting room spray by diluting essential oils in water and alcohol (optional) in a spray bottle. Spray the air in your living space or office to create a positive and uplifting environment.

10. Mindful breathing: Practice mindful breathing exercises with essential oils. Breathe deeply while holding the scent of the stress-relieving oil in your hands or on a cotton pad. Exhale slowly and focus on releasing tension and promoting relaxation.

Remember, essential oils are highly concentrated and should be used with caution. Always do a patch test before using them on your skin and stick to the proper dilution ratio to avoid skin sensitization. If you have any medical conditions or are pregnant or breastfeeding, please consult a qualified aroma-therapist or healthcare professional before using essential oils. Through these techniques, you can effectively integrate the benefits of stress-relieving and mood-enhancing essential oils into your daily life, resulting in a more balanced and positive attitude throughout the day.

H. Personalized Leisure Space

Creating a personalized relaxation space infused with essential oils is critical to increasing the effectiveness of relaxation practices and promoting overall health. Here are some key reasons why a relaxation space dedicated to essential oils can make a difference:

1. Encourage regular relaxation: Having a designated relaxation space encourages you to prioritize relaxation in your daily life. When you associate a specific area with relaxation, you're more likely to spend time there regularly relaxing and destressing.

2. Create an ambiance: A relaxing space infused with calming essential oils creates a tranquil and peaceful mood. The soothing aroma creates a peaceful environment, making it easier to get into a relaxed state of mind.

3. Reduce stress: In a personalized relaxation space, you can disconnect from the outside world and reduce stress. The combination of essential oils and a calming environment can significantly reduce cortisol levels and promote a sense of calm.

4. Enhance mindfulness practices: Dedicated relaxation spaces can support mindfulness practices such as meditation and yoga. The presence of essential oils can deepen your focus and help you stay present during these practices.

5. Improve sleep quality: Using essential oils in your relaxation space, especially before bed, can improve sleep quality. Calming scents signal your brain that it's time to relax, making it easier to fall asleep and stay asleep.

6. Boost your mood: Aromatherapy with mood-enhancing essential oils can lift your spirits and improve your overall mood. You can create a positive atmosphere to offset negative emotions in a personalized relaxation space.

7. Promote self-care: Have a dedicated relaxation space to encourage

self-care practices. Reading a book, practicing yoga, or simply taking a moment to breathe deeply into the oil's presence enhances the overall experience.

8. Create a retreat-like experience: Your personalized relaxation space can become your sanctuary — a retreat from the stresses of everyday life. This is a place where you can relax, recharge, and find solace.

9. Helps with stress management: Regularly spending time in a relaxing space using essential oils can be a valuable tool in managing stress. It provides an outlet to relax and cope with life's challenges.

10. Support overall health: By incorporating essential oils into your relaxing space, you can support your overall physical and emotional health. The calming fragrance and soothing environment promote a balanced and healthy lifestyle.

To create a personalized relaxation space, consider these tips:

1. Choose calming colors: Paint your walls in soothing colors like soft blues, greens, or neutrals to create a peaceful atmosphere.

2. Add comfortable seating: Invest in comfortable seating, such as a comfy armchair or a soft meditation cushion, where you can relax and unwind.

3. Use soft lighting: Choose soft, warm lighting to promote relaxation. Dimmable lights or candles can create a calming atmosphere.

4. Incorporate nature: Bring natural elements into your space, such as potted plants or natural materials, to increase a sense of tranquility.

5. Arrange mindfulness tools: Include items that support mindfulness practice, such as a meditation mat, yoga mat, or calming music.

6. Display essential oils: Use a diffuser to fill the space with calming scents to keep your favorite essential oils within easy reach.

7. Personalize your space: Add personal touches like inspirational quotes, artwork, or photos to bring joy and relaxation.

8. Limit distractions: Keep electronic devices and work-related items out of your relaxation space to create a digital detox zone.

By creating a personalized relaxation space infused with essential oils, you can enjoy the full benefits of relaxation practices and cultivate a more balanced and peaceful lifestyle. Here you can escape the stress of everyday life, reconnect with yourself, and find solace in the calming effects of aroma-therapy.

Creating a calming atmosphere with essential oils requires strategic diffuser placement, setting the right room mood, and incorporating the essential oil scent throughout the environment. Here are some tips to help you achieve a soothing and peaceful space:

1. Diffuser placement:

Place the diffuser in the center of the room to ensure even distribution of essential oil scents.

Keep the diffuser away from direct sunlight, as excessive heat can reduce the quality of the oil.

Consider using multiple diffusers in larger spaces to cover the entire area effectively.

2. Room atmosphere:

Choose soft, warm lighting to create a relaxing atmosphere. Dimmable lights or string lights can add a soft glow to a room.

Play calming music or nature sounds in the background to enhance the relaxing atmosphere.

Keep the room neat and organized to promote a feeling of peace and tranquility.

3. Essential oil blends:

Customize your blend using essential oils known for their calming properties, such as lavender, chamomile, and bergamot.

Experiment with different scent combinations to find the one that resonates most with you.

4. Inhalation technique:

Use the inhalation technique to enjoy the calming effects of essential oils instantly.

Inhale the scent directly from the bottle or use a personal inhalation wand to relax.

5. Linen and fabric spray:

Mix essential oils with water in a spray bottle to create a calming linen spray.

Gently mist sheets, pillows, curtains, and other fabric surfaces infuse a room with a relaxing scent.

6. Natural air freshener:

Make a natural air freshener by adding a few drops of essential oil to a bowl of dried flowers, potpourri, or cotton balls.

Place them in different room corners to release a gentle and lasting scent.

7. Calm bath soak:

Use essential oils in your bath water for a luxurious and calming soak.

Add a few drops of lavender, chamomile, or ylang-ylang to warm wash water before going in.

8. Essential oil pillow:

Apply a drop or two of calming essential oil to a cotton ball or piece of fabric and tuck it into your pillowcase.

The fragrance is slowly released to promote relaxation during sleep.

9. Scented candles:

Create a relaxing, aromatic atmosphere with scented candles made from essential oils.

Choose natural candles without synthetic fragrances or harmful chemicals.

10. Regular maintenance:

Clean your diffuser regularly to prevent any buildup or residue that may affect the quality of your scent.

Store essential oils in a cool, dark place to maintain their potency.

Remember that personal fragrance preferences may vary, so feel free to experiment and find the combination of essential oils that brings you the most relaxation and happiness. Creating a calming atmosphere with essential oils can greatly enhance your relaxation habits, promote better sleep, and foster a sense of well-being in your daily life.

This section summarizes the benefits and applications of essential oils for men's relaxation and calming purposes. We emphasize the role of essential oils in promoting tranquility, reducing stress, and creating an atmosphere of peace. By incorporating essential oils into relaxation practices and creating personalized calming blends, men can enhance their sense of well-being, manage stress more effectively, and experience moments of deep relaxation and tranquility.

5.2 Concentration and Concentration Support

In this chapter, we'll explore how essential oils can be used to support focus and focus in men. We discuss the cognitive benefits of essential oils and guide how to use them effectively to increase mental clarity, productivity, and focus.

A. Understand the Importance of Focus and Concentration

Focus and concentration play a vital role in all aspects of life, contributing to productivity, learning, and overall well-being. Here is their importance in different contexts:

1. Work and productivity:

* Focus enables individuals to bring their attention to tasks, thereby improving work quality and efficiency.
* Focused attention helps maintain a flow state where individuals are fully focused on their tasks and can achieve peak performance.
* Focusing on completing tasks reduces the need for multitasking, which can lead to errors and lost productivity.

2. Research and learn:

* Focused attention is essential for effective learning, leading to better retention and understanding of the material.
* Focused learning courses enable learners to master complex concepts and connect ideas, thereby improving problem-solving skills.
* Focused studying can improve test and assessment scores.

3. Daily tasks and decisions:

* Focus enhances decision-making by enabling individuals to consider all relevant information and weigh options thoughtfully.
* Maintaining focus and focus during daily activities improves the quality of experiences and interactions.
* Focused attention minimizes errors and oversights in daily tasks, making daily work smoother.

4. Creativity and problem-solving skills:

* Focus allows for deep exploration of ideas and brainstorming, resulting in innovative solutions.
* Focusing on the problem at hand helps individuals break it down into manageable pieces and develop effective strategies.

5. Reduce stress and health:

* Focus activities promote mindfulness and reduce stress and anxiety.
* Focusing on enjoyable activities, hobbies, and relaxation techniques improves overall health.

6. Relationships and communication:

* Being fully present in conversations and interactions enhances communication and fosters meaningful connections.
* Focusing on others' perspectives and feelings leads to empathy and effective communication.

Staying focused and focused can be challenging in a world full of distractions and information overload. However, some strategies and practices can help:

1. Time management: Break down tasks into smaller, manageable chunks and allocate dedicated time for focused work or study.

2. Minimize distractions: Create a distraction-free environment by muting notifications, closing irrelevant tabs, and finding quiet spaces.

3. Determine priorities: Identify and tackle your most important tasks

during peak attention periods.

4. Practice mindfulness: Cultivate mindfulness through techniques such as meditation, deep breathing, and grounding exercises to enhance present-moment awareness.

5. Rest: Regular breaks can help refresh your mind and prevent burnout.

6. Proper sleep and nutrition: Prioritize adequate sleep and nutritious meals to support cognitive function.

7. Limit multitasking: Focus on one task at a time to maintain quality and efficiency.

8. Set goals: Well-defined goals provide a sense of purpose and direction, making it easier to stay focused.

Developing focus and focus takes practice and consistency. Over time, improving your attention skills can increase productivity, reduce stress, and increase satisfaction in all aspects of your life.

Essential oils have been studied for their potential to improve cognitive function, increase mental clarity, and support overall brain health. While they are not a substitute for proper medical care or therapy, some essential oils may benefit focus, memory, and alertness. Here are some essential oils commonly associated with cognitive support:

1. Peppermint: Peppermint oil is known for its uplifting fragrance. Inhaling the aroma of peppermint may help increase alertness and concentration. Its cooling and stimulating properties can help improve mental clarity.

2. Rosemary: Rosemary oil is often associated with memory enhancement. Inhaling its aroma or using it in a massage blend can support focus and cognitive function.

3. Lemon: The citrus flavor of lemon oil is thought to have a mood-boosting effect. Inhaling lemon oil may help improve mental clarity and promote a positive mindset.

4. Eucalyptus: The fresh and eye-catching aroma of eucalyptus oil can help clear the mind and improve mental alertness when inhaled.

5. Basil: Basil oil is believed to have properties that support mental clarity and focus. Inhaling its aroma may help stimulate the mind.

6. Frankincense: Frankincense oil is associated with relaxing and calming effects. It may help reduce feelings of stress and promote mental clarity.

7. Lavender: The soothing scent of lavender oil can help reduce stress and anxiety, which can help improve mental clarity and focus.

Using essential oils for cognitive support:

1. Aromatherapy: Inhaling the aroma of essential oils through methods such as a diffuser, inhalation stick, or nasal inhaler can quickly achieve their beneficial effects.

2. Topical application: Massaging or rolling on the mixture can apply Diluted essential oils to the skin. Combining massage with aromatherapy can promote relaxation and focus at the same time.

3. Diffuse: Diffusing essential oils in your workspace or study area can create an environment that supports mental clarity and focus.

4. Personal inhaler: A portable inhaler containing essential oils can be taken with you, allowing you to inhale the aroma when you need a cognitive boost.

5. Mix: Creating a synergistic blend by combining different essential oils known for their cognitive support properties can enhance their overall effects.

While some people may benefit from using essential oils for cognitive support, it's important to note that reactions may vary, and not everyone will experience the same effects. Additionally, if you have an underlying health condition or are taking medications, it is best to consult with a healthcare professional before incorporating essential oils into your daily routine.

Remember to use high-quality, pure essential oils and always perform a patch test to check for any potential skin sensitivities. Essential oils should be used in moderation. If any adverse reactions occur, please stop using them immediately.

B. Essential Oils for Focus and Concentration

Essential oils known for their stimulating and cognitive-enhancing properties include:

1. Rosemary: Known for its uplifting fragrance, rosemary essential oil can help improve cognitive function, enhance memory, and increase mental clarity. It is often used in study or work meetings to improve focus and concentration.

2. Peppermint: Peppermint essential oil has a refreshing aroma that promotes alertness, mental sharpness, and wakefulness. It is commonly used to combat mental fatigue and improve cognitive performance.

3. Lemon: Lemon essential oil has a bright and uplifting fragrance that can improve mood, increase energy levels, and enhance mental clarity. It is often used to create a positive and focused atmosphere.

4. Basil: Basil essential oil has a fresh herbal aroma, which can help clear the mind and promote mental concentration. Its value lies in reducing mental exhaustion and increasing mental awareness.

These essential oils stimulate the senses and enhance cognitive function through inhalation, diffusion, or topical application. Here are some ways to use these oils to experience their stimulating effects:

1. Inhalation: Inhale the scent directly from the bottle or add a few drops of essential oil to a tissue and inhale deeply. This can provide a quick and direct way to experience the stimulating properties of the oil.

2. Aromatherapy diffuser: Use an aromatherapy diffuser to disperse essential oils into the air. Diffusing these oils in your workspace or study area can create a stimulating and focused environment.

3. Topical application: Dilute the essential oil in a carrier oil and apply it to pulse points such as the wrists or temples to experience its invigorating effects throughout the day.

4. Inhalation blends: Create stimulating inhalation blends by mixing two or more of these essential oils. For example, you can mix equal parts rose-

mary and peppermint to create a refreshing and stimulating mixture.

5. Focus roller blend: Make a roller blend by diluting these essential oils in a carrier oil and applying it to the back of your neck or wrists before a task that requires mental focus and concentration.

When using these oils topically, remember to start with a low dilution, especially if you have sensitive skin. Everyone may react differently to essential oils, so it's important to find the best concentration and method for you. These oils can be valuable tools for enhancing focus, mental clarity, and overall cognitive function.

Let's take a closer look at how rosemary, peppermint, lemon, and basil essential oils support mental focus, memory retention, and alertness:

1. Mental concentration:

Rosemary essential oil contains compounds such as 1,8 * eucalyptol, which has been shown to improve cognitive abilities and concentration. Inhaling rosemary oil can help stimulate the mind and improve mental clarity during tasks that require concentration.

Peppermint essential oil has uplifting properties that improve focus and concentration. Its menthol content increases alertness and helps combat mental fatigue, helping to stay on task and stay focused.

Basil essential oil is known for clearing mental fog and improving mental focus. It's refreshing aroma can help increase concentration and keep the mind sharp during challenging activities.

2. Memory retention:

Rosemary essential oil has been linked to memory enhancement. Inhaling rosemary oil can stimulate memory recall and retention, making it a valuable aid during study or learning activities.

The uplifting aroma of lemon essential oil can improve mood, promote cognitive function, and potentially enhance memory and information retention.

The stimulating effects of peppermint essential oil can extend to memory improvements, as it helps improve cognitive performance and alertness.

3. Alertness:

The energizing properties of peppermint essential oil can promote wakefulness and increase alertness. Inhaling peppermint oil can help individuals feel more alert and focused during tasks or activities that require concentration.

Lemon essential oil's fresh and energizing scent can boost energy levels and alertness, making it ideal for your morning routine or for times when you need to clear your mind.

Basil essential oil's ability to reduce mental fatigue may indirectly help improve alertness and concentration.

Instructions:

For enhanced mental focus and memory, consider diffusing a combination of rosemary, peppermint, and lemon essential oils in your study or workspace. This aromatic blend creates a stimulating and focused environment.

Before engaging in mentally demanding tasks, inhale the scent of an essential oil or two from a bottle or personal inhaler stick to increase alertness and mental clarity quickly.

For on-the-go support, mix these essential oils diluted in carrier oil and apply them to wrists or temples.

You can also try a refreshing and uplifting drink by adding a drop of lemon essential oil to a glass of water.

Remember to use essential oils with caution and follow proper dilution guidelines. While these oils may provide support for mental focus, memory retention, and alertness, individual responses may vary. If you have any sensitivities or concerns, please consult a qualified aromatherapist or healthcare professional before using essential oils.

C. Cognitively Supported Inhalation Techniques

Inhalation techniques using essential oils can be an effective way to provide cognitive support and enhance mental focus. The aroma of certain essential oils can directly stimulate the brain, triggering responses that promote mental clarity and cognitive function. Here are some inhalation techniques you can try:

1. Direct inhalation: This simple method involves inhaling the scent directly from the bottle or palm. Please follow these steps:

Open the cap of an essential oil bottle or place a few drops of your chosen essential oil in the palm of your hand.

Rub your hands together to heat the oil and release its aromatic compounds.

Cover your nose and mouth with your hands and take a series of slow, deep breaths, inhaling the scent deeply.

Pause between breaths to fully experience the scent and its effects.

2. Aromatherapy diffuser: Using an aromatherapy diffuser is an effective way to disperse essential oils into the air, creating an uplifting and focused environment. Please follow these steps:

Add water to the diffuser according to the manufacturer's instructions.

Add a few drops of your choice of essential oil or blend with the water.

Turn on the diffuser to release a fine mist infused with essential oil scents.

Sit or work near a diffuser to benefit from continuous inhalation.

3. Personal inhalation stick: Personal inhalers are portable and easy to use on the go. To create your inhaler stick:

Obtain an inhaler stick from a reputable supplier or health store.

Add a few drops of your chosen essential oil or blend to the cotton wick inside your inhaler.

Assemble the inhaler according to the instructions.

Breathe in from your inhaler whenever you need enhanced cognitive function or mental clarity.

4. Steam inhalation: This technique is especially useful for congestion relief and cognitive support. Please follow these steps:
Boil water in a pot and transfer to a heatproof bowl.

Add a few drops of desired essential oil or blend with hot water.

Create a tent by placing a towel over your head and leaning against the bowl, keeping a safe distance to avoid burns.

Breathe the steam deeply for a few minutes to allow the aromatic molecules to reach your nasal passages, promoting mental clarity.

When choosing essential oils for cognitive support, consider those with stimulating and clarifying properties, such as rosemary, peppermint, lemon, basil, or eucalyptus. Experiment with a single oil or create a blend that resonates with you. Remember that individuals may react differently to essential oils, so listen to your body and use essential oils in a comfortable and beneficial way. If you have any health concerns or conditions, it is best to consult a qualified aromatherapist or healthcare professional before incorporating essential oils into your daily life.

Direct inhalation:

Benefits: Direct inhalation provides a quick and direct way to experience the aromatic benefits of essential oils. Aromatic compounds directly stimulate the olfactory system and can have rapid effects on mood, concentration, and alertness.

Best Practice: When using direct inhalation, make sure to hold the oil bottle or hand a comfortable distance from your nose and take slow, deep breaths to inhale the aroma fully. Avoid putting the oil too close to your nose to prevent any potential irritation.

Aromatherapy diffuser:

Benefits: Diffusing essential oils causes a continuous release of aromatic molecules into the air, changing the mood of a room and promoting an environment of focus and upliftment.

Best practice: Follow the manufacturer's instructions for your diffuser and note the recommended amount of essential oil to add. Diffuse in a well-ventilated area and avoid diffusing for long periods, especially in small spaces.

Personal inhaler stick:

Benefits: Personal inhalers offer portability and convenience, allowing you to take the benefits of essential oils with you throughout the day. They offer a discreet and easy way to inhale essential oils on the go.

Best Practice: To create a personal inhaler, make sure the inhaler wand is clean and assembled correctly. Use an essential oil blend or single essential oil that suits your needs and preferences. Replace the cotton wick in your inhaler regularly to maintain the effectiveness of your scent.

General tips on inhalation technique:

1. Start with small inhalations and gradually increase as needed, especially if you are new to using essential oils.

2. Use high-quality, pure essential oils to ensure the best therapeutic effect and safety.

3. Store essential oils properly in dark glass bottles away from direct

sunlight and heat to maintain their potency.

4. If you experience any adverse reactions or sensitivity, discontinue use and seek the advice of a professional aromatherapist or healthcare provider.

5. Consider using essential oils in blends to create a synergistic effect and enhance their benefits for mental focus and cognitive support.

6. Choosing essential oils that resonate with you is crucial, as personal preference can play a role in the effectiveness of aromatherapy.

Remember, the use of essential oils should complement and enhance your relaxation or mindfulness practice, and practicing safety and moderation is crucial. People may react differently to essential oils, so it's always a good idea to do a patch test and consult a qualified aromatherapist or healthcare professional, especially if you have any pre-existing health conditions or concerns.

D. Create a Focus Mixture

Create custom focus blends using essential oils:

1. Choose your base note: Start by choosing a base note essential oil to serve as the base for your accent blend. Some popular tones for focus blends include:

* Rosemary: Known for its cognitive-enhancing properties and ability to promote mental clarity and alertness.
* Cedar Wood: Often used to enhance concentration, focus, and mental stability.
* Frankincense: Known for its grounding and calming effects, it helps improve focus and reduce distractions.

2. Add your heart note: Heart note essential oils add complexity and balance to your blend. They often have uplifting and harmonizing qualities that complement the tone. Some mid-note oils suitable for focus blends include:

* Peppermint: Known for its uplifting and refreshing scent, it stimulates mental clarity and increases energy levels.
* Lemon: A bright citrus oil that promotes mental focus and lifts mood.
* Eucalyptus: Can clear the mind and increase alertness, making it beneficial for focus-oriented blends.

3. Add your top notes: Top note essential oils provide the initial aroma and provide a refreshing and energizing element to your blend. They can help awaken the senses and keep the mixture alive. Consider these top-note oils as your focal point blend:

* Basil: has a stimulating and clarifying scent that enhances mental alertness and focus.
* Bergamot: Known for its uplifting and stress-reducing properties, it supports focus and a positive mindset.
* Lemon Verbena: An energizing and refreshing oil that promotes mental clarity and a sharp mind.

4. Mixing proportions: Creating a balanced and effective focus blend requires carefully blending essential oils. A common blending ratio is 2 drops of base note, 3 drops of middle note, and 1 drop of top note essential oil. However, feel free to adjust the proportions to suit your personal preference and desired scent intensity.

5. Dilution: Since focus mixtures are typically intended for inhalation or topical application, they must be diluted correctly. For topical use, a general guideline is to use a 2% dilution, which means adding approximately 12 drops of Focus Blend to 1 ounce (30 ml) of suitable carrier oil, such as jojoba or sweet almond oil.

6. Storage: Store your focus blend in a dark glass bottle away from direct sunlight and heat to maintain its potency.

7. Application: You can use focus blending in a variety of ways, such as:

Inhalation: Place a few drops of the mixture into a personal inhaler, diffuser, or tissue to provide focus support on the go.
Topical use: Apply the diluted mixture to pulse points, temples, or the back of the neck before tasks that require focus and concentration.

Remember, essential oils can uniquely impact an individual, and it's important to find the combination that works best for you. Experiment with different oils and ratios to create a customized focus blend to increase your mental clarity, focus, and productivity. If you have any specific health concerns or are pregnant, consider consulting with a certified aromatherapist or healthcare professional before using essential oils.

Proper mix ratio for enhancing focus:

Creating an effective focus-enhancing blend requires finding the right balance between different essential oils. Here are some mixing ratios to guide you:

1. Inhalation of the mixture:

Personal inhaler: 5 to 10 drops of essential oil in total, a balanced combination of base, middle, and top notes.

For a diffuser: 3 to 5 drops of essential oil, taking into account the size of the diffuser and the intensity of your desired scent.

2. Topical application mixture (2% dilution):

Add 12 drops of essential oil   to 1 ounce (30 ml) of carrier oil

Complementary scents for focus-enhancing blends:

To create a comprehensive focus-enhancing blend, consider combining essential oils from different categories:

1. Basic instructions:

Rosemary + Frankincense: A grounding and mentally stimulating combination.

Cedar + Vetiver: Promotes focus and a sense of tranquility.

2. Middle notes:

Mint + Lemon: A refreshing and uplifting blend for mental clarity.

Basil + Eucalyptus: Uplifting and clarifying, improving concentration.

3. Top notes:

Bergamot + Lemon Verbena: A bright, cheerful blend that lifts the mood and sharpens the mind.

Basil + Spearmint: An energizing and refreshing combination that enhances concentration.

How to apply the Focus Enhancement Blend:

1. Inhalation:

Personal Inhaler: Add the desired mixture to a personal inhaler and inhale as needed to improve focus and mental clarity quickly.

Diffuser: Use the blend in an aromatherapy diffuser to create a focused and productive environment in your workspace.

2. Local application:

Apply diluted focus mixture to pulse points, such as wrists and temples, before tasks that require concentration.

Massage the mixture into the back of your neck or shoulders to release tension and promote mental clarity.

3. Study or workspace:

Diffuse the focus-enhancing blend in your study or work area to create a conducive environment for productivity and focus.

Remember, when trying essential oils, start with a small amount to find the blend that best suits your preferences and needs. Additionally, essential oils affect individuals differently, so pay attention to how your body reacts to each blend. If you have any specific health concerns or are pregnant, consult a certified aromatherapist or healthcare professional before using essential oils to enhance your focus.

E. Use Essential Oils to Increase Productivity

Use essential oils to increase productivity and efficiency:

1. Rosemary: Rosemary essential oil is known for its cognitive-enhancing properties and can help improve memory and mental clarity. Diffuse rosemary oil in your work or study space to stay focused and alert.

2. Peppermint: Peppermint essential oil can increase energy levels and boost motivation, making it uplifting and refreshing. Inhale peppermint oil directly from the bottle or use a personal inhaler during breaks to rejuvenate and stay productive.

3. Lemon: Lemon essential oil has uplifting and mood-enhancing properties and can create a positive and inspiring atmosphere. Diffuse lemon oil in your workspace to promote feelings of optimism and focus.

4. Eucalyptus: Eucalyptus essential oil is known for its stimulating properties, which can enhance mental focus and clarity. Use it in a diffuser to keep your mind alert and focused while studying or working.

5. Sage: This essential oil can help reduce mental fatigue and promote relaxation while maintaining focus. Diffuse sage oil to balance productivity and stress relief.

Technology to improve productivity:

1. Pomodoro technique: Work in concentrated intervals of 25 minutes, followed by a short 5- 5-minute break. Use an essential oil diffuser during these intervals to create a supportive work environment.

2. Goal-oriented breaks: During breaks, inhale essential oils like peppermint or lemon to refresh and motivate yourself to complete tasks.

3. Personal inhaler: Keep your inhaler with Productivity Boosting Blend in your den or work bag for easy access whenever and wherever you need it.

4. Diffuse with music: Combine aromatherapy with background music to create an atmosphere that enhances creativity and productivity.

5. Aromatherapy roll-on: Make a roll-on mixture using essential oils such as rosemary and eucalyptus diluted in a carrier oil. Apply the roller ball to your temples or wrists when you need to focus quickly.

Individuals may respond differently to essential oils, so it's important to find the oils and techniques that work best for you. Consider using essential oils with effective time management strategies and healthy work habits to optimize productivity and efficiency in your work or study environment.

Tips for adding essential oils to your workspace aromatherapy:

1. Desktop diffuser: Place a compact essential oil diffuser on your desk to disperse pungent scents throughout your workspace. Use focus-enhancing oils like rosemary, peppermint, or lemon to uplift the atmosphere.

2. Aromatherapy jewelry: Wear diffuser jewelry, such as a necklace or bracelet designed to hold essential oils. This way, you can discreetly enjoy the

benefits of your chosen oil while working or studying.

3. Desktop spray: Make a DIY tabletop spray by mixing water and a few drops of your favorite essential oil in a small spray bottle. Gently mist the air around your workspace, infusing it with your chosen scent.

4. Cotton balls or paper towels: Add a few drops of essential oil to a cotton ball or paper towel and place it on your desk. Inhale the aroma when you need a quick mental boost.

5. Inhaler: Create your inhaler with a focus-enhancing oil blend. Carry it in your pocket or bag for quick access to your favorite scents anytime, anywhere.

6. Scent notepad: Dab a drop or two of essential oils into the corner of a notepad or notebook. As you take notes, the scent gently wafts up, providing a subtle stimulation.

7. Custom blends: Try different essential oil blends to find the one that resonates best with you to increase productivity and focus. Blending oils like rosemary, basil, and lemon create a refreshing, stimulating aroma.

8. Rotation and variety: Rotate the essential oils you use to prevent olfactory fatigue. Switch between different oils throughout the day or week to keep your senses engaged.

9. Timed diffuser: Set your desktop diffuser as a timer to release essential oils intermittently throughout your work or study session, keeping you alert and focused.

Remember to use essential oils with caution, as some people may be sensitive to certain scents. Start with a small amount of oil and adjust the concentration to your liking. Using essential oils in your workspace can create a positive and focused environment, increasing your productivity and overall health.

F. Mental Clarity and Memory Support

Essential Oils to Support Mental Clarity and Memory:

1. Cedarwood: Cedarwood essential oil has a grounding and calming

scent that can help improve focus and mental clarity. Its warm aroma is known to promote a sense of stability, making it beneficial for studying or handling complex tasks.

2. Frankincense: Frankincense is revered for its ability to enhance mental and mental clarity. Its woody and resinous scent can help calm the mind, reduce distractions, and improve concentration during meditation or focused work.

3. Sage: Sage has an herbal and slightly sweet aroma that promotes mental clarity and alertness. It is thought to support cognitive function and emotional balance, making it useful during stressful or demanding situations.

4. Rosemary: Rosemary essential oil is known for its stimulating properties, which can help improve memory and mental focus. Aromatherapy blends often use it to enhance cognitive abilities and improve mental clarity.

5. Peppermint: Peppermint essential oil has a refreshing and uplifting scent that awakens the mind and increases alertness. Inhaling peppermint oil can improve cognitive function and mental clarity.

6. Lemon: Lemon essential oil has a bright and uplifting aroma that promotes mental clarity and improves mood. Its fresh scent enhances focus and concentration, making it beneficial during study or work.

7. Basil: Basil essential oil has an herbal and uplifting fragrance that can help combat mental fatigue and promote clarity. It is thought to support mental alertness and cognitive function.

8. Vetiver: Vetiver essential oil has a deep, earthy aroma that provides grounding and stability. It is known for its calming effects and ability to improve focus and concentration.

Tips for using essential oils to improve mental clarity and memory:

1. Diffuse: Use an aromatherapy diffuser to disperse essential oils into the air of your workspace or study area. Inhaling aromatic molecules can enhance mental focus and clarity.

2. Inhale: Inhale the scent directly from the bottle or personal inhaler stick when you need a quick mental boost or for a stressful moment.

3. Topical application: Dilute the essential oil in a carrier oil, such as jojoba or sweet almond, and apply the mixture to your temples, wrists, or the back of your neck for a refreshing and invigorating experience.

4. Customize blends: Try different combinations of essential oils to create a personalized blend that suits your preferences and supports your mental clarity and memory.

5. Mindful breathing: Combine inhalation of essential oils with mindful breathing exercises to enhance the cognitive benefits of essential oils and improve focus during meditation or study.

6. Rotate: Rotate different essential oils for mental clarity and memory to prevent olfactory fatigue and keep the senses engaged.

As with any essential oil, it is important to follow safety guidelines, patch test skin sensitivities, and use essential oils in moderation. Incorporating these essential oils into your daily routine can support mental clarity, memory retention, and overall cognitive function, providing a natural and aromatic boost to your productivity and health.

Incorporating essential oils known for their cognitive-enhancing properties into your daily routine can help improve cognitive performance, mental clarity, and concentration. Here are some techniques and ideas for incorporating these oils into your daily life:

1. Aromatherapy diffuser: Start your day by diffusing essential oils like rosemary, peppermint, or lemon in your work or study area. Diffusing oils can create a stimulating and refreshing environment that promotes mental alertness and focus.

2. Morning inhalation: Inhale the scent of an uplifting oil like frankincense or sage directly from the bottle or personal inhaler stick in the morning to set a positive and focused tone for the day ahead.

3. Focus blending roller: Create a focus-enhancing blend by diluting a combination of your favorite cognitive support oils (like rosemary, basil, and vetiver) in a roller bottle with a carrier oil. Roll the mixture onto your wrists, temples, or the back of your neck when you need a boost of mental clarity throughout the day.

4. Meditate with oils: Incorporate essential oils into your meditation

practice. Apply a drop of frankincense or vetiver to your palms, rub them together, then bring your hands to your nose and inhale deeply during meditation. This can help clarify your thoughts and increase mindfulness.

5. Aromatherapy study break: Take a short aromatic study break during a study or work session. Inhale rejuvenating oils like peppermint or lemon before returning to your duties. This practice can help improve concentration and prevent mental fatigue.

6. Refreshing facial mist: Create a refreshing facial mist in a spray bottle by mixing water with a few drops of essential oil, such as rosemary or sage. Spray your face during the day for a quick pick-me-up and increased mental clarity.

7. Aromatherapy bath: Add a few drops of an uplifting oil like bergamot or lemon to your bath water at night. Enjoy a soak while inhaling aromatic steam to enhance mood and mental relaxation.

8. Scent your workspace: Place a cotton ball or small cloth with a drop of essential oil under your desk or near your workspace and enjoy a subtle scent throughout the day.

9. Bedtime ritual: Incorporate essential oils like lavender or cedarwood into your bedtime routine to promote relaxation and better sleep quality, which can positively impact cognitive function during the day.

Remember to choose high-quality essential oils and use them sparingly. When creating blends or incorporating oils into your daily routine, personal sensitivities and preferences must be considered. Additionally, rotating essential oils can prevent olfactory fatigue and maximize their benefits. By incorporating these techniques and essential oils into your daily life, you can support improvements in cognitive performance, mental clarity, and overall health.

G. Research and Study Skills

Integrating essential oils into study and study techniques can enhance focus, memory, and overall cognitive function. Here are some study and study strategies for combining essential oils for best results:

1. Aromatherapy diffuse: Diffuse essential oils like rosemary, lemon, or peppermint into your study area while reviewing notes or reading. Uplifting

scents can help improve concentration, focus, and information retention.

2. Scent association: Before studying or studying new material, inhale specific essential oils (such as peppermint) to create fragrance associations. The same oil triggers memory recall during study sessions and exams.

3. Focus blend inhalation: Use oils like rosemary, basil, and vetiver to create a focus-enhancing blend. Inhale the mixture from a personal inhaler stick or apply it to your wrist before and during the study to support mental clarity and focus.

4. Scented flashcards: Add a drop of essential oil to a cotton pad or cloth and place it near your study materials or flashcards. Inhaling aromas while studying can help create a positive connection with the material.

5. Memory-boosting room spray: Make a room spray with memory-boosting oils like lemon and rosemary. Spray it throughout your study area to enhance information retention and recall.

6. Scented study breaks: During study breaks, inhale stimulating oils like peppermint to rejuvenate your mind and keep you focused.

7. Mindful breathing: Practice deep breathing exercises infused with calming oils like lavender or frankincense before and after studying to reduce stress and enhance focus.

8. Aroma notes: While taking notes, place a drop of the focus-enhancing oil on your wrist or diffuser jewelry. This scent can help improve information retention and recall during exams.

9. Pre-exam inhalation: Inhale an essential oil blend before an exam to promote mental clarity and calm, reduce test anxiety, and improve performance.

10. Scented learning environment: Keep the learning space clean and orderly and integrate essential oils into the environment to create a positive and focused atmosphere.

Remember to use essential oils with caution and take a break if you notice any sensitivities. The goal is to enhance your learning experience and optimize cognitive function, so explore different technologies and find what works best for you. Additionally, regular exercise, adequate sleep, and a balanced diet play a vital role in supporting optimal cognitive function and learning.

Techniques such as scent association, diffusing scents during the study, and using oils during breaks can significantly increase mental recovery and improve cognitive performance. Let's explore each of these technologies in detail:

1. Fragrance learning session:

* Before studying, inhale specific essential oils, such as rosemary or peppermint.
* During your study period, diffuse the same essential oil in your study area or apply it to your inhaler.
* By creating scent associations, the aroma of essential oils can trigger memory recall during exams or later when reviewing material.

2. Diffuse during the study:

* Use an aromatherapy diffuser to disperse focus-enhancing essential oils like lemon, eucalyptus, or basil into the air.
* The aromatic molecules of these oils stimulate the brain while learning, increasing alertness and enhancing mental clarity.
* Keep a diffuser nearby and adjust settings to maintain a consistent and pleasant aroma throughout your study session.

3. Use oils during breaks to rejuvenate your mind:

* During your study break, take a moment to inhale an essential oil known for its uplifting and rejuvenating properties, such as peppermint or citrus oil.
* Inhaling these oils can help relieve mental fatigue, increase energy levels, and prepare you for your next study session.
* You can use a personal inhaler, take a few deep breaths straight from the bottle, or use a diffuser to create an energizing atmosphere.

Additionally, here are some tips to improve cognitive performance during the study:

4. Scent flashcards:

* Add a drop of essential oil to a cotton pad and place it near study

materials or flashcards.

* Inhale the aroma of essential oils while viewing materials to create a positive connection with the information.

5. Mindful breathing:

* Practice deep breathing exercises infused with a calming oil like lavender or frankincense before and after studying.
* Mindful breathing can reduce stress and anxiety, improving focus and information retention.

6. Aroma notes:

* While taking notes, place a drop of focus-enhancing essential oil on your wrist or diffuser jewelry.
* The scent of essential oils can help improve memory during exams or when reviewing notes.

Remember to consider your personal preferences and any sensitivities you may experience when selecting and using essential oils. The goal is to create a supportive and focused learning environment that complements your learning style and enhances your cognitive abilities.

H. Workplace Focus Strategies

Using essential oils to increase focus and concentration in the workplace can increase productivity and overall well-being. Here are some strategies for incorporating essential oils into your daily routine:

1. Personal inhaler:

Keep a personal inhaler at your desk with a blend of focus-boosting essential oils like rosemary and lemon.
Take a few deep breaths whenever you need to increase your focus or feel mentally fatigued.

2. Desktop diffuser:

Use the compact USB or battery-powered aromatherapy diffuser at your desk.
Choose oils like peppermint, eucalyptus, or basil to create a stimulat-

ing and focused atmosphere.

3. Rolling ball mixture:

Make a roll-on mixture using carrier oil and focus-enhancing essential oils like cedarwood and vetiver.
Apply the roller ball to your wrists or the back of your neck for a quick and easy way to boost focus.

4. Fragrance work area:

Spray a mixture of essential oils and water around your workspace to infuse the area with a concentrated and inspiring scent.
Consider using oils like frankincense, bergamot, or sage for clarity and mental acuity.

5. Aromatherapy jewelry:

Wear aromatherapy jewelry, such as a necklace or bracelet, containing focus-enhancing essential oils like lemon or rosemary.
The scent will stay with you all day long, providing sustained support for your focus.

6. Mindful rest:

Take short breaks during the day and practice mindful breathing infused with calming oils like lavender or chamomile.
Mindfulness exercises can help you refocus during a busy workday.

7. Custom blends:

Try to create a mix that suits your specific needs and preferences for focus and focus.
Combine essential oils like lemon, peppermint, and rosemary to create an uplifting and stimulating blend.

8. Focus during the meeting:

Diffuse essential oils in the meeting room before an important discussion or presentation.
Oils like rosemary or sage can help participants stay focused and engaged.

Everyone may react differently to different oils, so it's important to find the scent that works best for you. Always consider your colleagues' sensitivities and ensure your shared workspace is suitable for everyone. Creating a supportive environment using essential oils can significantly contribute to a positive work experience and increase your focus and productivity throughout the day.

Here are some tips for adding essential oils to improve focus and focus on the workplace:

1. Desktop diffuser:

Use a small tabletop diffuser to disperse essential oils like peppermint or lemon throughout your workspace.
The diffuser will create a refreshing and energizing environment, helping you stay alert and focused.

2. Scented stress ball:

Infuse a stress ball with a few drops of a focus-boosting essential oil, such as rosemary or basil.
Squeezing a scented stress ball can provide a quick pick-me-up during moments of stress or mental fatigue.

3. Mindful breathing exercises:

Take short breaks throughout the day to practice mindful breathing.
Inhale deeply through your nose, hold for a few seconds, and then exhale slowly through your mouth.
Combine this practice with inhaling calming oils like lavender or chamomile to increase relaxation and focus.

4. Personal aromatherapy inhaler:

Create a personalized aromatherapy inhaler using focus-enhancing oils like cedar wood or vetiver.
Keep your inhaler at your desk and use it when you need to improve mental clarity and focus.

5. Aromatherapy jewelry:

Wear essential oil diffuser jewelry, such as a necklace or bracelet, to enjoy the benefits of essential oils throughout the day.

Choose essential oils like frankincense or sage for clarity and mental focus.

6. Scent work area:

Use a spray bottle to spray a mixture of essential oil and water around your workspace regularly.

Oils like lemon or eucalyptus can create a stimulating and focused atmosphere.

7. Micro-breaks:

Practice the 20*20*20 rule: Every 20 minutes, take a 20-second break and look at something 20 feet away.

Combine this practice with deep inhalation of an invigorating oil like peppermint or rosemary to recharge your focus.

8. Calm moments:

Incorporate short periods of relaxation and mindfulness into your day to clear your mind and refocus.

Use soothing essential oils like lavender or bergamot during these moments to promote a sense of tranquility and mental clarity.

These techniques can help you incorporate essential oils into your daily routine to improve focus, concentration, and overall well-being. Remember to use oils that resonate with you and consider the sensitivities of your colleagues in the shared workspace. Careful use of essential oils can create a positive and productive work environment for everyone.

5.3 Solve Sleep Problems and Promote Restful Nights

In this chapter, we'll look at how you can use essential oils to address sleep issues and promote a restful night in men. We discuss the calming properties of essential oils and guide you on using them safely and effectively to improve sleep quality and establish healthy sleep patterns.

A. Understand the Importance of the Quality of Sleep

Quality sleep plays a vital role in overall health and well-being, affecting every aspect of physical, mental, and emotional well-being. Here are some key points that highlight the importance of sleep quality.

1. Body recovery: During sleep, the body goes through the basic physical recovery and repair process. Tissue and muscle are repaired, and the immune system is strengthened. Adequate sleep is essential for optimal immune function and can reduce the risk of infection and disease.

2. Clear thinking and cognitive functions: Sleep is closely related to cognitive functions such as memory consolidation, learning, and problem-solving. Getting enough restful sleep can enhance mental clarity, focus, and concentration, thereby increasing productivity and performance in daily activities.

3. Emotional health: Sleep profoundly impacts mood regulation and mental health. Adequate sleep helps stabilize mood, reduce irritability, and enhance emotional flexibility. On the other hand, chronic sleep deprivation can lead to increased stress, anxiety, and mood disorders.

4. Hormone balance: Sleep plays a vital role in regulating hormone levels. During sleep, the body releases hormones that control appetite, energy metabolism, and stress response. Proper sleep is essential for maintaining hormonal balance and preventing weight gain and hormonal imbalances.

5. Cardiovascular health: Lack of sleep has been linked to an increased risk of cardiovascular disease, including high blood pressure, heart disease, and stroke. Good quality sleep helps maintain a healthy cardiovascular system and blood pressure levels.

6. Metabolic health: Sleep plays a role in regulating glucose metabolism and insulin sensitivity. Poor sleep habits can lead to insulin resistance, weight gain, and an increased risk of type 2 diabetes.

7. Physical performance and sports recovery: Athletes and individuals involved in physical activity benefit greatly from quality sleep. Sleep promotes physical function and muscle recovery and reduces the risk of injury.

8. Immune function: A well-rested body has a stronger immune system and is more capable of fighting off infections and pathogens. Sustained

and restorative sleep is essential for maintaining a healthy immune response.

9. Cell repair and growth: Sleep is critical to cell repair and growth. During deep sleep, the body produces growth hormones critical for tissue repair, muscle growth, and overall regeneration.

10. Longevity: Chronic sleep deprivation is associated with an increased risk of premature death. Prioritizing quality sleep is essential to maintaining optimal health and longevity.

Quality sleep is a fundamental pillar of health, supporting various body functions and promoting overall health. Healthy sleep habits combined with relaxing practices, such as aromatherapy using calming essential oils, can help improve sleep quality and your health.

Men, like people of all genders, may face a variety of sleep issues that can significantly impact their daily lives and overall health. Some common sleep problems men face include:

1. Insomnia: Insomnia is a common sleep disorder characterized by difficulty falling asleep, staying asleep, or waking up prematurely and being unable to fall back asleep. Chronic insomnia can lead to daytime fatigue, decreased concentration, and irritability.

2. Sleep apnea: Sleep apnea is a sleep disorder in which a person's breathing is interrupted during sleep. The most common type is obstructive sleep apnea (OSA), in which the airways are blocked, causing brief awakenings throughout the night. Sleep apnea can cause loud snoring, poor sleep quality, and daytime sleepiness.

3. Restless legs syndrome (RLS): RLS is a neurological disorder that causes an irresistible urge to move the legs, often accompanied by an uncomfortable feeling. RLS can disrupt sleep and cause sleep deprivation.

4. Lack of sleep: Busy lifestyles, work-related stress, and modern demands often lead to a lack of sleep. Lack of sleep can impair cognitive function, reduce alertness, and increase the risk of accidents.

5. Shift work sleep disorder: Men who work irregular or night shifts may have difficulty establishing a regular sleep-wake cycle due to disrupting the body's natural circadian rhythm.

6. Snoring: While snoring is a common problem in both men and women, it may be more prevalent in men due to physiological factors. Snoring can cause sleep disturbance in both the snorer and his or her bed partner.

7. Sleep-disordered breathing: Conditions such as snoring and sleep apnea may fall under the category of sleep-disordered breathing, which can negatively impact sleep quality and lead to daytime fatigue.

The impact of these sleep problems on daily life can be significant and widespread. Men who experience sleep problems may face the following challenges:

Daytime fatigue: Lack of sleep can lead to ongoing daytime fatigue, leading to decreased productivity, impaired cognitive function, and increased irritability.

Impaired concentration and memory: Sleep problems can affect concentration, memory, and overall cognitive performance, affecting performance at work or school.

Mood changes: Disrupted sleep can lead to mood swings, irritability, and an increased risk of anxiety or depression.

Decreased physical function: Lack of sleep can impede physical function, affecting athletic ability and overall physical health.

Increased risk of chronic health conditions: Chronic sleep problems are associated with an increased risk of various health conditions, including cardiovascular disease, diabetes, and obesity.

Relationship tension: Sleep disturbances, such as loud snoring or restless leg movements, can disrupt a partner's sleep, leading to relationship tension and decreased intimacy.

Addressing these sleep issues and improving sleep quality is critical to men's overall health and well-being. Strategies such as establishing a consistent sleep schedule, creating a sleep-friendly environment, incorporating relaxation techniques, and using calming essential oils can all help promote better sleep and improve daily life. Consulting a healthcare professional for ongoing sleep problems is critical for proper diagnosis and personalized treatment.

B. Calming and Calming Essential Oils

Essential oils have long been recognized for their calming and calming properties, which can promote relaxation and improve sleep quality. Here are some key essential oils known for their calming and calming effects:

1. Lavender essential oil: Lavender is probably one of the most popular essential oils for promoting relaxation and sleep. Its soothing aroma helps reduce anxiety, calm the mind, and promote a sense of tranquility.

2. Chamomile essential oil: Chamomile is known for its calming properties. It can help reduce stress, anxiety, and restlessness, promote relaxation, and improve sleep.

3. Bergamot essential oil: Bergamot has a citrusy, uplifting aroma, but it also contains calming properties that can help relieve anxiety and induce a feeling of relaxation.

4. Sandalwood essential oil: Sandalwood has a rich, woody aroma and is known for its grounding and calming effects. It promotes inner peace and relaxation.

5. Ylang-ylang essential oil: Ylang-ylang has a sweet floral scent that can help reduce stress and anxiety. Its calming properties make it beneficial in promoting relaxation and restful sleep.

6. Vetiver essential oil: Vetiver has an earthy and grounding aroma that can effectively calm the mind and promote relaxation before bed.

7. Sage essential oil: Sage has a slightly sweet herbal scent that can help reduce tension and stress and promote a calm and peaceful atmosphere.

8. Marjoram essential oil: Marjoram is known for its warm, comforting aroma that can help relieve nervous tension and promote relaxation.

Using these essential oils in a variety of relaxation practices, such as aromatherapy diffusion, topical application, or bath rituals, can enhance their calming and calming effects and promote more restful sleep. It is important to use high-quality essential oils and follow proper dilution guidelines to ensure a safe and enjoyable experience. Additionally, incorporating these essential oils into your bedtime routine or relaxation ritual can create a calm and soothing atmosphere that supports better sleep and overall health.

Essential oils can profoundly impact the mind and mood, making them a valuable tool for promoting a relaxing and calm sleep environment. Here's how these essential oils can help achieve these effects:

1. Relax the mind: The aroma of essential oils can affect the limbic system, which is the part of the brain responsible for emotions and memory. When inhaled, the aroma molecules of essential oils stimulate the limbic system, promoting feelings of calm and relaxation. The soothing and gentle scents of oils like lavender, chamomile, and sandalwood can help calm a busy mind, ease thoughts, and create a more peaceful mental space.

2. Reduce anxiety: Essential oils contain natural compounds that interact with receptors in the brain, such as GABA receptors, to reduce anxiety and promote relaxation. Inhaling essential oils like bergamot and ylang-ylang can trigger the release of neurotransmitters, which have a calming effect on the nervous system and help relieve feelings of stress and anxiety.

3. Create a restful sleep environment: Diffusing essential oils in the bedroom or using them in a bedtime ritual can help create a restful sleep environment. The comforting scents of oils like vetiver, sage, and marjoram can signal to your brain that it's time to wind down and get ready for some rest. This connection between scent and sleep can help your brain regulate for a more restful and uninterrupted sleep.

4. Support a relaxing bedtime routine: Incorporating essential oils into your bedtime routine, such as massaging diluted essential oils into your skin or adding a few drops to a warm bath, can enhance relaxation and promote a sense of tranquility before bed. Engaging in these rituals can also signal to the body that it's time to relax and prepare for rest, further promoting better sleep quality.

5. Balance the nervous system: Some essential oils, like sage and lavender, have adaptogenic properties, which means they can help regulate the body's stress response and balance the nervous system. By reducing stress and promoting a state of calm, these oils help improve sleep patterns.

It's important to note that individuals may respond differently to essential oils, so it's important to find the oil and technique that works best for you. Also, always use high-quality, pure essential oils and dilute them appropriately to ensure safety and avoid skin irritation. Creating a relaxing bedtime routine with the help of essential oils can be a powerful tool for achieving better sleep and overall health.

C. Establish Sleep Habits

Consistent sleep habits are crucial to achieving better sleep quality and overall health. Here are some reasons why a regular sleep routine is important:

1. Regulate circadian rhythm: Our bodies have internal biological clocks, called circadian rhythms, that regulate the sleep * wake cycle. Going to bed and waking up simultaneously each day helps synchronize these rhythms, making it easier to fall asleep and wake up naturally.

2. Improve sleep quality: Consistency in sleep patterns allows the body to go through all necessary sleep stages, including deep sleep and REM (rapid eye movement) sleep, which are critical for physical and mental recovery. A regular sleep routine can promote more restorative sleep, leaving you feeling refreshed and energized during the day.

3. Improve sleep efficiency: With a consistent sleep schedule, your body becomes more efficient at initiating and maintaining sleep. It reduces the time it takes to fall asleep, reduces the likelihood of waking up during the night, and increases sleep time.

4. Supports the body's internal clock: Our bodies thrive on routine, and maintaining a consistent sleep schedule helps align the body's internal clock with the external environment. This synchronization can improve overall sleep quality and promote better health.

5. Reduce sleep disruptions: Inconsistent sleep schedules can lead to sleep disruptions and a condition called "social jet lag" The phenomenon. Social jet lag occurs when the body's internal clock does not match its external schedule, such as staying up late on the weekends and having difficulty adjusting to normal sleep habits during the work week. This can lead to fatigue and sleep-related problems.

Tips for establishing a consistent sleep routine:

1. Set a regular bedtime: Choose a bedtime that allows for at least 7 to 9 hours of sleep and stick to it, even on weekends.

2. Wake up at the same time every day: Aim to wake up at the same

time every day, including weekends, to regulate your body's internal clock.

3. Create a relaxing bedtime routine: Establish a calming bedtime routine to signal your body that it's time to wind down. This might include reading, listening to soothing music, or practicing relaxation techniques.

4. Limit screen time before bed: Reduce screen exposure (phones, tablets, computers, TVs) at least an hour before bed because blue light interferes with the production of the sleep hormone melatonin.

5. Avoid using stimulants before bed: Minimize consumption of caffeine and other stimulants in the hours before bed.

6. Make your sleeping environment comfortable: Keep your bedroom cool, dark, and quiet to create the best sleeping environment.

By establishing and maintaining a consistent sleep routine, you can improve the quality of your sleep, enhance your overall sense of well-being, and enjoy the many benefits of restorative sleep. Incorporating essential oils into your bedtime routine can further enhance relaxation and promote a peaceful transition to sleep.

Incorporating essential oils into your nightly ritual can be a soothing and effective way to signal your body to sleep. Here are some ways to use essential oils in your bedtime routine:

1. Diffuse: Use an aromatherapy diffuser in your bedroom to disperse calming essential oils like lavender, chamomile, bergamot, or sandalwood into the air. Start diffusing about 30 minutes before bed to create a relaxing atmosphere.

2. Pillow spray: Make a pillow spray by diluting a few drops of essential oil in water and transferring the mixture to a spray bottle. Gently apply a calming scent to your pillows and bedding before bed.

3. Bedtime bath: Add a few drops of your chosen essential oil to a warm bath before bed. The soothing aroma and warm water can help you relax and prepare for sleep.

4. Massage: Dilute the essential oil in a carrier oil, such as sweet almond or jojoba, and use the mixture for a calming bedtime massage. Focus on areas like the neck, shoulders, and feet, which tend to hold tension.

5. Aromatherapy inhaler: Create a personalized inhaler by adding a few drops of essential oil to a blank inhaler stick. Inhale the scent directly from your inhaler for quick and easy relaxation before bed.

6. Relaxation blends: Create your custom relaxation blend by combining 2 to 4 calming essential oils. Use 3 to 5 drops of the mixture in a diffuser, massage oil, or inhaler to help you relax and ease into a restful sleep.

7. Meditation or breathing exercises: Add essential oils to your meditation or deep breathing exercises before bed. Place a drop of the oil on your palms, rub them together, then hold them to your nose and inhale deeply the calming scent.

8. Bedtime tea: Add a drop of essential oil (such as chamomile or lavender) to a cup of herbal tea before bed. Warm drinks and soothing aromas can promote relaxation.

9. Soak your feet: Soak your feet with warm water and a few drops of calming essential oil. This can help relieve tension and promote overall relaxation.

Remember to choose high-quality, pure essential oils and always do a patch test before applying them to your skin to check for any sensitivities. Essential oils are potent, so a little goes a long way. Use them with caution and moderation for a safe and enjoyable bedtime experience. By incorporating these essential oil practices into your nightly ritual, you can create a calm and peaceful environment that signals your body for restful sleep.

D. Diffuse for Better Sleep

Diffusing essential oils in your bedroom can create a relaxing sleep environment with many benefits:

1. Calming aromas: Essential oils like lavender, chamomile, and bergamot have soothing properties that can help reduce feelings of stress and anxiety and promote relaxation before bed.

2. Improve sleep quality: The relaxing aroma of essential oils can help signal to the brain that it's time to wind down and prepare for sleep, resulting in improved sleep quality and a more restful night.

3. Reduce stress: Diffusing essential oils can reduce levels of cortisol, the stress hormone, helping you feel more relaxed and relaxed before bed.

4. Sleep associations: Consistent use of a specific essential oil or blend before bed can create sleep associations, and your brain begins to associate the scent with relaxation and bedtime, helping you transition to sleep more easily.

5. Enhance breathing: Some essential oils, such as eucalyptus or peppermint, can help clear the airways and promote better, more comfortable sleeping breathing.

6. Reduce nighttime wakings: The calming effects of essential oils help reduce nighttime wakings and interruptions, resulting in more uninterrupted sleep.

7. Tranquil sleeping environment: Diffusing essential oils helps create a peaceful and cozy atmosphere in the bedroom, making it a soothing and inviting space for rest.

8. Natural sleep aids: Essential oils are a natural alternative to traditional sleep aids, providing relaxation without the potential side effects often associated with medications.

9. Aromatherapy benefits: In addition to promoting sleep, diffusing essential oils also provides the broader benefits of aromatherapy, including mood enhancement, stress relief, and overall well-being.

To maximize the benefits of diffusing essential oils for a relaxing sleep environment, follow these tips:

A diffuser that disperses the oil effectively and safely.
About 30 minutes before bed to create a calming atmosphere in your bedroom.
Use calming essential oils or a custom blend designed to promote relaxation and sleep.
Adjust diffusion time and intensity to your personal preference and room size.
Keep your bedroom well-ventilated, especially if you're diffusing for a long time, so the scent doesn't overwhelm the space.
Be consistent with your bedtime routine and essential oil use to create a sleep association and increase the effectiveness of your relaxation exercises.

Remember that individuals may react differently to essential oils, so experiment with different essential oils or blends to find the one that works best for you. By diffusing essential oils in your sleep environment, you can create a calm and relaxing atmosphere that supports a restful night's rest and sets the stage for improved sleep quality and overall health.

Recommended oils for sleep support:

1. Lavender: Lavender is one of the most popular essential oils for sleep because of its calming and sedative properties. It helps promote relaxation and relieve anxiety, making it a great bedtime choice.

2. Chamomile: Chamomile essential oil is known for its soothing effects on the body and mind. It can help reduce stress, promote a sense of tranquility, and facilitate better sleep.

3. Bergamot: Bergamot oil has a unique citrus scent and has a calming effect. It can help relieve tension and create a restful sleep environment.

4. Sandalwood: Sandalwood has a grounding and relaxing effect, soothes the mind, and induces a sense of calm, making it a suitable oil before bed.

5. Vetiver: Vetiver essential oil has an earthy and grounding aroma that can help calm the mind and promote a more restful sleep.

Diffuser settings for optimal sleep support:

1. Timer: Set your diffuser to run on a timer, ideally starting around 30 minutes before bed. This allows the calming aroma to fill the room without running all night long, preventing potential sensory overload.

2. Intermittent mode: Some diffusers offer an intermittent mode that releases essential oils in a short period. This setup can be gentler on the senses while still providing the desired aromatherapy benefits.

3. Low diffusion rate: Choose a low diffusion rate for nighttime to create a subtle and calming fragrance in the bedroom.

4. Room size: Consider the size of your bedroom when choosing a diffuser. Larger rooms may require a diffuser with a higher output to disperse

the oil evenly.

Diffuser technology for best sleep support:

1. Single essential oil diffuser: Use a calming essential oil, such as lavender or chamomile, alone for a simple and effective sleep-inducing scent.

2. Bedtime blend: Create a custom bedtime blend by combining two or more calming essential oils to enhance their relaxing effects. For example, try blending lavender, chamomile, and bergamot for a soothing and comforting scent.

3. Pre-made sleep blends: Many essential oil companies offer pre-made sleep blends specifically designed to promote relaxation and restful sleep. These blends often combine various calming oils for maximum effect.

4. DIY diffuser blends: Try different essential oil combinations to find the best one for you. Start with 2 to 4 drops of each essential oil and adjust the ratio to your preference.

5. Aromatherapy jewelry: If you don't want to diffuse essential oils in your bedroom, consider wearing aromatherapy jewelry infused with calming oils to experience their benefits all night long.

Always follow the manufacturer's instructions for your diffuser and use high-quality, pure essential oils. If you have any respiratory conditions or sensitivities, ensure the room is well-ventilated when diffusing and discontinue use if any adverse reactions occur. Combining these recommended oils, diffuser settings, and diffusion techniques allows you to create an optimal sleep-supportive environment that promotes relaxation and restful sleep for better overall health and well-being.

E. Bedtime Bath and Body Products

Using essential oils in bath and body products can be a wonderful way to create a soothing pre-bed routine that promotes relaxation and prepares the body and mind for a restful sleep. Here are some bath and body products you can incorporate essential oils into:

1. Bath salts: Create a calming and aromatic bath by adding a few drops of your choice of sleep-supporting essential oil to Epsom salt or Hima-

layan pink salt. Dissolve salt in warm wash water and soak for 15 to 20 minutes to enjoy the soothing benefits of essential oils.

2. Bath bombs: Make your DIY bath bombs infused with essential oils like lavender or chamomile. These fizzing bath treatments release soothing scents as they dissolve in water, creating a luxurious and calming bathing experience.

3. Body oil: Make a relaxing body oil by blending your favorite sleep-enhancing essential oil with a carrier oil like jojoba, sweet almond, or coconut oil. Massage essential oils into your skin before bed to enjoy calming effects and skin-nourishing benefits.

4. Body lotion: Mix a few drops of calming essential oil into your favorite unscented body lotion to create a personalized sleep-inducing moisturizer. Gently apply lotion on your body before going to bed to make your skin smooth and fragrant.

5. Pillow spray: Make a DIY pillow spray by mixing water and a few drops of sleep-promoting essential oils in a spray bottle. Spray your pillows and sheets with a calming scent before bed to set the stage for a restful night.

The soothing scent will help you relax and unwind during your evening shower.

7. Massage oil: Mix sleep-supporting essential oils with a carrier oil like almond or grapeseed oil to create a relaxing massage oil. Give you a calming self-massage before bed, or ask your partner to massage to help you relax gently.

When using essential oils in bath and body products, always make sure to dilute appropriately and patch-test any new mixture to check for sensitivity. Choose high-quality, pure essential oils and avoid synthetic fragrances containing potentially harmful chemicals. Remember, essential oils are effective; a little goes a long way. Experiment with different oils and products to find the combination that best supports your bedtime routine and improves overall sleep quality.

Here are some simple and soothing recipes for making homemade sleep-inducing bath salts, body oils, and pillow sprays:

1. Calming Lavender Bath Salts:

Element:
* 1 cup Epsom salt
* 1/2 cup Himalayan pink salt (optional)
* 10*15 drops of lavender essential oil

Guide:
* In a mixing bowl, combine Epsom salt and Himalayan pink salt (if using).
* Add lavender essential oil to the salt mixture and stir evenly to distribute the fragrance evenly.
* Transfer the bath salts to a clean, airtight container for storage.
* When using, add a few tablespoons of bath salts to warm running water and soak for 15 to 20 minutes before going to bed.

2. Soothing Chamomile Body Oil:

Element:
* 1/4 cup carrier oil (such as sweet almond or jojoba)
* 5 ~ 10 drops of chamomile essential oil
* 5 drops of lavender essential oil
* 3 drops of bergamot essential oil

Guide:
* combine the carrier oil with the essential oil in a small dark glass bottle.
* Gently shake the bottle to mix the oil thoroughly.
* Before going to bed, massage a small amount of body oil into the skin, focusing on the neck, shoulders, and feet to achieve a calming effect.

3. Sweet Dreams Pillow Spray:

Element:
* 1/2 cup distilled water
* 1 tablespoon witch hazel or vodka (as emulsifier)
* 10 drops of lavender essential oil
* 5 drops of cedar essential oil
* 5 drops of ylang-ylang essential oil

Guide:
* combine distilled water and witch hazel (or vodka) in a small spray bottle.

* Add the essential oil to the water mixture and close the bottle tightly.

* Shake the bottle well before each use, then gently rinse the spray off pillows and sheets before bed.

These DIY recipes are designed to be customized to your personal preferences. You can adjust the number of essential oil drops to make the scent stronger or milder but always stick to the recommended dilution ratio. Additionally, high-quality, pure essential oils must be used for best results. Remember, aromatherapy works differently for everyone, so feel free to try different combinations of essential oils until you find something that helps you relax and improves your sleep quality.

F. Improvements in Bedding and Sheets

Essential oils can be important in enhancing bedding and linens to create a peaceful and soothing sleep environment. Here are some ways to incorporate essential oils into your bedding and sheets for a better sleep experience:

1. Linen spray: Create a DIY linen spray using essential oils known for their calming properties, such as lavender, chamomile, and bergamot. Mix a few drops of your chosen essential oil with water in a spray bottle and gently mist your bedding before bed. This will infuse your sheets and pillowcases with a relaxing scent, promoting restful sleep.

2. Aromatherapy diffuser jewelry: Consider using aromatherapy diffuser jewelry, such as a necklace or bracelet, to carry the soothing scent of essential oils throughout the day. This way, even when you're not in bed, you can experience the calming effects of essential oils, helping to reduce stress and anxiety, thus positively impacting the quality of your sleep.

3. Sleep-enhancing laundry: Add a few drops of essential oil to a damp cloth or wool dryer ball and toss it in the dryer with your bedding. The gentle heat from the dryer disperses oil, leaving your sheets and blankets with a subtle, cozy scent.

4. DIY sleeping bag: Make a small bag using a fabric bag filled with dried herbs and a few drops of essential oil. Lavender, chamomile, and cedar wood are great choices for sleep-inducing sachets. Place these sachets in your pillowcase or between layers of bedding to release their calming aroma.

5. Essential oil-infused pillowcases: You can apply a drop or two of

essential oil directly to your pillowcase before bed. This slowly releases the scent as you lower your head, promoting relaxation and sleep.

6. Calming eye pillow: Sew a small cloth bag and fill it with flax seeds and a few drops of calming essential oil. Place the eye pillow over your eyes while lying in bed to soothe and calm your senses and help you drift into a restful sleep.

Remember, use essential oils in bedding and linens cautiously, as some oils can stain fabrics. Always dilute essential oils correctly and spot-test them on a small area before applying them directly to linens. Also, remember that essential oils are potent, so a little goes a long way. High-quality oils and proper dilution ratios will ensure a safe and enjoyable sleep-enhancing experience.

Using essential oils in linen sprays, sachets, and aromatherapy-infused pillows can improve your sleep environment and promote a restful night's sleep. Let's explore each technology in more detail:

1. Linen spray:

Linen spray is a simple and effective way to infuse your bedding with the calming scent of essential oils. You'll need a small spray bottle and distilled water to make linen spray. Here's how to make it:

Fill a small spray bottle with distilled water, leaving some space at the top.
Add 5 to 10 drops of an essential oil of your choice, known for its relaxing properties, such as lavender, chamomile, or bergamot. Shake the bottle well to mix the oil with the water.
Gently rub your pillowcases, sheets, and blankets before bed.

Linen spray's soft fragrance creates a calming, soothing atmosphere to help you relax and prepare for a restful night's sleep.

2. Sleep-inducing sachet:

Sleep bags are small bags filled with dried herbs and essential oils. These pouches can be placed inside pillowcases or between bedding to release their calming aroma. Here's how to make it:

Choose a small cloth bag or a cloth bag.
Fill a bag with dried herbs known for their sleep-enhancing properties,

such as dried lavender flowers or chamomile buds.

Add a few drops of your favorite essential oil to the dried herbs. Lavender, chamomile, and cedar are popular choices.

Close the bag securely and place it near your pillow or a pillowcase.

The soothing scent of the sleep sachet will help promote relaxation and tranquility, setting the stage for a restful night's sleep.

3. Aromatherapy pillow:

Infusing your pillow with essential oils can create a subtle and calming sleep environment. To this end:

Place a few drops of essential oil on a cotton ball or small piece of cloth.

Stuff a cotton ball or cloth inside the pillowcase, close to the edge of the pillow.

The body and head movement heat will gently release the aroma throughout the night, encouraging relaxation and better sleep quality.

Aromatherapy-infused pillows are a great way to enjoy the benefits of essential oils while you sleep without having to come into direct contact with them.

By incorporating these tips into your nightly routine, you can create a personalized sleep sanctuary that promotes relaxation, reduces stress, and improves your overall sleep experience. Remember to use high-quality essential oils, and if you have any sensitivities or allergies, consider patch-testing a small area before using it on your bedding. Have a good dream!

G. Personalized Sleep Mix

Create a custom sleep blend using essential oils, allowing you to tailor the scent to your preferences and specific sleep needs. Here's a step-by-step guide to help you create a personalized sleep blend:

1. Choose your basic notes:

Start by choosing a base essential oil that will form the base of your blend. The base has a long-lasting, grounding scent that helps anchor the scent. Popular base oils for use in sleep blends include:

Sandalwood: Known for its calming and soothing properties.

Vetiver: Deeply relaxing and promoting a sense of tranquility.
Cedar Wood: Has a warm woody scent that induces relaxation.

2. Add medium oil:

The heart notes add complexity to the blend and help balance the aroma. They are generally sedative and have a medium-lasting scent. Some mid-note oils suitable for sleep blends are:

Lavender: Known for its calming and sleep-promoting properties.
Roman Chamomile: Has a mild, soothing aroma that relieves stress and tension.
Bergamot: Uplifting and stress-reducing, it complements the other oils in the blend.

3. Includes pre-conditioning oil:

Top note oils have a lighter, fresher scent and provide a pleasant initial aroma when you smell the blend. They tend to have longer-lasting effects. Consider adding one or both of the following top conditioning oils:

Sweet Orange: Bright and uplifting, it adds a hint of sweetness to the mix.
Citrus: Has a calming, fruity aroma that promotes relaxation.
Geranium: Balancing and soothing can help relieve anxiety and stress.

4. Create your mixture:

Once you've chosen your essential oils, it's time to create your sleep blend. Here's a simple recipe to get you started:

*3 drops of base oil of your choice
*5 drops of your favorite mid-tone oil
*2 drops to replenish the oil before use

Adjust the number of drops to your preference and the size of the bottle you use. You can also try combinations to find the perfect scent for your sleep needs.

5. Dilution and Application:

To use your sleep blend, dilute it in a carrier oil, such as sweet almond oil or jojoba oil, to the recommended dilution of 2 to 3 percent (approximately 12 to 18 drops of essential oil per 1 ounce of carrier oil). Combine the essential oils with the carrier oil in a small glass bottle, shake, and mix.

Apply the diluted mixture to your skin before bed by massaging it into your wrists, temples, or the back of your neck. You can also use the mixture in a diffuser or any previously mentioned sleep-enhancing techniques, such as linen spray or aromatherapy-infused pillows.

Remember to store essential oil blends in a cool, dark place out of direct sunlight to maintain potency.

Creating a custom sleep blend allows you to experience essential oils' relaxing and sleep-inducing properties tailored to your preferences and unique sleep needs. Enjoy a personalized blend of calming benefits to prepare you for a restful night's sleep.

Proper mixing ratios, soothing combinations, and application methods are crucial to addressing sleep-related issues effectively. Here are some guidelines for creating sleep blends based on specific sleep concerns:

1. General sleep support combination:

This blend is suitable for overall relaxation and promoting a restful sleep environment.

* Lavender: 4 drops
* Roman Chamomile: 3 drops
* Cedar: 3 drops

To dilute: Add the above essential oil mixture to 1 ounce (30 ml) of carrier oil, such as sweet almond oil or jojoba oil.

How to use: Massage a small amount of the diluted mixture onto your wrists, temples, and chest before bed. You can also use it in a diffuser or make a linen spray for your bedding.

2. Insomnia and insomnia mixed:

This blend is designed to calm the mind and provide better sleep for those with insomnia or difficulty falling asleep.

* Vetiver: 4 drops
* Bergamot: 3 drops

* Sandalwood: 3 drops

Dilute: Add the above essential oil mixture to 1 ounce (30 ml) of carrier oil.

How to use: Use a diluted mixture for a relaxing body massage or as a soothing bath oil before bed.

3. Relieve mixed stress and anxiety:

This blend helps reduce stress and anxiety, which can interfere with restful sleep.

* Ylang-ylang: 4 drops
* Frankincense: 3 drops
* Sweet orange: 3 drops

Dilute: Add the above essential oil mixture to 1 ounce (30 ml) of carrier oil.

How to use: Apply diluted mixture to your wrists and inhale deeply to help relieve stress and promote relaxation. You can also use it in an aromatherapy diffuser.

4. Nighttime mindfulness blend:

This blend is perfect for enhancing mindfulness before bed, promoting mental clarity, and calming racing thoughts.

* Sage: 4 drops
* Lavender: 3 drops
* Lemon: 2 drops

Dilute: Add the above essential oil mixture to 1 ounce (30 ml) of carrier oil.

Directions: Use the diluted mixture for a calming foot massage or apply it to the palms of your hands and cup your nose. Breathe deeply during mindfulness practice.

When making a sleep blend, always follow the proper dilution ratio (2 to 3% for most adults), as using undiluted essential oils can cause skin irritation. Also, before using the mixture more extensively, perform a patch test on a small skin area to check for any sensitivities or allergies.

Experiment with different essential oil combinations to find the one that best suits your sleep-related concerns. Remember to create a relaxing environment and maintain a consistent sleep routine to increase the effectiveness of your essential oil blend in improving sleep quality and overall health.

H. Solve Sleep Disorders

Essential oils can be a valuable addition to regular treatment for people with sleep disorders such as insomnia, sleep apnea, or restless legs syndrome. While essential oils alone may not cure these conditions, they can help promote relaxation, reduce anxiety, and create a more favorable sleep environment. Here are some ways essential oils can support people with sleep disorders:

1. Insomnia:

Essential oils with calming and sedative properties may be beneficial for people who suffer from insomnia. Lavender, chamomile, and vetiver are known for their sleep-inducing effects. Diffusing these oils or using them in a relaxing bedtime massage can help calm the mind and prepare the body for rest.

2. Sleep apnea:

Sleep apnea is a more complex sleep disorder that may require medical attention. However, essential oils can help relieve symptoms like snoring and improve overall sleep quality. Eucalyptus and peppermint oils can promote clearer breathing and reduce nasal congestion when diffused or applied topically (diluted).

3. Restless legs syndrome (RLS):

Restless legs syndrome causes discomfort and restlessness during sleep. Essential oils with soothing and relaxing properties, such as lavender, chamomile, and sage, can be used topically or in a warm bath before bed to help reduce symptoms and induce relaxation.

4. Aromatherapy massage:

Aromatherapy massage using essential oils is particularly beneficial for people with sleep disorders. Combining gentle massage and inhaling calming scents can promote deep relaxation and improve sleep quality.

5. Bedtime:

Incorporate essential oils into your bedtime routine to signal sleep. This might include using soothing oils when relaxing before bed or using a sleep-inducing pillow spray to create a restful sleep environment.

6. Personal inhaler:

For sleep disorder sufferers who are traveling or who don't have access to a diffuser, personal inhalers can conveniently carry the calming scent of essential oils.

It is important to consult with a healthcare professional before using essential oils as a complementary treatment, especially if you have been diagnosed with a sleep disorder. They can help identify any potential interactions with medications or other treatments and provide personalized guidance.

Additionally, consider personal sensitivities and preferences when using essential oils. Some people may find specific scents more relaxing, while others may be sensitive to certain oils. Always follow proper dilution guidelines and safety precautions to ensure a safe and effective experience when using essential oils for sleep support.

Here are some specific essential oils and techniques that can help relieve symptoms and improve sleep quality for people with sleep disorders:

1. Lavender: Lavender is one of the most popular essential oils to promote relaxation and improve sleep quality. Its calming and calming properties can help reduce anxiety and induce a sense of tranquility, making it beneficial for people with insomnia or restless legs syndrome. Diffusing lavender oil in your bedroom or adding a few drops to a warm bath before bed may help.

2. Chamomile: Chamomile essential oil is known for its soothing effects, making it useful for people suffering from insomnia or sleep disorders. It can be diffused, applied topically (diluted), or added to bedtime tea for relaxation.

3. Vetiver: Vetiver oil has grounding and calming properties, which can benefit people with insomnia, anxiety, or sleep apnea. Diffuse vetiver oil or mix it with carrier oil for a calming massage before bed.

4. Frankincense: Frankincense is traditionally used to promote relaxation and reduce stress. It can be diffused or used in massage blends to create a restful sleep environment.

5. Marjoram: Marjoram essential oil has a calming and comforting aroma that can help relieve nervous tension and promote relaxation. It can be diffused, added to a warm bath, or diluted with a carrier oil for a relaxing massage.

6. Bergamot: Bergamot oil has uplifting and mood-enhancing properties that can help reduce anxiety and stress and is beneficial for people with sleep disorders caused by emotional factors. Use bergamot oil in a massage blend to improve sleep quality.

Techniques for using essential oils to support sleep:

1. Diffuse: Use an aromatherapy diffuser in your bedroom to diffuse the calming scent of essential oils before and during bed. Diffusers with timers are particularly useful for controlling the duration of your diffuser.

2. Massage before bed: Dilute a few drops of essential oil in a carrier oil (such as sweet almond or jojoba) and massage your neck, shoulders, and back before bed for a relaxing and sleep-inducing experience.

3. Warm bath: Add a few drops of essential oils to a warm bath before bed to promote relaxation and create a soothing bedtime ritual.

4. Pillow Spray: Make a natural pillow spray by mixing water and a few drops of essential oil in a spray bottle. Spray lightly on pillows and bedding before bed.

Everyone may react differently to essential oils, so it's important to find the scent and technique that works best for you. Always use high-quality, pure essential oils, and consider potential sensitivities or allergies before using any new oils. If you have been diagnosed with a sleep disorder or medical condition, consult a healthcare professional for personalized guidance and to ensure that using essential oils is safe and appropriate for your specific situation.

Chapter 6

Essential Oils for Men's Hormone Health

Hormone balance is important for men's health. We dive into essential oils that can help balance testosterone levels, maintain sexual health, and address hormonal imbalances and symptoms.

6.1 Balance Testosterone Levels

In this chapter, we'll explore how essential oils can support the balance of testosterone levels in men. We discuss the importance of maintaining optimal testosterone levels for overall health and well-being and guide using essential oils to support hormonal balance.

A. Understand Testosterone and Its Importance

Testosterone is a hormone that plays a vital role in men's health and well-being. It is primarily produced in the testicles and has widespread effects on the body. Here are some key aspects of testosterone's role in men's health:

1. Muscle mass and strength: Testosterone is often associated with developing and maintaining muscle mass. It supports protein synthesis, which is essential for building and repairing muscles. Men with higher testosterone levels tend to have greater muscle mass and strength.

2. Bone health: Testosterone plays a role in maintaining bone density and strength. Low testosterone levels can lead to the risk of osteoporosis and fractures.

3. Sexual function: Testosterone is a key factor in male sexual development and function. It aids in developing male reproductive organs during puberty and maintains vitality throughout life. It also plays a role in achieving and maintaining an erection.

4. Emotional and mental health: Testosterone impacts emotional and mental health. Low testosterone levels are associated with symptoms such as irritability, mood swings, and, in some cases, depression.

5. Fat distribution: Testosterone helps regulate fat distribution in the body. Men with low testosterone levels may experience increased body fat, especially in the abdominal area.

6. Energy and vitality: Testosterone contributes to overall energy levels and vitality. Higher testosterone levels are often associated with increased energy and feelings of well-being.

7. Erythropoiesis: Testosterone stimulates the production of red blood cells in the bone marrow. This is important for oxygen transport throughout the body.

8. Cognitive functions: Some research suggests that testosterone may affect cognitive function, including memory and cognitive processing. However, the exact relationship is still under study.

9. Aging and decline: Testosterone levels naturally decline as we age, usually starting in our 20s or 30s. This decline is gradual but can lead to a variety of symptoms often referred to as " low testosterone " or " low T." These symptoms may include loss of muscle mass, decline, fatigue, mood changes, and difficulty concentrating.

10. Hormone balance: Testosterone is part of a complex hormonal sys-

tem that also involves other hormones such as estrogen and cortisol. Maintaining proper hormonal balance is vital to overall health.

It's important to note that testosterone levels vary widely between individuals and can be affected by factors such as genetics, lifestyle, diet, exercise, sleep quality, and stress. If you suspect you have low testosterone levels or develop symptoms related to for symptoms related to hormonal imbalance, it is recommended that you consult a healthcare professional. They can perform tests to assess your hormone levels and recommend appropriate treatment, if necessary, which may include lifestyle changes, hormone replacement therapy, or other medical interventions.

Testosterone levels can be affected by a variety of factors, and imbalances in testosterone levels can have a significant impact on a man's health and well-being. Here are some key factors that can affect testosterone levels and the potential effects of an imbalance:

1. Age:

Testosterone levels naturally decline with age. Starting around age 30, most men's testosterone levels gradually decrease at a rate of about 1% per year. This decline can lead to symptoms such as loss of muscle mass, decreased energy, and changes in sexual function.

2. Lifestyle factors:

* Diet: Poor nutrition, especially a diet high in processed foods and sugar, can negatively impact testosterone levels. Consuming enough vitamins, minerals, and healthy fats is important to maintain optimal hormone balance.
* Sports: Regular physical activity, especially resistance training and high-intensity interval training (HIIT), can help maintain healthy testosterone levels.
* Sleep: Poor sleep quality and insufficient sleep can disrupt hormonal balance, including testosterone production.
* Stress: Chronic stress can increase cortisol levels, which can lead to lower testosterone levels. It is important to manage stress through relaxation techniques and stress-reducing activities.

3. Body composition:

* Obesity: Excess body fat, especially abdominal fat, is associated with lower testosterone levels. Fat tissue can convert testosterone into estro-

gen, causing an imbalance between these hormones.

* Low body fat: Very low body fat, as seen in some athletes and body-builders, can also lead to low testosterone levels.

4. Medical conditions:

* Hypogonadism: This is a condition in which the testicles do not produce enough testosterone, either due to problems with the testicles themselves (primary hypogonadism) or problems with the hypothalamus or pituitary gland (secondary hypogonadism).

* Chronic disease: Certain chronic diseases, such as type 2 diabetes, obesity, and kidney disease, can cause low testosterone levels.

* Drugs: Some medications, such as corticosteroids and opioids, can affect testosterone production.

5. Hormone imbalance:

* Estrogen levels: An imbalance between testosterone and estrogen levels can occur, leading to symptoms such as gynecomastia (enlarged breasts) and other hormonal disorders.

* Cortisol levels: High cortisol levels caused by chronic stress can interfere with testosterone production.

6. Environmental factors:

* Endocrine disruptors: Exposure to certain chemicals, called endocrine disruptors, can interfere with the production and regulation of hormones. These chemicals are found in some plastics, pesticides, and other products.

7. Genetics:

Genetic factors can influence testosterone levels and the body's response to changes in hormone levels.

Impact of imbalance:

* Low Testosterone (Hypogonadism): Low testosterone levels can cause fatigue, fatigue, erectile dysfunction, reduced muscle mass and strength, mood changes, and reduced bone density.

* High Testosterone: High testosterone levels can lead to aggressive behavior, acne, and in extreme cases, polycystic ovary syndrome in women (PCOS) and other diseases.

It is important to note that testosterone levels may vary from person to person, and the effects of an imbalance may vary based on genetics, overall health, and other factors. If you suspect you have an imbalance in your testosterone levels or are experiencing symptoms related to hormonal changes, it is recommended that you Consult a health care professional. They can perform the appropriate tests, provide an accurate diagnosis, and recommend appropriate treatments or lifestyle changes to address any imbalances and optimize your health.

B. Essential Oils to Balance Testosterone

Certain essential oils are thought to have potential effects on hormonal balance and, in some cases, may support healthy testosterone levels. While research on the specific effects of essential oils on hormones is limited, some essential oils have traditionally been used for their potential benefits. Here are some essential oils that are often mentioned for their potential to support hormonal balance and promote healthy testosterone levels:

1. Ginger essential oil: Ginger is considered to have adaptogenic properties that may help support the body's overall hormonal balance. It is thought to help regulate cortisol levels and, when balanced, can indirectly support testosterone levels.

2. Sage essential oil: Sage is often cited for its potential to help balance hormones, including estrogen and testosterone. It is thought to have effects on the endocrine system and may help regulate hormone production.

3. Rosemary essential oil: Rosemary is thought to have a potential effect on cortisol levels, which can indirectly affect testosterone levels. Some studies have explored the effects of rosemary extract on testosterone levels in animals, but more research is needed to understand its effects on humans.

4. Ylang-ylang essential oil: Ylang-ylang is thought to have calming properties that can help reduce stress and cortisol levels. It may indirectly support hormonal balance by promoting relaxation and reducing stress.

It's important to note that essential oils should not be considered a primary treatment for hormonal imbalances or low testosterone. If you suspect you have a hormonal imbalance, it is recommended that you consult a health-care professional for proper diagnosis and guidance. Hormone imbalances can have a variety of underlying causes, and a healthcare provider can help determine the most appropriate treatment plan.

If you decide to use essential oils to reap their potential benefits, here are some tips:
* Uses high-quality pure essential oils from reputable sources.
* Be sure to properly dilute essential oils in a carrier oil before applying them to the skin.
* Perform a patch test to check for any skin sensitivities or allergies.
* Remember, essential oils should be used as part of a holistic approach to health and well-being, including a balanced diet, regular exercise, stress management, and medical guidance.

Additionally, it is important to use essential oils to support hormones with caution and to be realistic about their potential effects. Research in this area is ongoing, and individual reactions to essential oils may vary. Always consult a healthcare professional before using essential oils for any health-related purpose, especially if you have a pre-existing medical condition or are taking medications.

While essential oils are often thought to have the potential to support hormonal balance, it's important to note that the mechanisms by which they may affect hormones are not fully understood. Research in this area is limited, and the effects of essential oils on hormonal regulation may vary from person to person. Here are some ways to explore these essential oils to potentially support your body's natural hormone regulatory mechanisms:

1. Adaptogenic effects: Some essential oils, such as ginger and sage, are considered adaptogens. Adaptogens are thought to help the body adapt to stress and promote overall balance. These oils may indirectly affect hormonal regulation by reducing stress and supporting the body's response to stressors. Lowering stress levels can positively impact hormones like cortisol, which can have a cascading effect on other hormones.

2. Endocrine system support: Sage and rosemary are sometimes thought to have an impact on the endocrine system, which plays a vital role in the production and regulation of hormones. The exact mechanism by which these oils interact with the endocrine system is unknown, but some proponents believe they may help balance hormone levels.

3. Aromatherapy benefits: Aromatherapy with essential oils like ylang-ylang and rosemary can provide relaxation and stress-relieving benefits.

Reducing stress and promoting relaxation can positively impact the body's overall physiological balance, indirectly affecting hormone regulation.

4. Skin absorption: Some essential oils can be absorbed through the skin when properly diluted and used topically. Skin is a permeable barrier, and certain essential oil compounds may interact with receptors in the skin to affect hormone-related processes. However, the extent to which essential oils directly affect hormones when absorbed through the skin is still being studied.

It is important to use essential oils to support hormones with caution and to be realistic about their potential effects. Essential oils should not be used as a substitute for professional medical advice or treatment. If you are considering using essential oils to support hormonal balance, it is recommended that you consult a healthcare professional with experience in aromatherapy and integrative medicine. They can help you make informed decisions based on your personal health needs and circumstances.

C. Topical Application of Hormonal Support

When using essential oils to support hormonal balance potentially, safe and appropriate usage techniques must be followed. Here are some guidelines to consider:

1. Dilution: Essential oils are highly concentrated and can cause irritation or sensitization when applied directly to the skin. Always dilute essential oils in a carrier oil before applying them to your skin. A common dilution ratio is 2 to 3 drops of essential oil per teaspoon of carrier oil.

2. Patch test: Before applying a new essential oil to a larger area of skin, conduct a patch test. Apply a dilute mixture of essential oil and carrier oil to a small area of skin (such as the inner forearm) and wait 24 hours to check for any adverse reactions.

3. Targeted applications: If you're interested in hormonal balance, consider applying a dilute blend of essential oils to specific pulse points, such as your wrists, neck, and temples. Massaging the mixture into these areas can enhance absorption.

4. Frequently used: Consistency is key when potentially using essential oils to support hormonal balance. Incorporate them into your daily routine for a while, noting any changes or effects.

5. Personalization: Everyone's body chemistry is different. What works for one person may not work for another. Pay close attention to your body's reactions and adjust your usage accordingly.

6. Consult a professional: Before using essential oils to support hormones, it's best to consult a healthcare professional with experience in aromatherapy and integrative medicine. They can provide personalized guidance based on your health history and needs.

7. Avoid sensitive areas: Avoid applying essential oils near sensitive areas such as eyes, ears, or mucous membranes.

8. Pregnancy and medical conditions: If you are pregnant, nursing, or have any underlying medical conditions, it is especially important to consult a healthcare professional before using essential oils.

Here's a general approach to creating topical blends for potential hormonal support:

Element:

* 2 to 3 drops of selected essential oils (ginger, sage, rosemary, ylang-ylang)
* 1 teaspoon carrier oil (such as fractionated coconut oil, jojoba oil, or sweet almond oil)

Guide:

1. Choose an essential oil that you think may support hormonal balance. You can use it alone or mix it with another essential oil.
2. In a small glass container, add selected essential oil.
3. Add the carrier oil to the container and stir evenly.
4. Conduct a patch test on a small area of skin to ensure there are no adverse reactions.
5. If the patch test is successful, you can apply the diluted mixture to the pulse point or area of your choice.

Remember that essential oils are not a substitute for medical treatments, and their effects on hormonal balance may vary. If you experience any adverse reactions or are unsure about using essential oils, consult a healthcare professional for guidance.

Below is a more detailed discussion of appropriate dilution ratios, carrier oils, and targeted application methods for optimal absorption of essential oils:

Dilution ratio:

Dilution is critical to ensuring that essential oils are safe and effective when applied to the skin. Dilution rates are usually expressed as drops of essential oil per unit of carrier oil. A common dilution ratio for general use is 2 to 3% essential oil to carrier oil. This means that for every teaspoon (5 ml) of carrier oil, you will use 3 to 9 drops of essential oil.

Carrier oil:

Carrier oils are used to dilute essential oils and help apply them to the skin. They also provide moisturizing benefits and aid in the absorption of essential oils. Some popular carrier oils include:
* Fractionated Coconut Oil: Lightweight and absorbs quickly.
* Jojoba Oil: Like skin's natural oil, it absorbs well.
* Sweet Almond Oil: Nourishing, suitable for most skin types.
* Grapeseed Oil: Light and non-greasy.
* Avocado Oil: Rich and great for dry skin.
* Rosehip Seed Oil: Regenerating, great for mature skin.

Targeted application methods:

For enhanced absorption and efficacy, consider these targeted application methods:

1. Pulse point: Apply a diluted essential oil mixture to pulse points such as your wrists, neck, and temples. These areas have a higher concentration of blood vessels, which may enhance absorption and distribution.

2. Massage: Gently massage the mixture into the skin. Massage not only aids absorption but also promotes relaxation and circulation.

3. Feet: The pores on the soles of the feet are larger and are a good area for absorption. Additionally, reflex points on the feet are connected to various organs and systems in the body.

4. Chest and abdomen: The mixture is applied to the chest and ab-

dominal areas so it can be absorbed through the skin and inhaled through the breath.

5. Spine: Applying the mixture along the spine can promote absorption into the bloodstream and may affect the nervous system.

6. Local application: If you target a specific area (for example, muscle discomfort), apply the mixture directly to that area.

Everyone's skin sensitivity is different, so it's important to start with a low dilution and perform a patch test before applying a new mixture to a larger area. Plus, essential oils are powerful, so a little goes a long way.

For example, if you create 1 ounce (30 ml) of the mixture, a 2% dilution (safe for general use) would be approximately 12 drops of essential oil in 1 ounce of carrier oil. Adjust the amount of essential oil based on your comfort and specific needs.

Finally, it is crucial to consider the intended purpose of the mixture and the individual's health status. If you are using essential oils for a specific health concern or condition, it is recommended to consult a qualified aromatherapist or healthcare professional to ensure safe and effective use.

D. Hormone Support Blend

Here are some personalized hormonal support blends using essential oils:

Hormone Balancing Roller Balls:

* 10 ml roller bottle
* 8 drops of sage
* 6 drops of frankincense
* 4 drops of geranium
* 3 drops of lavender
* Filled with a carrier oil like jojoba or fractionated coconut oil.

Testosterone Support Massage Blend:

* 1 oz (30 ml) bottle
* 10 drops of ginger

* 8 drops rosemary
* 5 drops of ylang-ylang
* 5 drops of cedar
* Filled with a carrier oil such as sweet almond oil

Mood-Elevating Hormone Support Diffuser Blend:

* Essential oil diffuser:
* 3 drops of bergamot
* 3 drops of sage
* 2 drops of lavender
* 2 drops of frankincense

Hormone Balancing Bath Soak:

* 1 cup Epsom salt
* 5 drops of geranium
* 4 drops of sage
* 3 drops of lavender
* Mix essential oils with Epsom salt and add to bath water

Monthly Hormone Support Inhaler:

* Aromatherapy inhaler stick
* 8 drops of sage
* 6 drops of bergamot
* 4 drops of frankincense

Remember to adjust the number of drops based on the size of the mixture you are making and your personal preference. These blends are designed to provide a starting point that you can customize to suit your needs. Always conduct a patch test before applying any new mixture to a larger area, and consult a health care professional if you have a specific health concern or condition. Also, remember that essential oils can have powerful effects, so it's important to use them in moderation and dilute them appropriately.

Here are some application techniques for replenishing essential oil combinations and balancing testosterone levels:

1. Testosterone Support Massage Blend:

* 1 oz (30 ml) carrier oil (such as jojoba or sweet almond)

* 8 drops of ginger
* 6 drops of sage
* 4 drops of rosemary
* 3 drops of ylang-ylang
* Mix essential oils with a carrier oil for a relaxing massage. Suitable for areas such as the lower abdomen, lower back, and inner thighs.

2. Hormone Balancing Diffuser Blend:

* Essential oil diffuser
* 3 drops of frankincense
* 3 drops of cedarwood
* 2 drops of bergamot
* Diffuse this blend into your living space for a calming and hormone-balancing scent.

3. Daily Hormone Support Roll-On:

* 10ml roller bottle
* 8 drops of geranium
* 6 drops of sage
* 4 drops of lavender
* 2 drops of rosemary
* Add a carrier oil and apply to pulse points like wrists and neck for hormonal support.

4. Relaxing Hormone Balancing Bath Blend:

* 1 cup Epsom salt
* 6 drops of ylang-ylang
* 4 drops of bergamot
* 3 drops of sandalwood
* Mix essential oils with Epsom salts and add to a warm bath to relax.

5. Hormone Balancing Inhaler:

* Aromatherapy inhaler stick
* 6 drops of sage
* 4 drops of frankincense
* 4 drops of bergamot
* Breathe from the inhaler as needed throughout the day for mood support and hormonal balance.

Remember, everyone's body reacts differently to essential oils, so it's important to start with a patch test and observe any reactions. Additionally, consistent use over time is key to experiencing the potential benefits. If you have any underlying health conditions or concerns about hormone balance, it is recommended that you consult a healthcare professional before incorporating essential oils into your daily routine.

E. Lifestyle Factors for Hormonal Balance

Lifestyle factors play an important role in maintaining hormonal balance, including testosterone levels. Here are some strategies to help maintain hormonal balance:

1. Diet and nutrition:

* BALANCED DIET: Eat a balanced diet rich in whole foods, including lean protein, healthy fats, complex carbohydrates, and a variety of fruits and vegetables.
* Nutrient-rich foods: Certain nutrients, such as zinc, vitamin D, and omega-3 fatty acids, are associated with healthy testosterone levels. Include foods such as seafood, eggs, nuts, seeds, and green leafy vegetables.
* Limit sugar and processed foods: Excessive sugar intake and processed foods can lead to insulin resistance and hormone imbalances.

2. Physical activity:

* Exercise regularly: Regularly exercise, including resistance training and cardiovascular exercise. Exercise can help maintain a healthy weight and improve hormonal regulation.
* Strength training: Resistance training, especially compound exercises like squats and deadlifts, can increase testosterone levels.

3. Stress management:

* Reduce stress: Chronic stress can cause elevated cortisol levels, affecting hormonal balance. Practice stress-reduction techniques such as deep breathing, meditation, yoga, and mindfulness.

4. Sleep quality:

* Prioritize sleep: Aim for 7 to 9 hours of quality sleep every night. Sleep is essential for the production and regulation of hormones, including testosterone.

5. Healthy living habits:

* Limit alcohol consumption: Excessive alcohol consumption can hurt hormonal balance. Moderate drinking is recommended.
* Avoid smoking: Smoking is associated with reduced testosterone levels. Quitting smoking can have a positive impact on hormonal health.
* Maintain a healthy weight: Obesity and underweight can disrupt hormonal balance. Aim for a healthy weight range.

6. Environmental toxins:

* Reduce Exposure: Minimize exposure to endocrine-disrupting chemicals found in plastics, pesticides, and personal care products.

7. Hydration:

* Stay hydrated: Drink enough daily water to support overall body functions, including hormone regulation.

8. Mindfulness and relaxation:

* Practice relaxation: Practice relaxation exercises such as deep breathing, meditation, and time in nature to lower stress levels.

9. Avoid overtraining:

* Balance exercise: Overtraining and overexercising can cause stress hormones to rise and affect testosterone. Balance vigorous exercise with adequate rest and recovery.

10. Professional guidance:

* Speak to a professional: If you suspect a hormonal imbalance, work with a healthcare professional, such as an endocrinologist or registered dietitian, to develop a personalized plan.

Remember, maintaining hormonal balance is a holistic approach that involves many aspects of your lifestyle. Using these strategies consistently over time can support overall health and hormonal health. If you are considering making major changes to your lifestyle, it is recommended that you consult with a healthcare professional to ensure they are appropriate for your personal needs and health condition.

Of course, addressing these issues in the context of maintaining hormonal balance, including testosterone levels, is critical to men's health and well-being:

Nutrition:

* Balanced diet: Eat a diet rich in whole foods, including lean protein, healthy fats, complex carbohydrates, and a variety of fruits and vegetables.
* Essential nutrients: Prioritize foods rich in zinc, vitamin D, omega-3 fatty acids, and antioxidants, as these nutrients are associated with hormonal balance.
* Limit sugar and processed foods: High sugar intake and processed foods can lead to insulin resistance and affect hormone regulation.

Exercise:

* Strength training: Perform strength training exercises regularly as they increase testosterone levels. Focus on compound movements like squats, deadlifts, and bench presses.
* Cardiovascular exercise: Includes cardiovascular activities to support overall health and maintain a healthy weight.
* Moderateness: Avoid excessive exercise, which may cause elevated cortisol levels and affect hormonal balance.

Stress management:

* Reduce stress: Practice stress management techniques such as deep breathing, meditation, yoga, and mindfulness to lower cortisol levels and support hormonal balance.
* Prioritize relaxation: Create a regular relaxation routine to counteract the effects of chronic stress.

Sleep hygiene:

* Consistent sleep schedule: Maintain a regular sleep schedule by going to bed and waking up at the same time every day.
* Sleeping environment: Ensure a comfortable sleeping environment

in a dark, quiet, and cool room.

* Limit screen time: Avoid using electronic devices before bed, as blue light disrupts sleep hormones.

Hydration:

* Adequate fluid intake: Stay hydrated throughout the day, as dehydration can affect hormone regulation.

Mindfulness and happiness:

* Mindful eating: Practice mindful eating to improve digestion and support overall health.
* Mental Health: Prioritize mental health through activities you enjoy, social connections, and seeking professional help when needed.

Alcohol and smoking:

* Alcohol consumption in moderation: Limit alcohol consumption as excessive drinking can affect hormone levels.
* Quit smoking: If you smoke, consider quitting because smoking disrupts the hormonal balance.

Professional guidance:

* Consult a healthcare professional: If you suspect a hormone imbalance or have a health problem, consult an endocrinologist or registered dietitian for personalized guidance.

Remember, consistency is key when implementing lifestyle changes. Focus on incremental improvements and a balanced approach in each area. It's important to consult a healthcare professional before making major changes to your lifestyle, especially if you have an existing health condition or are taking medications. They can provide personalized guidance and ensure that any changes are tailored to your needs.

F. Stress Reduction and Testosterone

The relationship between stress and testosterone levels is complex and bidirectional. Stress can significantly impact testosterone levels, and testosterone levels can influence the body's response to stress. Here is an overview of this relationship:

Effects of stress on testosterone:

* Cortisol release: When the body is under stress, it releases the hormone cortisol. High levels of cortisol interfere with testosterone production and signaling.
* Hypothalamic-pituitary-testicular axis: Chronic stress can disrupt the normal function of the hypothalamic-pituitary-testicular axis that controls testosterone production.
* Reduced testosterone production: Chronic stress can cause reduced testosterone production in the testicles, potentially leading to imbalances and related health problems.

Effects of testosterone on stress response:

* Stress resilience: Adequate testosterone levels are associated with improved stress resilience and coping with challenging situations.
* Mood regulation: Testosterone plays a role in regulating mood and emotion. Low testosterone levels can lead to mood disorders and increased stress.
* Feedback loop: Testosterone can influence the body's response to stress by regulating the release of stress hormones such as cortisol.

Manage stress to support testosterone:

* Stress reduction tips: Engaging in stress-reduction techniques such as meditation, deep breathing, and yoga can help lower cortisol levels and support testosterone balance.
* Exercise regularly: Exercise can reduce stress and boost testosterone production but overdoing it without proper recovery can have the opposite effect.
* Get enough sleep: Prioritize quality sleep, as insufficient sleep can increase stress and disrupt hormonal balance.
* Balanced diet: Eat a balanced diet rich in nutrients that support hormone regulation.
* Social support: Maintaining strong social connections can provide emotional support and help buffer the effects of stress.

Chronic stress and long-term effects:

Chronic stress, if not managed, can negatively affect overall health, including hormonal balance. Chronically elevated cortisol levels can lead to a variety of health problems, including inflammation, immune system dysfunction, and metabolic imbalances.

Personal changes:

It's important to note that individuals may respond differently to stress and changes in testosterone levels. Some people may be more sensitive to stress, while others may maintain testosterone levels better under stress.

Consult a health care professional:

If you are concerned about the effects of stress on testosterone levels or are experiencing symptoms of a hormonal imbalance, it is recommended that you consult a healthcare professional. An endocrinologist or healthcare provider can evaluate your hormone levels, discuss your stress management strategies, and provide personalized recommendations.

Remember: A holistic approach to stress management and overall health is essential to maintaining healthy testosterone levels and promoting overall health.

G. Support Sleep and Promote Hormonal Health

Sleep and hormonal balance, including testosterone production, are closely related. The quality and quantity of sleep play an important role in maintaining healthy hormone levels, including testosterone. Here's how sleep and hormonal balance are related:

Testosterone production and sleep:

* During sleep: Testosterone is primarily produced during the body's deep sleep stages, specifically during rapid-eye movement (REM) and slow-wave sleep. These stages, including hormone regulation, are critical to the body's recovery process.
* Circadian rhythm: Testosterone production follows a circadian rhythm, with the highest levels produced in the early morning. Disturbed sleep patterns, such as an irregular sleep schedule or insufficient sleep, can disrupt this rhythm and affect testosterone production.
* Sleep duration: Chronic sleep deprivation or poor sleep quality can cause testosterone levels to drop. Research shows that even a few

nights of sleep deprivation can cause testosterone levels to drop.

Effects of sleep disorders:

* Sleep apnea: Sleep apnea is a disorder characterized by interruptions in breathing during sleep and is associated with reduced testosterone levels. Repeated hypoxia and sleep disruption can negatively impact hormone production.
* Insomnia: Chronic insomnia can lead to hormonal imbalances, including disruption of testosterone production. Difficulty sleeping is associated with higher cortisol levels, affecting hormone regulation.

Bidirectional relationship:

The relationship between sleep and hormonal balance is a two-way street. While sleep affects hormone production, hormonal imbalances can also affect sleep quality and patterns. For example:
* Low testosterone and sleep disorders: Low testosterone levels are associated with sleep disorders, such as difficulty falling asleep, staying asleep, or having a restful sleep.
* Hormonal imbalances and insomnia: Hormone imbalances, including disruptions in cortisol and melatonin levels, can lead to insomnia and difficulty sleeping.

Optimize sleep to balance hormones:

* A consistent sleep schedule: Maintaining a regular sleep schedule helps regulate circadian rhythms, which supports hormone production and balance.
* Sleep hygiene: Adopting healthy sleep hygiene habits, such as establishing a relaxing bedtime, minimizing screen time before bed, and maintaining a comfortable sleep environment, can improve sleep quality.
* Adequate sleep time: Prioritize 7 to 9 hours of quality sleep each night to support hormonal balance and overall health.
* Manage sleep disorders: If you suspect a sleep disorder, such as sleep apnea or insomnia, seek medical care and treatment.

Consulting and management:

If you are experiencing symptoms of a hormonal imbalance, such as changes in mood or energy levels, and suspect this may be related to disrupted sleep, it is recommended that you consult a healthcare professional. A medical provider can evaluate your hormone levels, sleep patterns, and overall health to provide appropriate guidance and treatment options.

Sleep and hormonal balance, including testosterone production, are intricately linked. Maintaining optimal hormone levels and overall health is crucial to prioritizing healthy sleep habits.

Using essential oils to support quality sleep and improve hormonal regulation can be a helpful and natural approach. Here are some tips and techniques for using essential oils for this purpose:

1. Evening aromatherapy ritual:

Create a calming evening routine that incorporates essential oils to signal sleep. Consider the following approaches:
* Diffuse: Diffuse calming oils like lavender, chamomile, and bergamot in your bedroom 30 minutes to an hour before bed.
* Topical application: Dilute a sleep-inducing essential oil, such as lavender or cedarwood, in a carrier oil and apply it to your feet' pulse points or soles.

2. Bath before going to bed:

Enjoy a relaxing bath infused with sleep-inducing essential oils:
* Bath salts: Add a few drops of lavender, chamomile, or sandalwood essential oil to Epsom salts and add to your bath water.
* Bath oil: Mix essential oils with carrier oil and add a few drops to your bath.

3. Pillow and linen spray:

Use homemade pillows or linen spray to create a peaceful atmosphere in your bedroom:
* DIY spray: Mix distilled water and a few drops of your choice of essential oil in a spray bottle. Spray pillows and bedding before bed.

4. Relaxation techniques:

Combine essential oils with relaxation techniques to enhance their effectiveness:
* Deep breathing: Inhale calming essential oils while practicing deep breathing. This combination triggers the body's relaxation response.

* Meditation: Use essential oils during meditation to promote mental peace and mindfulness.

5. Night massage:

Enjoy a gentle massage before bed using essential oils known for their calming properties:
* Carrier oil blend: Blend sleep-inducing essential oils with a carrier oil like jojoba or sweet almond oil. Massage your neck, shoulders, and back with this mixture.

6. Personal inhaler:

Create a personal inhaler with your favorite sleep-inducing essential oils. Inhale the aroma whenever you need to relax or unwind.

7. Aromatherapy diffuser jewelry:

Wear diffuser jewelry infused with the sleep-supporting essential oil of your choice to experience its benefits throughout the day.

8. Consistency is key:

To support hormonal regulation, maintain a consistent sleep schedule and use essential oils as part of your nightly routine. Repetition helps signal to your body that it's time to wind down.

9. Personal preference:

Try different essential oils to find the one that works best for you. Everyone may respond differently to aromatherapy, so choosing essential oils that resonate with you is important.

10. Professional consultation:

If you are dealing with specific sleep or hormonal issues, consider consulting a healthcare professional, such as a doctor or aromatherapist, for personalized guidance and advice.

Remember safety:

* Please dilute essential oils appropriately before applying them to

your skin.
    * Perform a patch test to check for any adverse reactions.
    * Avoid using oils that may irritate or cause sensitivity before bed.
    * Follow safety guidelines for using essential oils, especially if you have allergies, skin sensitivities, or underlying health conditions.

Incorporating essential oils into your sleep routine can be a great way to support hormonal regulation and improve sleep quality naturally. Experiment with different methods and blends to find what works best for you and promotes a restful night's sleep.

H. Healthy Lifestyle Habits for Testosterone

Supporting testosterone balance goes hand in hand with maintaining a healthy lifestyle. Here are some additional healthy habits that can help maintain optimal testosterone levels:

1. Maintain a healthy weight:

Being overweight or underweight can disrupt hormonal balance, including testosterone levels, so aim for a balanced diet and regular physical activity to achieve and maintain a healthy weight.

2. Balanced diet:

Eat a diet rich in nutrients that support hormonal health:
    * Includes lean protein, healthy fats, and a variety of fruits and vegetables.
    Include foods rich in zinc (such as nuts, seeds, and lean meats) and vitamin D (fatty fish, fortified dairy products, and sun exposure).

3. Limit alcohol consumption:

Excessive drinking can disrupt hormonal balance and affect testosterone levels. Aim for moderate drinking or consider eliminating it.

4. Manage stress:

Chronic stress can cause elevated cortisol levels, which can negatively impact testosterone. Practice stress-reduction techniques such as meditation, yoga, deep breathing, and mindfulness.

5. Exercise regularly:

Regular physical activity, especially resistance training and high-intensity interval training, can increase testosterone levels. Be sure to incorporate cardiovascular and strength training exercises into your workout routine.

6. Quality sleep:

As mentioned before, prioritize quality sleep by maintaining a consistent sleep schedule, creating a comfortable sleep environment, and incorporating relaxation techniques and essential oils.

7. Hydration:

Drink plenty of water throughout the day to stay well hydrated. Proper hydration supports overall health and may indirectly affect hormonal balance.

8. Avoid excessive sugar intake:

High sugar consumption can lead to insulin resistance, which may negatively impact testosterone levels. Minimize your intake of sugary foods and drinks.

9. Manage chronic health conditions:

If you have underlying health conditions such as diabetes or thyroid disease, work with your healthcare provider to manage them effectively, as these conditions can affect hormonal balance.

10. Avoid endocrine disruptors:

Limit exposure to endocrine-disrupting chemicals found in some plastics, pesticides, and household products. Choose natural cleaning and personal care products whenever possible.

11. Maintain hygiene and avoid toxins:

Be cautious about using personal care products that contain harmful chemicals like parabens and phthalates. Choose natural alternatives to reduce toxin exposure.

12. Regular inspection:

Schedule regular physical exams to monitor your overall health and hormone levels. Discuss any questions with a healthcare professional.

13. Consult a health care professional:

If you suspect a hormonal imbalance, consult a healthcare provider or endocrinologist for appropriate evaluation and guidance tailored to your specific needs.

Remember: Hormone balance is affected by many factors, and individual needs may vary. Taking a holistic approach to health and wellness by incorporating these healthy lifestyle habits can contribute to overall hormonal balance and well-being. Always consult a healthcare professional before making major changes to your lifestyle or if you have specific health problems.

After this chapter, we summarize the benefits and applications of essential oils in balancing testosterone levels in men. We emphasize the role of essential oils in supporting hormonal balance, promoting overall health, and enhancing vitality. By incorporating essential oils into their lifestyle and developing healthy habits, men can take proactive steps to optimize testosterone levels and improve physical and mental health.

6.2   Support and Sexual Health

In this chapter, we'll explore how essential oils can be used to support men's sexual and sexual health. We discuss factors that may affect sexual performance and provide guidance on using essential oils to enhance and increase sexual arousal and promote overall sexual health.

A. Understand Sexual Health

Sexual health plays an important role in a man's overall well-being and relationships. Here's why they're important:

1. Good health:

Health and sexual function are indicators of overall physical health. and sexual function problems can sometimes be early signs of underlying health problems, such as cardiovascular disease, diabetes, hormonal imbalances, or neurological disorders. Staying healthy encourages men to pay attention to their overall health and seek medical advice when necessary.

2. Emotional health:

A satisfying sex life contributes to emotional well-being. Engaging in sexual activity releases endorphins, known as the " feel good " hormones. These hormones can reduce stress, anxiety, and depression, thereby improving mood and emotional resilience.

3. Relationship satisfaction:

Sexual intimacy is an important part of a romantic relationship. A fulfilling sex life can strengthen the emotional bond between partners, promote intimacy, and increase overall relationship satisfaction. Open communication about and preferences is critical to cultivating healthy and fulfilling relationships.

4. Self-esteem and confidence:

Being healthy and sexually confident can positively impact a man's self-esteem and body image. Feeling desired and experiencing sexual success can boost self-confidence and self-worth.

5. Stress reduction:

Sexual activity is associated with stress reduction. Engaging in sexual activity can help lower stress hormones and induce relaxation, leading to a calmer mind.

6. Hormone balance:

Healthy usually indicates balanced hormone levels, including testosterone. Hormonal imbalances can affect not only sexual health but also energy levels, mood, and physical vitality.

7. Quality of life:

A satisfying sex life contributes to overall well-being and quality of life. It enhances vitality, energy, and enjoyment of daily activities.

8. Age-related changes:

As men age, sexual function may change due to factors such as hormonal changes, stress, and health conditions. As men age, taking a proactive approach to these changes can lead to a better quality of life.

9. Communication:

Discussing sexual health and preferences with your partner can promote open communication and understanding. This can lead to a more fulfilling and satisfying sexual experience for both parties.

10. Holistic approach:

Men's well-being includes physical, emotional, and interpersonal aspects. Including sexual health and wellness as part of an overall well-being strategy can lead to a more rounded and fulfilling life.

Overall, staying healthy and resolving any issues related to sexual health is vital to a man's overall well-being, happiness, and the health of his relationships. Open communication, living a healthy lifestyle, and seeking medical advice, when needed, are key components of supportive health.

Several factors can affect a man's sexual performance. It is important to realize that sexual health is affected by a combination of physical, psychological, and lifestyle factors. Here are some key factors that may affect sexual performance:

1. Hormonal changes:

Testosterone is an important hormone for male sexual health. As men age, testosterone levels naturally decline, which can lead to a decrease in erectile function. Hormone imbalances or medical conditions that affect hormone production can also affect sexual health.

2. Stress and anxiety:

Stress and anxiety are common factors in sexual problems. High levels of stress can lead to decline and difficulty maintaining an erection. Performance anxiety, fear of failure, and concerns about sexual performance can also affect sexual confidence and enjoyment.

3. Relationship dynamics:

The quality of a relationship affects performance and performance. Relationship problems, lack of emotional intimacy, or unresolved conflicts can lead to decreased sexual satisfaction. On the other hand, healthy communication and emotional connection can enhance sexual health.

4. Health status:

Certain health conditions, such as diabetes, cardiovascular disease, obesity, and neurological disorders, can affect blood flow, nerve function, and hormonal balance, affecting sexual health. Medications used to treat these conditions may also have side effects that affect sexual function.

5. Lifestyle factors:

Unhealthy lifestyle habits such as excessive drinking, smoking, and drug use can hurt sexual health. A sedentary lifestyle and poor dietary choices can lead to obesity and other health problems that affect sexual performance.

6. Mental health:

Depression, anxiety, and other mental health disorders can lead to decreased sexual enjoyment. Antidepressant medications may also have side effects that affect sexual function.

7. Fatigue and sleep disorders:

Lack of sleep and chronic fatigue can lead to decreased energy levels and reduced interest in sexual activity. Sleep disorders such as sleep apnea can disrupt hormonal balance and lead to sexual problems.

8. Body image and self-esteem:

Negative body image and low self-esteem can affect sexual confidence. Feeling insecure about one's body can lead to reluctance to engage in sexual activity.

9. Pornographic uses:

Excessive consumption of pornography may lead to unrealistic expectations about sexual performance, which may affect real-life sexual experiences.

10. Aging:

As men age, sexual function may change due to factors such as hormonal changes, reduced blood flow, and changes in sensitivity.

11. Culture and religious beliefs:

Cultural or religious beliefs about sex can influence a person's attitudes toward sexual activity. These beliefs can influence feelings of guilt or shame associated with sexual experiences.

12. Communication and intimacy:

A lack of communication with your partner about your preferences and concerns can lead to misunderstandings and unsatisfactory sexual experiences.

Solving and manifesting problems often requires a comprehensive approach considering physical health, mental health, relationship dynamics, and lifestyle habits. Consulting a healthcare professional, such as a doctor or therapist, can provide guidance and support in resolving these issues and improving overall sexual health and satisfaction.

B. Enhanced Essential Oils

Of course, essential oils are believed to have aphrodisiac properties and may help enhance and. Here are some essential oils known for their potential aphrodisiac properties:

1. Ylang-ylang: Ylang-ylang is often used for its sensual and exotic aroma. It is thought to help reduce anxiety and promote relaxation, contributing to a more receptive state of mind in intimate relationships.

2. Sage: Sage has a calming and euphoric scent that may help relieve stress and anxiety, creating a more relaxing environment for intimacy.

3. Cinnamon: Cinnamon stimulates blood flow and circulation, helping to enhance sensation. Its warm and spicy fragrance may also evoke feelings of comfort and sensuality.

4. Sandalwood: Sandalwood has a rich, woody aroma that is both grounding and calming. It is often used to promote relaxation and emotional balance, creating a conducive atmosphere for intimacy.

5. Patchouli: The earthy and musky scent of patchouli is thought to affect mood fundamentally. It is thought to help relieve anxiety and stress and foster a more receptive mood.

6. Rose: Rose essential oil is associated with romance and love. Its floral and sweet aroma is thought to have uplifting and aphrodisiac properties, making it a popular choice for enhancing intimacy.

7. Jasmine: Often called the " King of Flowers, " Jasmine is known for its sexy fragrance. Its sweet and floral aroma is thought to help increase feelings of desire and passion.

8. Ginger: Ginger essential oil is believed to have warming properties that can stimulate blood flow and circulation, potentially enhancing body sensations.

It's important to note that the effects of essential oils may vary from person to person, and the benefits of aromatherapy largely depend on personal preference and experience. Additionally, while these essential oils have been linked to aphrodisiac properties, their effects on health and wellness have not been scientifically proven and may be more related to the psychological and sensory effects of aromatherapy.

When using essential oils to enhance intimacy, consider personal sensitivities, preferences, and any potential allergies. Dilution and proper application methods are critical to ensure a safe and positive experience. As with any health-related matter, it's best to consult a qualified healthcare professional before using essential oils for aphrodisiacs, especially if you have an underlying medical condition or are taking medications.

The potential effects of essential oils on stimulating the senses, increasing blood flow, and promoting healthy sexual responses are primarily based on their aromatic and physiological properties. While these effects are not universally guaranteed, some essential oils are believed to have qualities that may lead to these results:

1. Aroma stimulation: Essential oils have unique aromas that can evoke memories, emotions, and feelings. Scents stimulate the limbic system,

which is involved in emotions and memory. Stimulating scents can create a relaxed and accepting state of mind, helping to set the mood for intimacy.

2. Relax and reduce anxiety: Many essential oils, including those with aphrodisiac properties, have calming and relaxing effects. By reducing anxiety and stress, these oils can create a more comfortable and open environment for intimacy.

3. Improve blood circulation: Some essential oils, such as cinnamon, ginger, and rose, are thought to have vasodilatory properties, meaning they may help dilate blood vessels and improve blood circulation. This effect may enhance physical sensations.

4. Emotional connection: The use of essential oils promotes a sense of ritual and mindfulness. Creating a calm and inviting atmosphere with soothing scents can promote an emotional connection between partners.

5. Sensory stimulation: Essential oils can stimulate the senses through their unique aroma and texture. Adding essential oils to a massage or sensual experience can enhance touch and heighten pleasure.

6. Mind-body connection: The mind-body connection plays an important role in sexual response. Scents can affect emotional states, which in turn can affect physical reactions. Essential oils can indirectly promote a healthy sexual response by promoting relaxation and positive emotions.

It's important to use essential oils to enhance your sexual experience and understand that individual reactions may vary. What works for one person may not work for another. When incorporating essential oils into intimate moments, it's crucial to communicate with your partner about preferences and sensitivities.

Proper dilution and appropriate application methods are crucial when using essential oils for this purpose. It is recommended to perform a patch test on a small area of the skin to check for any allergic reactions or sensitivities before applying the oil more widely. As always, it is recommended that you consult a healthcare professional, especially if you have any underlying health conditions or concerns.

C. Sensual Massage and Aromatherapy

The use of essential oils in sensual massage and aromatherapy can enhance intimacy and sexual pleasure by creating a sensual and relaxing atmosphere, stimulating the senses, and promoting emotional and physical connection. Here are some ways you can incorporate essential oils into these experiences:

1. Sensual massage:

Sensual massage involves using touch, scent, and relaxation techniques to create heightened intimacy. Essential oils can be mixed into massage oil to enhance the experience. The specific operation method is as follows:

* Choose a carrier oil: Start by choosing a carrier oil, such as jojoba, coconut, almond, or grapeseed oil. These oils provide lubrication to the massage and help spread the oil evenly on the skin.

* Choose essential oils: Choose essential oils known for their aphrodisiac or sensual properties. Some options include ylang-ylang, sage, jasmine, rose, and sandalwood.

* Create the massage oil mixture: Add a few drops of your chosen essential oil to a carrier oil. A typical dilution ratio is 1 to 2% essential oil to carrier oil for sensual massage. This means that for every teaspoon (5 ml) of carrier oil, add 3 to 6 drops of essential oil.

* Patch test: Before using the mixture on a larger area, conduct a patch test on a small area of skin to check for any adverse reactions or sensitivities.

* Heating oil: Place the bottle in warm water and gently heat the massage oil mixture. Test the temperature on the inside of your wrist to make sure your partner is comfortable.

* Massage Technique: Use slow, deliberate movements and varying pressure to provide a relaxing and sensual experience. Focus on areas such as shoulders, neck, back, and feet.

2. Intimate aromatherapy:

Aromatherapy involves diffusing essential oils into the air to create the desired atmosphere and mood. Here are ways to use aromatherapy to enhance your intimacy:

* Choose an essential oil diffuser: Choose an aromatherapy diffuser that suits your preferences. Ultrasonic diffusers are popular and disperse essential oils in a fine mist.

* Choose essential oils: Choose essential oils that have aphrodisiac, soothing, or relaxing properties. Create a blend that you and your partner both find attractive.

* Diffusion technology: Diffuse the essential oil blend into rooms where you plan to spend intimate time together. Start diffusing for a while before interacting to establish the desired ambiance.

* Create a relaxing atmosphere: Dim the lights, light candles, and play soft music to prepare for a relaxing and intimate experience.

Important notes:

* Always make sure you and your partner are not allergic to or irritable to the essential oils you choose. Do a patch test and use an oil that is safe for topical use.

* Communicate openly with your partner about their preferences and any sensitivities they must scent or touch.

* Remember, the goal is to create a comfortable and enjoyable experience for both parties. Consent, respect, and clear communication are key.

* Essential oils are effective and should be used in moderation. Avoid applying essential oils directly to sensitive areas.

* If you or your partner have any medical conditions or are pregnant, please consult a healthcare professional before using essential oils for sensory purposes.

Essential oils should be used with caution and with each partner's comfort in mind when using them in an intimate setting. It's about strengthening the connection and enjoyment between partners while ensuring safety and respect.

Creating a sensory experience with essential oils involves choosing the right oil, using the appropriate dilution ratio, and using gentle and intimate massage techniques. The specific operation method is as follows:

Choose the right oil:

* Aphrodisiac oils: Choose essential oils known for their aphrodisiac properties, such as ylang-ylang, sage, jasmine, rose, sandalwood, and patchouli.

* Sexy scent: Choose an oil with an alluring, alluring scent that appeals to you and your partner's liking.

* Personal preference: Make sure you and your partner both enjoy the scent of your chosen oil, as scents are highly personal.

Dilution ratio:

* For sensual massage, use a 1 to 2% dilution ratio of essential oil to carrier oil. This means adding about 3 to 6 drops of essential oil per teaspoon (5 ml) of carrier oil.

Massage techniques:

1. Gentle: Use your palms with long, sweeping strokes to spread the oil evenly and create a relaxing feeling.

2. Petrification: Gently knead and squeeze the muscles with your fingertips and palms. This helps release tension and increases relaxation.

3. Circular Strokes: Use your fingers, thumb, or palm in circular motions to target specific areas. This is especially sensual on the back and shoulders.

4. Feathering: Use your fingertips to glide across the skin gently with soft, feathery strokes. This can create a subtle and pleasant feeling.

5. Pressure points: Gently explore pressure points, such as those on your neck, shoulders, and back. Apply gentle pressure and hold for a few seconds to increase relaxation.

Create experiences:

* Set the mood: Dim the lights, play soothing music, and consider using candles for soft lighting.

* Warmth: Make sure the room is comfortable and warm. You can also warm the massage oil slightly by placing the bottle in warm water.

* Communicate: Continuously communicate with your partner about their comfort levels and preferences. Ask for feedback and adjust your technique accordingly.

* Relaxation: Focus on creating a relaxing environment where you and your partner can both relax and enjoy the experience.

Important notes:

* Always perform a patch test to check for any sensitivities or allergies to your chosen essential oil.

* Avoid using essential oils directly on sensitive areas or mucous membranes.

* Pay attention to your partner's comfort level and any feedback they provide during the massage.

* If you are new to massage, consider researching or taking a basic massage class to learn effective techniques.

* Consent and clear communication are crucial. Always prioritize your partner's comfort and boundaries.

* Enjoy the experience and focus on connecting with your partner meaningfully and emotionally.

Creating a sensual experience with essential oils can enhance your connection with your partner and create an unforgettable and intimate moment. Everyone's preferences are unique, so feel free to explore different oils, techniques, and methods to find the ones that work best for you and your partner.

D. Create Sexy Mixtures

Here are some personalized sensory blends using essential oils that can be used for massage, aromatherapy, or to enhance intimacy:

Sexy Massage Oil:

Element:
* 1 tablespoon carrier oil (such as sweet almond, jojoba, or coconut oil)
* 4 drops of ylang-ylang essential oil
* 3 drops of sandalwood essential oil
* 2 drops of jasmine essential oil

Guide:
1. In a small glass bottle, combine the carrier oil and the designated number of drops of each essential oil.
2. Close the bottle and shake gently to mix the oil.
3. Before use, conduct a patch test on a small skin area to ensure no allergic reaction.
4. When ready to use, warm a small amount of the mixture with your hands and gently massage it into your partner's skin.

Sensory Aromatherapy Diffuser Blend:

Element:
* 3 drops of sage essential oil
* 3 drops of bergamot essential oil
* 2 drops of patchouli essential oil

Guide:
1. Drop the specified amount of each essential oil into your aromatherapy diffuser.
2. Fill the diffuser with water according to the manufacturer's instructions.
3. Turn on the diffuser and enjoy the sensual aroma that fills the room.

Intimate Atmosphere Spray:

Element:
* 1 oz (30 ml) distilled water
* 2 ~ 3 drops of ylang-ylang essential oil
* 2 ~ 3 drops of rose essential oil
* 1 drop vanilla essential oil (sweetness optional)

Guide:

1. In a small spray bottle, add the specified amount of each essential oil.

2. Fill the rest of the bottle with distilled water and close the cap.

3. Shake well before each use.

4. Spray a fine mist around the room or on the sheets to create a romantic atmosphere.

Remember, choosing oils that resonate with you and your partner's preferences is the key to creating a personalized blend. Feel free to adjust the number of drops or oil combinations to create a scent that you both find appealing and alluring. As with any new blend, it's best to do a patch test to make sure there are no sensitivities or allergies to the oils used. Enjoy the sensory experience and intimacy that essential oils can enhance.

Essential oils to create alluring and sensual blends require balanced fragrance and the right dilution ratios. Here are some mixing techniques, combinations, and applications to enhance your sexual experience:

Mixing ratio:
* For massage oils and body blends, a common dilution ratio is about 1 to 2% essential oil to carrier oil (about 10 to 20 drops of essential oil per 1 ounce of carrier oil).
* For a diffuser blend, start with a total of 5 to 10 drops of essential oil in the diffuser.

Tempting essential oil combinations:
1. Ylang-Ylang, patchouli, jasmine: A classic combination known for its sexy and floral fragrance.
2. Sandalwood, rose, bergamot: The earthy scent of sandalwood combines with the romantic aroma of rose and the uplifting aroma of bergamot.
3. Sage, orange blossom, frankincense: A blend that combines the relaxing properties of sage with the exotic and calming scent of orange blossom and the spiritual depth of frankincense.
4. Cinnamon, vanilla, cardamom: A warm and spicy combination that creates a cozy and inviting atmosphere.

Instructions:
1. Massage oil: Dilute the essential oil of your choice in a carrier oil for sensual massage. Focus on areas with more muscle and tissue, such as the back, neck, and shoulders.
2. Aromatherapy diffuser: Create an intimate atmosphere by diffusing a sensual blend in the bedroom before or during intimate moments.

3. Sexy bath: Add a few drops of essential oil of your choice to a warm bath for a relaxing and romantic soak.

4. Sensual atmosphere spray: Use distilled water and essential oils to make a spray. Spray the mixture on sheets, pillows, or around the room to create a charming ambiance.

5. Sexy massage candle: Make your massage candle using soy wax and your favorite essential oils. While the candle melts, warm oil can be used for massage.

Patch test:
Before using any new mixture, a patch test must be performed on a small area of the skin to check for allergies or sensitivities.

Communicate:
Always have open communication with your partner about the scents and blends you plan to use. Everyone's preferences are unique, so make sure the scents you choose are mutually enjoyable.

Safety measures:
* Never apply undiluted essential oils directly to the skin.
* Choose high-quality, pure essential oils from reputable sources.
* Pregnant women, people with certain medical conditions, or people taking certain medications should consult a healthcare professional before using essential oils, especially for intimate purposes.

Remember, sensual and intimate experiences are personal and should be treated with sensitivity and respect for both parties' comfort levels. Experiment with different mixes and techniques to find what works best for you and your partner, creating a space of connection and intimacy.

E. Emotional Connection and Intimacy

Essential oils can play an important role in promoting emotional connection and intimacy between partners. Their aromatic and therapeutic properties can enhance the overall sensory experience, deepen emotional bonds, and create a nurturing environment for intimacy. Here's how essential oils promote emotional connection and intimacy:

1. Aromatherapy and mood enhancement: Certain essential oils can enhance mood, reduce stress, and create a relaxing atmosphere. Emotionally connecting and cultivating intimacy becomes easier when both parties have a

calm and positive frame of mind.

2. Shared sensory experience: Scent can evoke memories, emotions, and feelings. By using essential oils that resonate with positive memories or emotions, couples can create a shared sensory experience that deepens their emotional connection.

3. Reduce stress: Stress and anxiety can hinder emotional connection. Essential oils like lavender, bergamot, and chamomile have calming properties that can help reduce stress and create a peaceful environment in which emotional intimacy can thrive.

4. Aphrodisiac properties: Certain essential oils are considered aphrodisiacs because of their ability to stimulate the senses and heighten feelings of desire. Oils such as ylang-ylang, sage, and jasmine are traditionally associated with sensual and romantic experiences.

5. Physical contact and massage: Giving or receiving a massage using essential oils promotes physical intimacy and relaxation. Touch, combined with the aroma of the oil, can deepen the emotional connection between partners.

6. Open communication: The process of selecting and blending essential oils encourages open communication between partners. Discussing preferences, choosing scents together, and applying essential oils can foster understanding and connection.

7. Creation ritual: Creating rituals that involve essential oils, such as preparing a relaxing bath together, diffusing oils during shared moments, or applying them before bed, can create a sense of routine and anticipation that enhances intimacy.

8. Mindfulness and presence: Aromatherapy can promote mindfulness and living in the present moment. When partners are fully engaged and present to each other, it enhances emotional connection and intimacy.

9. Enhance sensuality: Essential oils heighten the senses, making touch, taste, and smell more vivid. This heightened sensory experience facilitates deeper senses and connections.

10. Personalize the experience: Selecting and blending essential oils can be a personal and intimate activity. Tailoring the blend to each partner's

preferences and creating a unique experience can help strengthen emotional bonds.

It's important to remember that everyone's preferences and sensitivities are different, so communication and consent are key when using essential oils to enhance emotional connection and intimacy. Creating a safe, comfortable, and respectful space is essential for both parties to enjoy and benefit from the aromatic experience fully.

Of course, several essential oils are known for reducing stress, creating a romantic atmosphere, and enhancing the connection between partners. These oils can help set the mood, evoke positive emotions, promote relaxation, and ultimately help create a deeper connection between partners. Here are some essential oils that are particularly effective for these purposes:

1. Lavender: Lavender is known for its calming and relaxing properties. It can help reduce stress and anxiety and create an atmosphere of peace and tranquility. Its soft floral scent is often associated with comfort and tranquility.

2. Ylang-Ylang: Ylang-ylang is considered an aphrodisiac oil that stimulates sensuality and promotes feelings of warmth and connection. Its sweet, exotic scent is often used to create a romantic atmosphere.

3. Bergamot: Bergamot has a fresh and uplifting aroma that can help relieve stress and anxiety. It creates a cheerful atmosphere, making it ideal for enhancing romantic settings.

4. Jasmine: Jasmine is known for its alluring and sexy fragrance. It can evoke feelings of intimacy and romance and is often used to create passionate moods.

5. Rose: Rose essential oil is associated with love and beauty. Its sweet and floral scent can help create an atmosphere of love and affection, making it a popular choice for romantic occasions.

6. Sandalwood: Sandalwood has a warm, woody aroma that promotes relaxation and a sense of grounding. It is often used to create a calm and meditative atmosphere.

7. Patchouli: Patchouli has an earthy and exotic scent and is sometimes considered an aphrodisiac. It can help create a warm and sensual atmosphere.

8. Neroli: Neroli essential oil comes from the flowers of the bitter orange tree. Its sweet floral scent can help reduce anxiety and create a soothing atmosphere.

9. Sage: Sage has sedative and aphrodisiac properties. It can help relieve tension and promote relaxation, making it suitable for enhancing emotional intimacy.

10. Vanilla: The sweet and comforting scent of vanilla is often associated with warmth and comfort. It can evoke feelings of nostalgia and relaxation.

When using essential oils to enhance the connection between partners, consider creating a personalized blend that combines essential oils with complementary scents. For example, a blend of ylang-ylang and bergamot is both relaxing and romantic. A blend of rose and sandalwood promotes love and calm. Try different combinations to find something that resonates with you and your partner.

Remember to use proper dilutions when applying essential oils to your skin, and make sure you are both happy with the oil you choose and its scent. Open communication and consent are key to creating a positive and enjoyable aroma experience for both parties.

F. Solve Sexual Dysfunction

Essential oils can provide support for common sexual problems, such as erectile dysfunction and performance anxiety. However, it is important to note that while essential oils may provide some benefits, they should not be considered a substitute for professional medical advice and treatment. If you or your partner are experiencing sexual problems, it is recommended that you consult a qualified healthcare professional for proper diagnosis and guidance.

Some essential oils are believed to have properties that can help address these issues:

1. Ginger: Ginger is thought to have stimulating properties that may help increase blood circulation, which may be beneficial in resolving erectile dysfunction.

2. Rosemary: Rosemary is thought to have potential circulatory benefits and may help improve blood flow in certain areas.

3. Frankincense: Frankincense is known for its calming and grounding effects, which may help reduce performance anxiety and promote relaxation.

4. Sandalwood: Sandalwood is often used to promote relaxation and reduce stress, which may help manage performance anxiety.

5. Lavender: The relaxing properties of lavender may help relieve anxiety and promote a calm and focused mind.

6. Ylang-ylang: Ylang-ylang is known for its aphrodisiac properties and may help create a sensual and romantic atmosphere.

7. Bergamot: Bergamot's uplifting and mood-enhancing properties help reduce stress and promote positive emotions.

8. Orange blossom: The calming effects of orange blossom may help relieve anxiety and tension and may contribute to a more relaxed state.

When using essential oils to address sexual issues, it's important to treat them with care:

1. Consult a professional: If you or your partner is experiencing ongoing sexual problems, consult a health care professional for an appropriate diagnosis and treatment plan.

2. Patch test: Before using essential oils more extensively, conduct a patch test on a small area of skin to check for any adverse reactions.

3. Proper dilution: Properly dilute essential oils in a carrier oil before applying them to your skin. Dilution helps prevent skin irritation or sensitivity.

4. communicate: Open and respectful communication between partners is crucial. Discuss essential oils' use and potential effects to ensure both parties are comfortable.

5. Personal reaction: Remember that individuals may respond differently to essential oils. What works for one person may not work for another.

6. Holistic approach: Addressing sexual problems often requires a ho-

listic approach that includes lifestyle changes, emotional support, and potentially medication. Essential oils can be part of this approach but shouldn't be the only solution.

7. Use with caution: Avoid applying essential oils to sensitive or intimate areas without proper dilution and professional guidance.

Always prioritize safety and communication when using essential oils in an intimate setting. If sexual problems persist, seeking guidance from a qualified healthcare provider is the best course of action.

While essential oils can be used in complementary ways to support sexual function and confidence, it's important to approach these issues with sensitivity and realize that individual responses may vary. Here are some essential oils and techniques that may help improve sexual function and confidence:

1. Sage: Known for its potential to balance hormones and reduce stress and anxiety, Sage may help create a more relaxed and confident state of mind.

2. Ginger: Ginger's warming and stimulating properties may increase circulation and increase energy, potentially enhancing arousal.

3. Black pepper: Black pepper oil has warming and uplifting qualities that help improve blood flow and energy.

4. Cinnamon: Cinnamon is believed to have aphrodisiac properties and may help increase desire and energy.

5. Patchouli: Patchouli's earthy and exotic aroma is thought to have aphrodisiac properties and promote self-confidence.

6. Bergamot: The uplifting scent of bergamot can help relieve anxiety and lift your mood, leading to a more confident state.

7. Rose: Rose oil is associated with love and sensuality. Its scent may contribute to a romantic atmosphere and increased self-esteem.

8. Personal inhaler: Create a personal inhaler by adding a few drops of essential oil (or a mixture) to a cotton wick. Breathe deeply from your inhaler before intimate moments to promote relaxation and confidence.

9. Diffuse: Diffuse essential oils with aphrodisiac or mood-enhancing properties in your bedroom before intimate occasions to create a sensual atmosphere.

10. Sensual massage: Add diluted essential oils to a sensual massage to promote relaxation, connection, and a heightened sense of confidence.

11. Self-care rituals: Perform self-care rituals before intimate moments. This may include a warm bath with essential oils, deep breathing, and positive affirmations to boost confidence.

12. Open communication: Discuss using essential oils and other methods with your partner to ensure you are both comfortable and consistent with your intentions.

Remember, essential oils should be used as part of a holistic approach that includes emotional, mental, and physical health. Addressing sexual function and self-confidence issues often involves a combination of factors, including communication, emotional connection, and overall health.

Additionally, individual reactions to essential oils may vary. Some people may find certain scents or techniques beneficial, while others may not. It's important to approach the use of essential oils with an open mind and be willing to explore what works best for you and your partner. If you or your partner have any concerns or medical conditions, consider consulting a healthcare professional before using essential oils in this situation.

G. Communication and Relationship Building

Open communication and relationship building are important foundations for a satisfying and fulfilling sexual experience. Here are some points to consider:

1. Trust and comfort: Establish a safe and open environment where both parties feel comfortable expressing their desires, concerns, and boundaries.

2. Mutual understanding: Take the time to listen to each other's needs and preferences. Understand that everyone's desires and comfort levels may be different.

3. Respect boundaries: Respect each other's boundaries and communicate openly and honestly about what feels comfortable and what doesn't. Consent is crucial at every stage of an intimate relationship.

4. Emotional connection: Building emotional intimacy and trust can enhance physical intimacy. Share your feelings, fears, and desires to create a deeper connection.

5. Reduce stress: Stress and anxiety can affect sexual satisfaction. Openly discussing stressors and finding ways to alleviate them can help make the experience more relaxing.

6. Explore together: Explore new experiences, technologies, and ideas together. Keep an open mind and encourage each other to share fantasies or curiosities.

7. Acknowledge change: Bodies and desires change over time. Discuss any changes openly and work together to find ways to adapt and continue to enjoy intimacy.

8. Empathy and support: If one partner is facing challenges related to sexual functioning or self-confidence, be understanding and supportive. Find solutions together.

9. Express love: Regular expressions of love, whether physical or emotional, can strengthen the bond between partners.

10. Quality time: Spend quality time together outside the bedroom to nurture your emotional connection and maintain a healthy relationship.

11. Professional help: If issues related to intimacy or sexual satisfaction persist, consider seeking guidance from a therapist or counselor who specializes in relationship and sexual health.

Remember, a satisfying sexual experience involves both parties feeling respected, valued and heard. Open communication is key to understanding each other's desires and creating a deeper connection. It's important to create an atmosphere where both parties can freely express their feelings, needs, and desires without fear of judgment. This method not only enhances the physical aspects of intimacy but also strengthens the emotional bond between partners.

Essential oils can play a subtle yet impactful role in facilitating communication, promoting relaxation, and creating a supportive environment for sexual exploration in a relationship. Here's how to use them:

1. Relaxing aromatherapy: Certain essential oils, such as lavender, chamomile, and ylang-ylang, are known for their relaxation-inducing properties. Diffusing these essential oils into the bedroom or using them during a relaxing massage can help both parties relax and feel relaxed.

2. Enhance the sensory experience: Essential oils with aphrodisiac properties, such as ylang-ylang, sage, and sandalwood, can be used to create a sensual atmosphere. Diffusing or incorporating these oils into massage oil can enhance mood and stimulate the senses.

3. Set the mood: Essential oils help create a specific atmosphere. Use oils like rose, jasmine, or bergamot to create a romantic and inviting atmosphere in your bedroom.

4. Open communication: Create a safe space for open dialogue by adding essential oils that encourage communication and emotional connection. Oils like frankincense, cedarwood, and rose can help cultivate a sense of trust and vulnerability.

5. Aromatherapy diffuser: Use an aromatherapy diffuser to disperse essential oils to promote relaxation and connection. Diffusing oils can help set the tone for intimate conversations and experiences.

6. Sensual massage: A sensual massage with essential oils can be an intimate experience that promotes relaxation and emotional connection. Choose an oil that resonates with your partner's preferences for smell and feel.

7. Partner involvement: Involve your partners in selecting essential oils to experience. This collaborative approach allows both parties to have a say in the atmosphere they want to create.

8. Create a ritual: Create a ritual that involves using essential oils together, such as applying them before bed or in the bath. These rituals can be a way to connect regularly.

9. Intimacy and trust: Certain oils can help cultivate feelings of intimacy and trust, which are essential for open communication and exploration. Essential oils like sandalwood, rose, and jasmine can help evoke these emotions.

10. Explore together: Experiment with different oils and methods of use. Openly discuss your experiences and preferences to create an atmosphere of mutual exploration and understanding.

Remember, essential oils are meant to complement and enhance experiences, including those related to intimacy and communication. They can contribute to well-being and a holistic approach to relationships, but they are only one piece of the puzzle. Open communication, respect, and a genuine desire to connect with your partner are core to creating a supportive environment for exploration.

Conclusion: In the conclusion of this chapter, we summarize the benefits and applications of essential oils in supporting male and sexual health. We emphasize the role of essential oils in enhancing, promoting intimacy, and cultivating a satisfying sexual experience. By incorporating essential oils into their sexual health routine and promoting open communication with their partners, men can enhance their sexual health and enjoy more fulfilling and intimate relationships.

6.3 Address Hormonal Imbalances and Symptoms

In this chapter, we'll explore how essential oils can be used to address male hormonal imbalances and relieve related symptoms. We discuss common hormonal imbalances that men may experience and provide guidance on using essential oils to support hormonal regulation and promote overall health.

A. Understanding Male Hormonal Imbalances

Hormonal imbalances can have a significant impact on men's health. Here are some explanations for common hormonal imbalances:

1. Low testosterone:

* Testosterone is the primary male sex hormone responsible for muscle development, bone density, and mood.
* Low testosterone (hypogonadism) can lead to fatigue, loss of muscle mass, depression, erectile dysfunction, and mood changes.
* Age, medical conditions, obesity, stress, and certain medications can cause it.

2. Estrogen dominance:

* Estrogen is generally thought of as a female hormone, but men also have it in small amounts. Estrogen dominance occurs when estrogen levels are disproportionately high relative to testosterone.
* This imbalance can lead to weight gain, mood swings, decline, and potential prostate problems.
* Factors contributing to estrogen dominance include excess body fat, exposure to environmental estrogen (xenoestrogens), and hormonal imbalances.

3. Adrenal insufficiency:

* The adrenal glands produce hormones such as cortisol (the stress hormone) and DHEA (the precursor to testosterone).
* Adrenal gland dysfunction, often due to chronic stress, can lead to imbalances in cortisol and DHEA levels and affect energy, sleep, and hormone regulation.

4. Thyroid imbalance:

* The thyroid gland produces hormones that regulate metabolism. Imbalances, such as hypothyroidism (an underactive thyroid gland) or hyperthyroidism (an overactive thyroid gland), can affect energy levels, weight, and mood.

5. Insulin resistance:

* Insulin is a hormone that regulates blood sugar levels. Insulin resistance occurs when the body's cells become less responsive to insulin, leading to high blood sugar.
* It may lead to obesity, inflammation, and disruption of hormone production.

6. Cortisol imbalance:

* Cortisol is a hormone released in response to stress. Chronic stress can lead to excessive cortisol production, affecting metabolism, immune function, and hormone balance.

7. Growth hormone deficiency:

* Growth hormone (GH) regulates growth, metabolism, and muscle development. A deficiency can reduce muscle mass, increase body fat, and lower energy levels.

8. Prolactin imbalance:

* Prolactin is responsible for milk production in women. In men, elevated prolactin levels (hyperprolactinemia) can lead to decline, erectile dysfunction, and underlying hormonal disturbances.

9. Progesterone imbalance:

* Progesterone is a female hormone found in small amounts in men. Imbalances can affect mood, sleep, and hormonal harmony.

10. Sex hormone binding globulin (SHBG) imbalance:

*SHBG is a protein that binds to sex hormones, affecting their availability. Imbalances in SHBG levels can affect hormone activity.

These imbalances can often be controlled through lifestyle changes, dietary modifications, stress reduction, exercise, and sometimes medical intervention. If you suspect you have a hormonal imbalance, be sure to consult a healthcare professional for proper diagnosis and guidance.

Hormonal imbalances can cause a wide range of symptoms and potential health effects in men. Here is an overview of some common symptoms and their corresponding health effects for various hormonal imbalances:

1. Low Testosterone (Hypogonadism):

* Symptoms: Fatigue, loss of muscle mass, hypotension, erectile dysfunction, mood changes, hair loss, reduced bone density.
* Health effects: Reduced muscle strength, increased risk of osteoporosis, impaired sexual function, mood disorders, increased cardiovascular risk.

2. Estrogen dominance:

* Symptoms: Weight gain, mood swings, decline, gynecomastia (breast enlargement), bloating, prostate problems.
* Health effects: Increased risk of cardiovascular disease, potential effects on prostate health, disruption of hormonal balance.

3. Adrenal dysfunction (cortisol and DHEA imbalance):

* Symptoms: Chronic fatigue, difficulty managing stress, sleep disturbance, weight gain, weakened immune function.
* Health effects: Increased susceptibility to infections, impaired stress response, disrupted sleep patterns.

4. Thyroid imbalance:

* Symptoms (Hypothyroidism): Fatigue, weight gain, sensitivity to cold, dry skin, hair loss, depression.
* Symptoms (hyperthyroidism): weight loss, rapid heartbeat, anxiety, heat sensitivity, hand tremors.
* Health Effects: Metabolic disorders, mood disorders, potential effects on heart health.

5. Insulin resistance:

* Symptoms: Weight gain (especially around the abdomen), increased hunger, fatigue, frequent urination, and difficulty losing weight.
* Health effects: Increased risk of type 2 diabetes, cardiovascular disease, inflammation.

6. Cortisol Imbalance:

* Symptoms (Chronic Stress): Fatigue, insomnia, anxiety, irritability, weight gain, weakened immune response.
* Health Effects: Increased risk of chronic disease, immune system suppression, and hormonal disorders.

7. Growth hormone deficiency:

* Symptoms: Loss of muscle mass, increase in body fat, low energy, decreased exercise capacity.
* Health Effects: Decreased muscle strength, reduced bone density, potential effects on overall vitality.

8. Prolactin imbalance:

* Symptoms: Decline, erectile dysfunction, infertility, mood changes.
* Health effects: Impaired sexual function, potential effects on repro-

ductive health.

9. Progesterone imbalance:

* Symptoms: Mood swings, irritability, sleep disruption, decline.
* Health effects: Mood disorders, sleep disorders, hormonal imbalances.

10. Sex hormone binding globulin (SHBG) imbalance:

* Symptoms: Altered hormonal activity, changes, potential mood changes.
* Health effects: Disruption of hormonal balance, potential effects on reproductive health.

It's important to note that hormonal imbalances can vary greatly in their manifestations and effects. If you are experiencing persistent or severe symptoms that may be related to a hormonal imbalance, it is recommended that you consult a healthcare professional for proper diagnosis and personalized treatment recommendations.

B. Hormone Balancing Essential Oil

Of course, essential oils can play a role in supporting hormonal regulation and balance. Here are some essential oils known for their potential to support hormonal balance:

1. Sage: Sage is often associated with women's hormonal health but may also benefit men. It is known for its potential to balance estrogen levels and support overall hormonal harmony.

2. Frankincense: Frankincense essential oil has been studied for its potential to modulate hormonal pathways and promote balance in the endocrine system. It is also known for its calming and grounding properties.

3. Geranium: Geranium oil is considered to have adaptogenic properties, meaning it can help the body adapt to stress and promote overall balance. It can support hormonal regulation and emotional health.

4. Lavender: Lavender oil is known for its calming effects on the nervous system, which can indirectly support hormonal balance. It may have a

positive impact on hormonal health by reducing stress and promoting relaxation.

5. Bergamot: Bergamot oil has been studied for its potential mood-enhancing effects. It may indirectly help with hormonal balance by promoting a positive mood and reducing stress.

6. Ylang-ylang: Ylang-ylang is known for its potential to balance hormones, reduce stress, and promote emotional health. It is thought to have a calming effect on the nervous system.

7. Rosemary: Rosemary oil is thought to have a positive effect on the adrenal glands, which play a role in hormone production. It is also known for its uplifting aroma.

8. Sandalwood: Sandalwood oil has been studied for its potential to support testosterone production and hormonal balance. It is also known for its grounding and soothing properties.

When using essential oils to support hormones, it is important to remember that they should be used as a complementary measure, not as a replacement for medical treatment. Essential oils can be incorporated into relaxation exercises, massages, diffusers, or personal care products to promote overall well-being.

Individuals may react differently to essential oils, so it's a good idea to conduct a patch test before using an essential oil widely. Additionally, if you have specific concerns about hormonal imbalance, it is recommended that you consult with a healthcare professional to determine the best approach for your unique situation.

Essential oils are thought to provide a variety of benefits that can help regulate hormone production, relieve symptoms, and promote overall hormonal health. Here's how some of the essential oils mentioned earlier can help in these areas:

1. Sage: Sage is thought to have estrogen-like properties that may help balance hormone levels in both men and women. It may help reduce symptoms of hormone imbalance, such as mood swings, cramps, and hot flashes.

2. Frankincense: Frankincense oil's potential to modulate hormone pathways may aid in overall hormone balance. Its calming effects also help

reduce stress-related hormonal fluctuations.

3. Geranium: The adaptogenic properties of geranium oil are thought to help the body cope with stress, which can support hormonal balance. It can also relieve symptoms such as mood swings and fatigue.

4. Lavender: The relaxation-inducing properties of lavender can help reduce stress, promote better sleep, and indirectly support hormonal health. Adequate sleep is essential for proper hormonal regulation.

5. Bergamot: The mood-enhancing effects of bergamot can help relieve stress and anxiety, which can affect hormonal balance. Managing stress is important to maintaining healthy hormone levels.

6. Ylang-ylang: Ylang-ylang's calming properties may help regulate cortisol levels, the body's primary stress hormone. By reducing stress, it supports hormonal balance and emotional health.

7. Rosemary: Rosemary oil's potential effects on the adrenal glands can help with hormonal balance. It also improves blood circulation, which has a positive impact on hormones.

8. Sandalwood: Sandalwood oil's potential to support testosterone production and balance estrogen levels may contribute to overall hormonal health. Its soothing aroma also helps reduce stress.

It's important to note that essential oils work best as part of a holistic approach to hormonal health. Lifestyle factors such as nutrition, exercise, stress management, and sleep play an important role in maintaining hormonal balance. Essential oils can be integrated into a variety of wellness practices, such as aromatherapy, massage, and relaxation techniques, to enhance a holistic approach.

Keep in mind that individual reactions to essential oils may vary. When using essential oils to support hormones, it is recommended to use high-quality oils, dilute them appropriately, and consider any personal sensitivities or allergies. If you have specific hormonal issues, consulting with a healthcare professional can provide personalized guidance on incorporating essential oils into your wellness routine.

C. Topical Application of Hormonal Support

Topically applied essential oils may be an effective way to address hormonal imbalances. Here are some guidelines on how to use essential oils safely and effectively for this purpose:

1. Dilute: Essential oils are highly concentrated and should always be diluted before applying to the skin. A common dilution ratio is 1 to 2% of essential oil and carrier oil. For each teaspoon (5 ml) of carrier oil, add 3 to 6 drops of essential oil. This helps prevent skin irritation and sensitivity.

2. Carrier oil: Choose a carrier oil that suits your skin type and preferences. Common carrier oils include jojoba oil, coconut oil, sweet almond oil, and grapeseed oil. Carrier oils also have beneficial properties that can enhance the effects of essential oils.

3. Patch test: Before applying the essential oil mixture to a larger area, conduct a patch test on a small area of skin to check for any adverse reactions or sensitivities. Wait 24 hours to ensure there are no negative responses.

4. How to use: Apply the diluted essential oil mixture to areas with relatively thin skin and good blood vessels. For hormonal support, you can target areas such as the wrists, inner thighs, lower abdomen, and base of the neck.

5. Massage: Massage the diluted mixture into the skin using gentle circular motions. This not only aids absorption but also promotes relaxation and stress reduction, which can aid in hormonal balance.

6. Consistency: Consistency is key. Hormonal imbalances may take time to correct, so regular and consistent use of essential oil blends is important.

7. Avoid sensitive areas: Avoid applying essential oils to sensitive areas such as eyes, ears, and mucous membranes. Also, be careful when applying to broken or irritated skin.

8. Consult a professional: If you are dealing with a severe hormonal imbalance, it is best to consult a healthcare professional, especially if you are taking medications or have a medical condition. They can guide you in selecting the most appropriate essential oils and dilution ratios for your situation.

9. Monitor reactions: Pay attention to how your body reacts to es-

sential oils. If you experience any discomfort, irritation, or adverse reactions, discontinue use and consult a health care professional.

10. Personalize: Everyone's body is different, so what works for one person may not work for another. It may take some experimentation to find the essential oil blends and methods of use that work best for you.

Remember, addressing hormonal imbalances is a holistic process that involves lifestyle changes, nutrition, stress management, and more. Essential oils may be an important part of this approach, but they are not a substitute for professional medical advice and treatment. If you have underlying health conditions, it is recommended that you work with your healthcare provider to develop a comprehensive plan to address hormonal imbalances.

Here are more details on proper dilution ratios, carrier oils, and targeted application methods for using essential oils to address hormonal imbalances:

Dilution ratio:

Dilution is critical to ensuring the safety and effectiveness of essential oils. A general guideline for dilution is to dilute essential oils 1 to 2% into a carrier oil, which means using 3 to 6 drops of essential oil for every 3 teaspoons (5 ml) of carrier oil. For hormonal support, you may prefer a 2% dilution.

Carrier oil:

Choosing the right carrier oil is important for two reasons: Carrier oils help dilute the essential oils, carry them into the skin, and have healing properties. Here are some commonly used carrier oils:

* Jojoba Oil: Suitable for all skin types, jojoba oil closely resembles the skin's natural sebum and is easily absorbed.
* Coconut Oil: Coconut oil is known for its moisturizing properties and is a good choice for a hormone-support blend.
* Sweet Almond Oil: A versatile carrier oil with nourishing benefits suitable for most skin types.
* Grapeseed Oil: Grapeseed oil is lightweight, easily absorbed, and often used in massage blends.

Targeted application methods:

1. Lower abdomen: Apply the diluted mixture to the lower abdomen where the reproductive organs are located. Massage gently in a clockwise direction, following the natural flow of your digestive system.

2. Inner thighs: The skin on the inner thighs is thinner and has good blood circulation. Apply the mixture here to absorb.

3. Wrists and inner forearms: The skin in these areas is thinner and can be effective sites for essential oil applications.

4. Bottom of the neck: Apply to the bottom of the neck and can be inhaled and absorbed through the skin.

5. Pulse points: Suitable for pulse points such as wrists and behind ears. The blood vessels in these areas are close to the surface, aiding absorption.

6. Back of neck: Applying here can support the endocrine system and promote relaxation.

7. Spine: Some aromatherapists recommend applying a diluted mixture along the spine for hormonal support.

8. Massage: Consider using the diluted mixture for a gentle self-massage for an overall calming effect and better absorption.

Remember to patch test before widespread use and use caution around sensitive areas and broken skin. The effectiveness of an essential oil blend will also depend on individual response and consistency of use.

If you're new to using essential oils to support hormones, consider starting with a lower dilution and working your way up based on your comfort and response. Additionally, if you have any pre-existing medical conditions or are taking medications, please consult a healthcare professional before incorporating essential oils into your daily life.

D. Hormone Support Blend

Here are some recipes and suggestions for using essential oils to create a personalized hormonal support blend. Remember to use proper dilution ratios and carrier oils to ensure safe and effective use:

Balancing Hormone Blend:

* 4 drops of sage
* 3 drops of lavender
* 3 drops of geranium
* 2 drops of frankincense
* 1 oz (30 ml) jojoba oil

Testosterone Balancing Blend:

* 4 drops of ginger
* 3 drops of sandalwood
* 2 drops of cedarwood
* 1 drop of ylang-ylang
* 1 oz (30 ml) sweet almond oil

Estrogen Harmony Blend:

* 3 drops of sage
* 3 drops of geranium
* 2 drops of frankincense
* 2 drops of lavender
* 1 oz (30 ml) grapeseed oil

Stress Reducing Hormone Blend:

* 4 drops of lavender
* 3 drops of bergamot
* 2 drops of frankincense
* 1 drop of Roman Chamomile
* 1 oz (30 ml) coconut oil

Adrenal Support Blend:

* 4 drops of rosemary
* 3 drops of mint
* 2 drops of lemongrass
* 2 drops of lavender
* 1 oz (30 ml) jojoba oil

Guide:

1. Choose a 1 oz (30 ml) glass bottle for your mix.
2. Drop the specified amount of each essential oil into the bottle.
3. Fill the rest of the bottle with the carrier oil of your choice (jojoba, sweet almond, grapeseed, coconut, etc.).
4. Close the bottle and gently roll or shake to mix the oil.
5. Conduct a patch test before widespread use to avoid adverse reactions.
6. Apply mixture to target areas daily or as needed (as described above).

You can adjust the number of drops according to your preference and sensitivity. It's important to note that essential oils work gradually and consistently over time. Consistency is key to experiencing the potential benefits of a hormonal support blend.

Remember, essential oils work holistically, and their effects may vary from person to person. If you have an existing health condition, are taking medications, or are pregnant / nursing, it is recommended that you consult a healthcare professional before using essential oils for hormonal support.

Here are some supplement oil combinations and application techniques for specific hormonal issues:

Low testosterone:

* Blend ginger, sandalwood, cedarwood, and ylang-ylang.
* How to use: Make a massage mixture using a carrier oil and apply it to the lower abdomen, inner thighs, and wrists.

Estrogen dominance:

* Blend sage, geranium, frankincense, lavender.
* Instructions: Dilute and use for abdominal massage, lower back, and pulse points.

Adrenal insufficiency:

* Blend rosemary, mint, lemongrass, lavender.
* Instructions: Make a diluted massage oil and apply it to the lower back, adrenal area, and soles of the feet.

Stress and cortisol imbalance:

* Blend lavender, bergamot, frankincense, and Roman chamomile.
* Instructions: Diffuse in your relaxation space, use in a personal inhaler, or add to your bath before bed.

Thyroid imbalance:

* Blend myrrh, lemongrass, frankincense, and lavender.
* Instructions: Dilute and massage the thyroid area (front of the neck) and soles of feet.

Insulin sensitivity support:

* Blend cinnamon, coriander, bergamot, myrrh
* Instructions: Dilute and apply to the belly and wrists or diffuse to create a relaxing atmosphere.

Everyone's body reacts differently, so it's important to experiment and find the combinations and application techniques that work best for you. Always ensure proper dilution and conduct a patch test before using a new mixture on a larger area.

In addition to using essential oils, consider maintaining a healthy lifestyle through proper nutrition, exercise, stress management, and getting enough sleep to support hormonal balance. If you are dealing with specific hormonal issues, it is recommended that you consult a healthcare professional to ensure a comprehensive and personalized approach to your health.

E. Lifestyle Factors Affecting Hormonal Health

Lifestyle factors play an important role in maintaining hormonal balance. Here are some strategies to consider promoting optimal hormone levels:

1. Diet:

* Balanced nutrition: Eat a diet rich in whole foods, including vegetables, fruits, lean proteins, healthy fats, and whole grains.
* Manage sugar intake: Avoid excessive consumption of refined sugars and processed foods to prevent insulin spikes and imbalances.
* Omega 3 fatty acids: Include sources of omega 3 fatty acids, such as

fatty fish, flax seeds, and walnuts, which support hormone production.

2. Exercise:

* Regular activity: Get regular physical activity to help regulate insulin sensitivity, increase testosterone levels, and manage stress.
* Strength training: Incorporate strength training exercises to support muscle mass and testosterone production.

3. Stress management:

* Mindfulness techniques: Practice mindfulness, meditation, deep breathing, or yoga to reduce chronic stress and cortisol levels.
* Get enough sleep: Prioritize quality sleep to support hormone production, especially growth hormone and testosterone.

4. Sleep hygiene:

* A consistent sleep schedule: Maintain a regular sleep schedule, aiming for 7 to 9 hours of uninterrupted sleep every night.
* Sleep environment: Create a dark, quiet, and comfortable sleeping environment to enhance melatonin production.

5. Avoid environmental toxins:

* Reduce Exposure: Minimize exposure to endocrine-disrupting chemicals found in some plastics, pesticides, and personal care products.

6. Manage weight:

* Maintain a healthy weight: Both excess and insufficient body fat can disrupt hormonal balance. Maintain a healthy weight through balanced nutrition and regular exercise.

7. Hydration:

* Adequate fluid intake: Stay properly hydrated to support overall body functions, including hormone production.

8. Limit alcohol and caffeine:

* Moderation: Limit alcohol and caffeine intake, as excessive intake

can affect hormone levels.

9. Supportive supplements:

* Speak to a Professional: Talk to your healthcare provider before adding supplements like vitamin D, magnesium, or adaptogenic herbs to your daily routine.

10. Hormone testing:

* Speak to an expert: If you suspect a hormonal imbalance, consider consulting with a healthcare provider specializing in hormonal health for accurate testing and personalized guidance.

11. Professional guidance:

* Hormonal specialist: If you experience ongoing symptoms of a hormonal imbalance, consult a healthcare professional who specializes in hormonal health.

Remember, maintaining hormonal balance is a holistic endeavor that involves many aspects of your lifestyle. Over time, consistency in healthy habits can significantly help achieve and maintain optimal hormone levels. Always consult a healthcare professional before making major changes to your lifestyle or starting any new supplements.

Of course, addressing these issues is crucial to maintaining hormonal balance. Here's a breakdown of how each aspect affects hormonal health:

1. Nutrition:

* Eat a balanced diet: Eating a balanced diet rich in whole foods, lean protein, healthy fats, and a variety of vegetables and fruits supports overall health and hormone production.
* Macronutrient ratios: Make sure you get the right balance of carbohydrates, proteins, and fats to support energy levels and hormone synthesis.
* Avoid Processed Foods: Minimize processed foods that are high in refined sugars, unhealthy fats, and artificial additives, as they can disrupt hormonal balance.

2. Exercise:

* Regular physical exercise: Regular exercise helps regulate insulin levels, supports metabolism, and promotes healthy hormone levels.

* Strength training: Incorporating resistance or strength training can increase testosterone levels and support muscle mass.

3. Stress management:

* Reduce stress: Chronic stress can cause elevated cortisol levels, disrupting hormonal balance. Stress management techniques such as meditation, deep breathing, and yoga can help alleviate this condition.

4. Avoid toxins:

* Environmental toxins: Minimize exposure to endocrine-disrupting chemicals found in some plastics, pesticides, and personal care products.

* Organic foods: Choose organic produce and hormone-free animal products whenever possible to reduce exposure to pesticides and synthetic hormones.

5. Sleep hygiene:

* Get enough sleep: Prioritize quality sleep to support hormone production, especially growth hormone and testosterone. Maintain a regular sleep schedule and create an environment conducive to sleep.

6. Hydration:

* Proper hydration: Staying adequately hydrated supports various body functions, including hormonal balance.

7. Alcohol and caffeine intake:

* Control: Try to control alcohol and caffeine intake, or even reduce it to 0.

8. Nutrient intake:

* Vitamins and Minerals: Make sure you get enough essential vitamins and minerals, such as vitamin D, zinc, magnesium, and omega-3 fatty acids, which can support hormone production.

9. Fiber intake:

* Fiber-rich foods: Include fiber-rich foods like whole grains, legumes, and vegetables in your diet to support digestive health and estrogen metabolism.

10. Adaptogenic herbs:

* Ask a professional: Certain adaptogenic herbs like ashwagandha, Rhodiola, and maca are thought to support hormonal balance. Check with your healthcare provider before adding these to your daily routine.

11. Hormone testing:

* Professional Guidance: If you suspect a hormonal imbalance, consult a healthcare provider specializing in hormonal health. Hormone testing can provide insight into your specific needs.

Remember, individual needs may vary, and it's important to consult a healthcare professional before making major changes to your diet, exercise routine, or supplements. A holistic approach that combines these factors helps maintain healthy hormone levels and overall health.

F. Managing Stress and Cortisol Levels

Stress and cortisol levels significantly impact hormonal balance, particularly in the context of adrenal gland function and the body's stress response. Here's how stress, cortisol, and hormonal imbalances are related:

Stress and HPA axis:

The hypothalamic-pituitary-adrenal (HPA) axis regulates the body's stress response. When you feel stressed, your hypothalamus releases corticotropin-releasing hormone (CRH), which releases adrenocorticotropic hormone to the pituitary gland (ACTH) signal. ACTH then triggers the adrenal glands to produce cortisol, often called the " stress hormone. "

The role of cortisol:

Cortisol is essential for managing stress and maintaining various body functions, such as regulating blood sugar levels, immune response, and metabolism. During short-term stressful situations, cortisol helps mobilize resources to cope with challenges.

Chronic stress and imbalance:

However, chronic stress can lead to persistently elevated cortisol levels. Over time, chronic activation of this stress response can disrupt the delicate balance of hormones, causing hormonal imbalances. High cortisol levels can suppress the production of other important hormones, such as testosterone and thyroid hormone.

Effects on reproductive hormones:

In men, chronic stress and elevated cortisol levels can lead to reduced testosterone production. High cortisol levels may also interfere with the production and release of the hypothalamic gonadotropin-releasing hormone (GnRH), critical for regulating reproductive hormones.

Insulin resistance and weight gain:

Chronic stress can lead to insulin resistance and weight gain, disrupting hormonal balance. Insulin resistance causes an imbalance in blood sugar levels and insulin production, affecting hormones such as insulin and leptin.

Adrenal fatigue:

Long-term exposure to chronic stress can lead to a condition called adrenal fatigue, or dysfunction, in which the adrenal glands struggle to produce adequate amounts of cortisol and other hormones. This can further exacerbate hormonal imbalances and affect overall health.

Hormonal feedback loop:

Hormones in the body are intricately connected through feedback loops. An imbalance in one hormone can affect the production and function of other hormones. For example, elevated cortisol levels suppress the production of hormones such as thyroid and sex hormones.

Manage stress to balance hormones:

To promote hormonal balance, it is crucial to manage stress effectively:

* Incorporate stress-reduction techniques like meditation, deep breath-

ing, yoga, and mindfulness into your daily life.

    * Get regular physical exercise, which helps regulate stress hormones.

    * Make getting enough sleep a priority, as poor sleep quality and quantity can exacerbate stress and cortisol levels.

    * Consider counseling, therapy, or support groups to address underlying emotional stressors.

By managing stress effectively and maintaining a balanced lifestyle, you can help prevent the negative effects of chronic stress on hormonal balance and overall health. If you suspect a hormonal imbalance, consider seeking guidance from a healthcare professional experienced in hormone regulation.

Essential oils and relaxation techniques can play an important role in reducing stress and promoting healthy hormone production. Here's how to use essential oils and relaxation techniques to reduce stress and balance hormones:

1. Stress-reducing essential oil:

    * Lavender: Lavender oil is known for its calming properties, which can help reduce stress and promote relaxation.

    * Roman chamomile: This oil has soothing properties and can help relieve stress and anxiety.

    * Bergamot: Bergamot oil has a citrus aroma that uplifts mood and reduces stress.

    * Frankincense: Frankincense is often used in meditation and can help create a sense of tranquility and calm.

    * Ylang-ylang: Known for its floral scent, ylang-ylang can promote relaxation and reduce tension.

2. Aromatherapy diffuser:

Using an aromatherapy diffuser to disperse essential oils into the air can create a soothing atmosphere. Diffuse stress-reducing oils like lavender, chamomile, or bergamot into your living space, bedroom, or workspace.

3. Relaxation techniques:

    * Deep breathing: Practice deep, slow breathing exercises to activate your body's relaxation response and lower stress hormones.

    * Meditation: Regular meditation can help calm the mind and reduce stress. Use calming essential oils during meditation to enhance the experience.

    * Yoga: Combine yoga poses and stretches to release body tension and

calm the nervous system.

    * Progressive muscle relaxation: This technique involves tensing and relaxing different muscle groups to promote physical and mental relaxation.

    * Guided imagery: Visualize peaceful scenes or scenarios to distract you and reduce stress.

4. Massage and self-care:

    * Consider self-massage with diluted essential oils. Massage helps release muscle tension and promotes relaxation.

    * Add a few drops of stress-relieving essential oils to your bath water for a calming bath ritual.

5. Bedtime ritual:

    * Use essential oils known for their calming properties during your bedtime routine to signal rest.

    * Apply relaxing oil to your bedroom before bed.

6. Mindfulness and gratitude:

    * Practice mindfulness techniques to stay present and reduce anxious thoughts.

    * Keep a gratitude journal and focus on the positive aspects of your life, which can lower stress levels.

7. Regular sleep habits:

    * Prioritize consistent sleep patterns and create a relaxing bedtime.

    * Diffuse or apply essential oils that promote relaxation and sleep.

Remember to choose high-quality, pure essential oils and do a patch test before applying them to your skin. Dilute essential oils with a carrier oil to ensure safe use. Incorporating these techniques into your daily life can help reduce stress and support healthy hormone production. If you experience ongoing stress or hormonal imbalances, consult a healthcare professional for personalized guidance.

G. Supports Detoxification and Liver Health

The liver plays a vital role in hormone metabolism and overall hormonal balance. It is responsible for processing and metabolizing hormones, including sex hormones such as estrogen and testosterone. Here is an overview of the role of the liver and how to support its hormonal balancing function:

The role of the Liver in hormone metabolism:

1. Detoxification: The liver detoxifies hormones by breaking them down into forms that can be excreted from the body. This prevents the accumulation of excess hormones, which can lead to imbalances.

2. Estrogen metabolism: The liver helps metabolize estrogen into various forms, including " good " and " bad" metabolites. Balanced estrogen metabolism is critical to preventing estrogen dominance.

3. Testosterone regulation: The liver helps regulate testosterone levels by breaking down and eliminating excess testosterone from the body.

Supports liver function and promotes hormonal balance:

1. Healthy diet: Eat a balanced diet rich in fiber, antioxidants, and nutrients. Include cruciferous vegetables (broccoli, cauliflower, cabbage) that support liver detoxification.

2. Hydrate: Drink plenty of water to support the liver's detoxification process.

3. Limit alcohol consumption: Excessive alcohol consumption can strain the liver and interfere with hormone metabolism. Moderate drinking is recommended.

4. Reduce sugar: High sugar intake can lead to fatty liver and affect hormone metabolism. Choose natural sweeteners and limit refined sugars.

5. Exercise regularly: Physical exercise supports overall liver health and metabolic processes.

6. Minimize toxins: Reduce exposure to environmental toxins, as the liver also helps process these toxins. Use natural cleaning products and limit exposure to contaminants.

7. Herbal support: Certain herbs, such as milk thistle and dandelion root, are known for their liver-supporting properties. Consult a healthcare pro-

fessional before using herbal supplements.

8. Liver support essential oils:
* Lemon: Lemon oil is known for its detoxifying properties and can support liver function.
* Rosemary: This oil may help improve blood circulation and liver function.
* Geranium: Geranium oil can have a positive impact on liver health.

9. Stress management: Chronic stress can affect liver function and hormone balance. Practice stress-reduction techniques such as meditation, deep breathing, and relaxation.

10. Quality sleep: Adequate sleep supports overall body function, including liver health and hormonal regulation.

11. Limit processed foods: A high intake of processed foods can stress the liver. Focus on whole foods to provide essential nutrients.

12. Avoid excess fat: Maintain a healthy weight to prevent fatty liver disease, which affects liver function.

13. Medical Guidance: If you suspect liver problems or hormonal imbalances, please consult a healthcare professional for appropriate evaluation and guidance.

Remember, supporting liver health is a holistic approach that involves multiple lifestyle factors. Balancing hormones and maintaining a healthy liver contribute to overall health and vitality.

Essential oils and techniques can play a supportive role in detoxifying and promoting liver health. Here are some essential oils and methods that can help with this process:

1. Lemon essential oil:

Lemon oil is known for its detoxifying properties. It supports the liver by promoting bile production and aiding in the breakdown of toxins. You can use lemon oil in a variety of ways:
* Aromatherapy: Diffuse lemon oil in your living space to create a fresh and uplifting atmosphere.
* Ingestion: Add one drop of therapeutic-grade lemon oil to a glass

of water or herbal tea. Make sure the essential oil is safe for internal use, and consult a healthcare professional before ingesting any essential oil.

2. Peppermint essential oil:

Peppermint oil can support digestion and liver function by promoting bile flow. It has a cooling and uplifting aroma that also helps reduce nausea.
* Aromatherapy: Inhale peppermint oil directly from the bottle or use a personal inhaler wand for a quick pick-me-up.

3. Rosemary essential oil:

Rosemary oil has been shown to have hepatoprotective properties, which means it may help protect the liver from damage and support its overall health.
* Topical application: Dilute rosemary oil with carrier oil and apply it topically to the abdominal area above the liver.

4. Juniper essential oil:

Juniper berry oil is thought to have detoxifying properties and may support kidney and liver function.
* Aromatherapy: Diffuse juniper berry oil to create a purifying and cleansing atmosphere.

5. Castor oil pack:

Castor oil packs are a traditional way to support liver detoxification. Apply a castor oil-soaked cloth to the abdominal area over the liver, cover it with plastic wrap, and apply a warm compress over it. Leave it on for about an hour. Consult a healthcare professional before using this method.

6. Dry brushing:

Dry brushing stimulates lymph flow and helps remove toxins. Before showering, use a dry brush to gently brush your skin upward toward your heart before showering.

7. Detox bath:

Add a few drops of detoxifying essential oils such as lemon, lavender, or juniper berry to a warm bath. The combination of warm water and essential oils promotes relaxation and detoxification.

8. Hydration:

Staying hydrated is essential for liver health and detoxification. Drink plenty of water throughout the day to support liver function.

9. Whole foods:

Support liver health by eating a diet rich in whole foods, antioxidants, and nutrients. Include foods like leafy greens, cruciferous vegetables, and herbs like cilantro.

10. Consultation:

Consult a health care professional before using essential oils or any detoxification technique, especially if you have a pre-existing medical condition or are taking medications.

Remember, while essential oils can provide support, they should not replace medical advice or treatment. A holistic approach that includes a balanced diet, regular exercise, hydration, and stress management is essential to promoting liver health and overall well-being.

After this chapter, we summarize the benefits and applications of essential oils in addressing male hormonal imbalances and alleviating related symptoms. We emphasize the role of essential oils in supporting hormone regulation, reducing symptoms, and promoting overall health. By incorporating essential oils into their lifestyle and developing healthy habits, men can take proactive steps to address hormonal imbalances and improve physical and mental health.

Chapter 7

Men's Pain Essential Oil

M en often experience pain. Here, we explore essential oils to relieve headaches and migraines, soothe back and neck discomfort, and address sports injuries and muscle soreness.

7.1 Relieve Headaches and Migraines

In this chapter, we will explore the topic of headache and migraine relief for men. We discuss the causes and types of headaches and their impact on daily life and guide on using natural remedies, including essential oils, to relieve headache symptoms and promote relief.

A. Understanding Headaches and Migraines

Headaches are a common health problem that varies in intensity, duration, and underlying causes. Here are some explanations of common headache types:

1. Tension headache:

Tension headaches are the most common type and are usually caused by neck, shoulders, and scalp muscle tension. They feel like tight bands around the head, usually mild to moderate intensity. Tension headaches are often triggered by stress, poor posture, eye strain, dehydration, and lack of sleep.

2. Migraine:

Migraines are more severe and are often accompanied by other symptoms such as sensitivity to light and sound, nausea, and sometimes vision disturbances (called auras). Migraines are thought to involve changes in blood flow and chemicals in the brain. They can last from hours to days and significantly interfere with daily activities. Migraines can be triggered by a variety of factors, including certain foods, hormonal changes, stress, weather changes, and more.

3. Cluster headache:

Cluster headaches are the least common but most severe type. They occur in periodic patterns or clusters, often hitting one side of the head and causing severe pain around the eyes or temples. Cluster headaches often accompany other symptoms, such as nasal congestion, watery eyes, and restlessness. They can be very painful and may last only a short time but may occur multiple times a day during a cluster.

4. Sinus headache:

Sinus headaches are often mistaken for migraines but are related to sinus congestion and inflammation. They often cause pain in the forehead, cheekbones, and bridge of the nose. Sinus headaches are caused by sinus infections or allergies that cause pressure and inflammation in the sinus cavities.

5. Hormone-related headaches:

Some people, especially women, experience headaches related to hormonal changes. These may include menstrual migraines, which occur before or during a woman's menstrual cycle, and hormone-related headaches during pregnancy or menopause.

6. Rebound headache:

Rebound headaches, also called medication overuse headaches, can occur when pain relievers or migraine medications are overused. As the effects of the medication wear off, these headaches tend to occur more frequently, leading to a cycle of more medication and more headaches.

Each type of headache has its characteristics, triggers, and management strategies. It is important to accurately identify the type of headache you are experiencing to determine the most appropriate treatment. If you frequently experience severe or debilitating headaches, it is recommended that you consult a healthcare professional for proper diagnosis and guidance on managing and preventing headaches.

Headaches and migraines can have a variety of triggers and contributing factors, which vary from person to person. Here are some common triggers and factors that can cause headaches and migraines in men:

1. Stress and emotional factors:

Stress, anxiety, and tension are well-known triggers of tension headaches and migraines. Emotional factors can cause muscle tension and changes in blood flow, which can contribute to the development of headaches.

2. Diet triggers:

Certain foods and drinks are common triggers of migraines. These may include aged cheese, processed meats, chocolate, caffeine, alcohol (especially red wine), and artificial sweeteners. It is important to identify any specific dietary triggers through a process of elimination.

3. Dehydration:

Not drinking enough water can lead to dehydration, a known trigger of headaches. Staying properly hydrated is important to prevent headaches, especially during hot weather or after physical activity.

4. Lack of sleep:

Poor sleep quality, insufficient sleep, or disrupted sleep patterns can trigger or worsen existing headaches. Maintaining a regular sleep schedule and practicing good sleep hygiene can help prevent this trigger.

5. Hormonal changes:

Hormonal fluctuations, such as those that occur during menstruation, pregnancy, and menopause, can trigger migraines in some people. However, this trigger is more relevant to women than men.

6. Environmental factors:

Bright or flashing lights, strong odors, loud noises, and weather changes can trigger tension headaches and migraines.

7. Physical factors:

Poor posture, tight neck and shoulder muscles, and eye strain from prolonged use of a computer or screen can all contribute to tension headaches.

8. Caffeine intake:

While caffeine can relieve some headaches, sudden withdrawal can trigger others. Moderating caffeine intake and avoiding sudden changes can help.

9. Drinking alcohol:

Alcohol, especially red wine, beer, and certain spirits, can trigger migraines in some people. It is recommended to observe how different types of alcohol affect you.

10. Skipping meals:

Skipping meals or long periods without eating can lead to low blood sugar levels, triggering headaches.

11. Physical exertion:

Strenuous physical activity or sudden exertion can trigger exertion-related headaches, especially in people who are prone to such headaches.

12. Drugs:

Some medications, including vasodilators and certain blood pressure medications, may trigger headaches or worsen existing medications. If you suspect that your medication is causing your headaches, talk to your healthcare professional.

Everyone's triggers may be different, and it's important to identify and manage your specific triggers to help prevent headaches and migraines. Keeping a headache diary can help identify patterns and triggers. If headaches are frequent, severe, or interfere with your quality of life, it is recommended to consult a healthcare professional for appropriate evaluation and management.

B. Essential Oils for Headache Relief

Several essential oils are known for their potential to relieve headaches and migraines. Here are some essential oils commonly used for their headache-relieving properties:

1. Mint:

Peppermint essential oil contains menthol, which has cooling and analgesic properties. It can help relax tense muscles, improve blood flow, and provide a cooling sensation that can relieve headaches.

2. Lavender:

Lavender essential oil is known for its calming and relaxing effects. It can help reduce stress and anxiety, which are common triggers of headaches and migraines. The soothing aroma of lavender helps relieve headaches.

3. Eucalyptus:

Eucalyptus essential oil has a refreshing aroma and contains compounds that increase blood circulation and help relieve sinus congestion. It may be particularly useful for tension headaches associated with sinus problems.

4. Rosemary:

Rosemary essential oil has analgesic and anti-inflammatory properties. Its scent can help improve concentration and mental clarity, making it a good choice for headaches caused by tension or stress.

5. Chamomile:

Chamomile essential oil has anti-inflammatory and calming properties. It may help reduce tension and promote relaxation, both of which can help relieve headaches.

6. Frankincense:

Frankincense essential oil has soothing and anti-inflammatory properties. It can help relieve headaches by promoting relaxation and reducing inflammation.

7. Basil:

Basil essential oil is known for its muscle-relaxing and tension-reducing properties. It may be beneficial for headaches caused by muscle tension or stress.

8. Helichrysum:

Helichrysum essential oil has anti-inflammatory and analgesic properties. It may help reduce inflammation and pain associated with headaches.

9. Sweet marjoram:

Sweet marjoram essential oil is known for its calming and muscle-relaxing effects. It may help relieve tension and promote relaxation, which may help relieve headaches.

When using essential oils for headache relief, it's important to dilute them appropriately in a carrier oil before applying them to your skin, especially if you're applying them to your forehead or temples. Essential oils can also be diffused to create a calming atmosphere and support headache relief. Keep in mind that individuals may react differently to essential oils, so it's best to test a small area of skin before using it extensively to make sure you don't have any adverse reactions. If you have frequent or severe headaches, it is recommended that you consult a healthcare professional for appropriate diagnosis and management.

The essential oils mentioned have a variety of mechanisms by which they may provide relief from headaches and migraines. These mechanisms generally involve its analgesic, anti-inflammatory, and sedative properties:

1.Analgesic properties:

Many essential oils contain compounds that have analgesic or analgesic properties. These compounds can help reduce the perception of pain by interacting with receptors in the body. For example, peppermint essential oil contains menthol, which has a cooling effect that can help relieve headaches by numbing the area and reducing pain signals.

2. Anti-inflammatory properties:

Inflammation can lead to headaches, especially in the case of tension headaches or headaches related to sinus congestion. Essential oils like eucalyptus, rosemary, and helichrysum contain anti-inflammatory compounds that can help reduce inflammation and relieve headaches.

3. Calming and relaxing properties:

Stress and tension are common triggers of headaches and migraines. Essential oils like lavender, chamomile, and sweet marjoram have calm and relaxing properties that can help relieve stress, anxiety, and muscle tension. Their aroma can also have a positive impact on the nervous system, promoting a sense of calm.

4. Improve blood circulation:

Some essential oils, such as peppermint and rosemary, can help improve blood circulation. Better circulation relieves tension and promotes the delivery of oxygen and nutrients to the affected area, potentially reducing headache discomfort.

5. Aromatherapy effect:

Aromatherapy is an integral part of using essential oils to relieve headaches. Inhaling the aroma of certain essential oils can stimulate the olfactory system and affect areas of the brain that regulate pain perception and emotion. This can help with a feeling of relief and relaxation.

6. Muscle relaxation:

Essential oils with muscle-relaxing properties, such as basil and sweet marjoram, can help relieve tension headaches by reducing muscle tightness and promoting relaxation.

It's important to note that while essential oils can relieve headaches and migraines, their effectiveness may vary from person to person. What works for one person may not work for another. Additionally, some headaches may have an underlying medical cause that requires appropriate diagnosis and treatment. If you experience chronic or severe headaches, it is recommended that you consult a healthcare professional for appropriate guidance and management.

C. How to Use

There are several ways to use essential oils to relieve headaches effectively. Each method has its advantages and can be customized to your preferences and needs:

1. Local application:

* To create a safe and effective blend, Dilute your essential oil of choice in a carrier oil (such as coconut, almond, or jojoba).
* Apply the diluted mixture to the temples, forehead, and back of the neck, massaging gently in circular motions.
* You can also apply the mixture to your wrists or pulse points.

2. Inhalation:

* Inhaling essential oils can quickly and immediately impact your senses and mood.
* Add a few drops of your chosen essential oil to a tissue or handkerchief and inhale deeply.
* You can also add a few drops to a bowl of hot water, lean over the bowl, and cover your head with a towel to create a temporary steam inhalation.

3. Aromatherapy diffuser:

* Use an aromatherapy diffuser to disperse essential oils into the air, providing a lasting yet gentle scent.
* Fill a diffuser with water and add a few drops of essential oil.
* Turn on the diffuser and let it create a calming atmosphere.

4. Aromatherapy inhaler:

* Portable inhalers are a convenient way to take your chosen essential oil blend with you.
* Fill the essential oil blend into the aromatherapy inhaler tube and inhale through the nose as needed.

5. Hot compress:

* Apply heat to the forehead or back of the neck.
* Add a few drops of essential oil to the dressing for relief.

6. Soaking:

* Add a few drops of essential oil to your bath water for a soothing bath.
* Warm water and aromatic oils help relieve tension and promote relaxation.

7. Massage:

* Use dilutes essential oil for gentle massage. Massaging the neck, shoulders, and back can help relieve muscle tension and promote relaxation.

When topically applying essential oils, remember to start with a low dilution (usually 1 to 2%), especially for sensitive skin. Additionally, if you are new to using essential oils or are trying new ones, consider doing a patch test to check for any adverse reactions.

It's worth trying different methods to find what works best for you. A combination of the right essential oils, chosen application methods, and your personal preferences can significantly impact headache relief. If you experience chronic or severe headaches, it is recommended that you consult a healthcare professional for proper diagnosis and management.

Each method of using essential oils for headache relief has benefits and considerations. Knowing these can help you choose a method that suits your preferences and provides effective relief:

1. Local application:

* Benefits: Direct application allows the essential oil to be absorbed through the skin, potentially providing topical relief. Massaging the mixture

into the skin can also help relax tense muscles.

* Note: Dilution is essential to prevent skin irritation, especially for people with sensitive skin. Always conduct a patch test before applying to a larger area.

2. Inhalation:

* Benefits: Due to direct interactions with the olfactory system, inhaling essential oils can directly impact mood and headache symptoms.
* Caution: Although inhalation provides quick relief, the effects may be temporary. It's important to have essential oils available when needed.

3. Aromatherapy diffuser:

* Benefits: The diffuser provides continuous, gentle diffusion of essential oils, creating a calming atmosphere throughout the room.
* Caution: The aroma may not provide immediate relief from severe headaches. However, it may help relax and prevent stress-related headaches.

4. Aromatherapy inhaler:

* Benefits: The inhaler is portable and discreet for on-the-go relief. They provide concentrated doses of essential oils.
* Caution: Inhalers may not be effective for severe headaches. They are best used for mild headaches or as a preventive measure.

5. Hot compress:

* Benefits: Applying hot compresses with essential oils can help soothe tense muscles and provide localized relief.
* Note: This method may not be practical when you are away from home. It is best suited for relaxing at home during a headache attack.

6. Soaking:

* Benefits: Aromatherapy baths provide overall relaxation and help relieve muscle tension.
* Note: This method requires more time and may not be feasible during the day. It's more suitable for relaxing in the evening.

7. Massage:

* Benefits: Massage can provide overall relief by combining the benefits of touch and essential oils. It helps relax muscles and promotes overall health.

* Note: A professional massage therapist can provide more targeted relief, but self-massage can still be effective.

When choosing a method, consider your headache's severity, immediate environment, and personal preference. For acute headaches, inhalation or topical application may provide faster relief. For preventive care or relaxation, diffusers and baths are excellent options.

It's important to remember that individual reactions may vary. If you're new to using essential oils to treat headaches, start with a small amount and see how your body reacts. If you have a pre-existing medical condition or are taking medications, consult a healthcare professional before using essential oils. Additionally, maintain proper dilution ratios and follow safety guidelines to ensure a safe and effective experience.

D. Create a Soothing Mixture

Here are some headache relief blend recipes and suggestions using essential oils and carrier oils. Remember to patch-test any new mixture before applying it to a larger area of skin, and always dilute essential oils correctly.

1. Mint Cooling Mix:

* 2 drops of peppermint essential oil
* 2 drops of lavender essential oil
* 2 drops of eucalyptus essential oil
* 2 teaspoons carrier oil (such as jojoba or sweet almond oil)

Mix essential oils with a carrier oil in a roller bottle. Apply the mixture to your temples, forehead, and back of your neck. Gently massage the mixture into the skin.

2. Soothing Lavender Blend:

* 3 drops of lavender essential oil
* 2 drops of frankincense essential oil
* 2 teaspoons carrier oil

Mix essential oils with a carrier oil in a roller bottle. Apply the mixture to your temples, forehead, and wrists. Take a deep breath and enjoy the calming aroma.

3. Citrus Refreshing Blend:

* 2 drops of bergamot essential oil
* 2 drops of lemon essential oil
* 2 drops of peppermint essential oil
* 2 teaspoons carrier oil

Mix essential oils with a carrier oil in a roller bottle. Apply the mixture to your temples, forehead, and pulse points. The bright and uplifting aroma can help relieve tension.

4. Floral Relaxing Blend:

* 2 drops of chamomile essential oil
* 2 drops of ylang-ylang essential oil
* 2 drops of lavender essential oil
* 2 teaspoons carrier oil

Mix essential oils with a carrier oil in a roller bottle. Apply the mixture to your temples, forehead, and behind your ears. This blend is particularly calming and relaxing.

5. Customizable Mixing:

Feel free to customize your blend and choose the essential oils that resonate with you. Some options include ginger, rosemary, basil, and sage. Mix 2 to 3 essential oils with a carrier oil and use as needed.

Carrier oil options:
* Jojoba oil
* Sweet almond oil
* Coconut oil
* Grape seed oil

Application tips:
* Apply mixture to clean skin for better absorption.
* Gently massage the mixture into the temples, forehead, and other affected areas.

* Use a roller bottle for easy use on the go.
* Try different blends to find the one that works best for you.

Remember, the key is finding the blend that provides the most relief. Be patient and watch how your body reacts. If you experience any irritation, discontinue use and consult a healthcare professional.

E. Complementary Therapies for Headache Relief

Complementary therapies can be a great addition to using essential oils for headache relief. Here are some techniques you can consider using with essential oils:

1. Acupressure method:

Acupressure involves applying pressure to specific body areas to relieve pain and promote relaxation. There are a few acupuncture points that can help relieve headache symptoms. The most common acupoints for headaches are LI4 (between thumb and index finger) and GB20 (base of the skull). Gently massage these points and a headache-relieving essential oil blend for extra benefits.

2. Scalp and neck massage:

Gentle scalp and neck massage can help relax tense muscles and improve blood circulation. Apply a small amount of the headache relief mixture to your fingertips and massage in circular motions onto your scalp, temples, and neck. The combination of massage and essential oils can provide soothing relief.

3. Hot and cold therapy:

Applying hot or cold compresses to the affected area can help relieve headaches. You can use warm or cold washcloths, gel packs, or even a bag of frozen vegetables wrapped in a cloth. Apply your preferred temperature to the forehead, temples, or back of the neck. Add an essential oil blend of your choice to enhance the therapeutic effects.

4. Breathing techniques:

Deep breathing and relaxation techniques can help relieve headache symptoms by reducing stress and promoting relaxation. Practice slow, deep breathing as you inhale the aroma of the headache relief essential oil blend. Focus on each breath to calm the nervous system and relieve tension.

5. Hydrate and rest:

Staying hydrated and getting enough rest are crucial to managing headache symptoms. Drink plenty of water throughout the day, and make sure you get enough sleep. Combine these practices with your essential oil blends for a comprehensive approach to headache relief.

6. Yoga and stretching:

Gentle yoga poses and stretches can help release tension and improve blood flow. Incorporate poses that focus on stretching your neck, shoulders, and back. Enhance your yoga practice by diffusing your headache-relief essential oil blend around the room.

Remember, everyone's body responds differently to various treatments, so it's important to find the combination of techniques that works best for you. Pay attention to your body's signals and see a healthcare professional if your headache symptoms are severe or persistent.

Complementary therapies can enhance the effects of essential oils and help with relaxation and pain relief. When these approaches are combined, a synergistic effect addresses multiple aspects of headache symptoms. Here's how these treatments complement the use of essential oils:

1. Multimodal approach:

Headaches often have a variety of triggers and factors that contribute to their onset. A multimodal approach that combines essential oils with complementary therapies allows you to target different aspects of your headache symptoms. For example, while essential oils provide aromatherapy benefits and pain relief, acupressure or massage can help release muscle tension and improve circulation.

2. Enhance relaxation:

acupressure, massage, and cold / heat therapy promote relaxation by stimulating the body's natural relaxation response. The relaxing effect can be amplified when used with essential oils known for their calming properties, such as lavender and chamomile. This combination helps reduce stress and tension, which are common triggers of headaches.

3. Improve blood flow and circulation:

Massage, acupressure, and yoga/stretching techniques can improve blood flow and circulation. When combined with essential oils like peppermint or rosemary, which have vasodilatory properties, blood vessels can relax and dilate more effectively. This can relieve tension and reduce the severity of headaches.

4. Address physical and emotional issues:

Headaches can have physical and emotional components. Essential oils can address the emotional aspect by promoting relaxation and reducing stress and anxiety. Complementary therapies, on the other hand, directly target physical tension and discomfort. You can create a holistic approach to headache relief by addressing both of these areas.

5. Personalized relief:

Everyone responds to treatment differently. By combining essential oils with various supplementation techniques, you can customize the best approach for you. This customization increases the likelihood of finding effective relief that suits your unique needs.

6. The effect is longer lasting:

While essential oils can provide immediate relief through aromatherapy, the effects of complementary therapies can often have a longer-lasting impact. Techniques like acupressure and massage can help release muscle tension and promote prolonged relaxation, helping to provide lasting relief.

It is important to note that these complementary therapies should be used in a way that is consistent with your preferences and any health concerns you may have. If you are unsure about incorporating any of these therapies, it is recommended that you consult a healthcare professional before making any major changes to your daily routine. By combining the power of essential oils with these complementary techniques, you can create a comprehensive and holistic approach to managing and relieving headache symptoms.

F. Lifestyle Changes and Prevention

Lifestyle changes and preventive measures are important in managing headaches and reducing their frequency. Here are some key aspects to consider:

1. Stress management:

Stress is a common trigger of headaches. Practicing stress-reduction techniques such as meditation, deep breathing, progressive muscle relaxation, and yoga can help manage stress and reduce the likelihood of headaches. Essential oils such as lavender and frankincense can complement these practices by promoting relaxation.

2. Hydration:

Dehydration can lead to headaches, so staying well hydrated is crucial. Make sure you drink enough water throughout the day, and consider infusing your water with a drop or two of citrus essential oils like lemon or orange for added flavor and potential benefits.

3. Sleep hygiene:

Lack of sleep can trigger headaches in some people. Establishing regular sleep habits, maintaining a comfortable sleep environment, and avoiding caffeine and electronic devices before bed can improve sleep quality. Essential oils like lavender and chamomile can be used in aromatherapy or as part of a nighttime routine to promote better sleep.

4. Dietary precautions:

Certain foods and additives can trigger headaches in susceptible people. Common culprits include processed foods, caffeine, alcohol, and artificial sweeteners. Keeping a food diary to identify potential triggers and eating a balanced, whole-food diet can help manage headaches.

5. Regular physical exercise:

Regular physical activity can help reduce the frequency and severity of headaches. Exercise promotes better blood flow, releases endorphins (natural painkillers), and helps manage stress. Essential oils with uplifting scents, such as peppermint, can be used before or after exercise to enhance the experience.

6. Avoid known triggers:

Identifying and avoiding specific triggers that have caused headaches in the past can significantly reduce their occurrence. These triggers can vary from person to person and may include specific foods, strong odors, bright lights, and certain environmental factors.

7. Caffeine management:

While caffeine can temporarily relieve some headaches, it can trigger or worsen headaches in others due to withdrawal or overuse. Moderation is key. If you regularly consume caffeine, consider gradually reducing your intake to avoid potential withdrawal headaches.

8. Regular eye care:

Eyestrain can lead to tension headaches. Make sure you have proper lighting when reading or working on a screen, take regular breaks to rest your eyes, and consider using a blue light filter if you spend much time on electronic devices.

9. Mindful breathing and relaxation:

Practicing mindful breathing exercises throughout the day can help reduce tension and stress and help prevent headaches. Essential oils such as lavender or bergamot can be added to these practices to increase relaxation.

10. Professional help:

If your headaches are frequent or severe, consult a healthcare professional to rule out underlying conditions and get personalized guidance.

Remember, preventive measures may take time to show results, so patience and consistency are key. Integrating essential oils and relaxation techniques into these lifestyle changes can create a holistic approach to managing headaches and improving overall health.

Essential oils can be valuable in supporting overall health and preventing headaches. Their natural properties can help address various factors contributing to headaches and promote balance and relaxation. Here's how essential oils can help with headache prevention and health:

1. Relax and reduce stress:

Many essential oils, such as lavender, chamomile, and frankincense, are known for their calming and stress-relieving properties. Inhaling these oils through a diffuser, personal inhaler, or aromatherapy can help reduce stress and tension, common triggers of headaches.

2. Improve sleep quality:

Essential oils like lavender, cedarwood, and bergamot can be used to create a soothing bedtime environment to promote better sleep. Adequate sleep is vital to overall health and can significantly affect headache frequency.

3. Relieve pain and relax muscles:

Essential oils like peppermint and eucalyptus contain compounds with analgesic and anti-inflammatory properties. Applying diluted oils to tense muscles or using them in a massage can help relieve muscle tension and discomfort that may lead to headaches.

4. Mood enhancement:

Citrus oils like lemon, orange, and grapefruit are known for their uplifting and mood-enhancing effects. Creating a positive environment with these oils helps with emotional well-being and reduces the likelihood of stress-induced headaches.

5. Improve blood circulation:

Essential oils like rosemary and ginger have properties that can improve blood circulation. Enhanced blood circulation can help prevent blood vessel-related headaches by ensuring proper blood flow to the brain.

6. Inhalation technique:

Inhalation methods, such as inhaling directly from the bottle or using a personal inhaler, can provide quick relief during a headache attack. Oils like peppermint and eucalyptus have a cooling sensation and can help relieve discomfort.

7. Aromatherapy diffuser:

Diffusing essential oils in your living or workspace can create a calming and supportive atmosphere. Applying oils like lavender or a headache-relieving blend regularly can help create an environment that minimizes stress and tension.

8. Regular self-care:

Incorporating essential oils into your self-care routine, such as through a relaxing bath, massage, or mindfulness practice, can aid overall health. Taking time for yourself can reduce stress and prevent headaches.

9. Mind-body connection:

Aromatherapy and essential oils can promote a mind-body connection that encourages relaxation and self-awareness. This connection can help you identify and address triggers before they lead to headaches.

10. Consistency:

Consistently using essential oils in your daily routine can help with long-term health and prevent headaches. Consider incorporating them into your morning and evening rituals or use them during stressful times throughout the day.

Remember that individuals may respond differently to essential oils, so finding the oil and method that works best for you is important. Additionally, if you are experiencing chronic or severe headaches, it is recommended to consult a healthcare professional to rule out underlying conditions.

After this chapter, we highlight the potential benefits of using natural remedies, such as essential oils, to relieve headaches and migraines in men. By incorporating essential oils into their headache management strategy, men can find relief from headache symptoms, reduce their impact on daily life, and improve their overall health. However, it is important to remember that individual experiences may vary, and consultation with a healthcare professional is recommended for persistent or severe headaches.

7.2 Relieve Back and Neck Discomfort

In this chapter, we will explore the topic of soothing back and neck discomfort in men. We discuss common causes of back and neck pain, its impact on daily life, and guide on using natural remedies, including essential oils, to relieve discomfort and promote relief.

A. Understanding Back and Neck Discomfort

Back and neck pain in men can stem from a variety of factors, and understanding these common causes is crucial to effectively addressing and managing discomfort:

1. Muscle tension: Prolonged sitting, repetitive movements, and over-exertion can cause back and neck muscle tension, causing pain and discomfort.

2. Poor posture: Poor posture when sitting or standing can strain the muscles and ligaments in the back and neck, causing pain and stiffness.

3. Physical strain: Lifting heavy objects, making sudden movements, or engaging in activities without proper form can strain muscles and ligaments, causing pain.

4. Stress: Emotional stress and tension can cause back and neck muscle tightness and discomfort.

5. Inactive lifestyle: Lack of regular exercise and physical activity can weaken the muscles that support the back and neck, leading to pain.

6. Age-related changes: As men age, the spine's discs and joints degenerate, leading to pain and reduced flexibility.

7. Injuries: Accidents, falls, or sports injuries can cause trauma to the back and neck, causing pain.

8. Medical conditions: Conditions such as a herniated disc, spinal stenosis, or arthritis can cause chronic back and neck pain.

9. Occupational factors: Certain occupations that involve repetitive movements, lifting weights, or sitting for long periods can cause back and neck pain.

10. Sleeping habits: Using an unsupportive pillow or mattress or sleeping in awkward positions can lead to neck pain.

Identifying the underlying cause of back and neck pain is important to determine the most appropriate relief and prevention methods. Combining strategies, including exercise, proper ergonomics, stress management, and targeted therapy, can help effectively relieve and manage pain.

Back and neck discomfort can significantly impact every aspect of a man's daily life and overall health. Here are some of the ways this discomfort can affect individuals:

1. Physical limitations: Back and neck pain can limit a person's range of motion, making it difficult to perform daily tasks such as bending, lifting, and even turning the head. This can affect a person's ability to carry out work, household chores, and recreational activities.

2. Productivity: Chronic back and neck pain can lead to decreased productivity at work due to difficulty concentrating, moving around, or sitting for long periods. This can impact job performance and career progression.

3. Sleep quality: Pain can disrupt sleep patterns and make finding a comfortable sleeping position challenging. Poor sleep quality can lead to fatigue, irritability, and an overall decreased sense of well-being.

4. Emotional health: Ongoing pain can take a toll on mental health, causing feelings of depression, anxiety, and stress. Emotional stress may further exacerbate the perception of pain.

5. Physical fitness: Pain can prevent men from engaging in physical activity, leading to reduced fitness and potential weight gain. This, in turn, can lead to a cycle of reduced mobility and increased discomfort.

6. Social activities: Persistent pain can make participating in social gatherings, hobbies, and recreational activities difficult. This can lead to social isolation and reduced quality of life.

7. Relationships: Back and neck pain can strain relationships because pain management may affect a person's mood and ability to participate in shared activities or responsibilities.

8. Self-esteem: Chronic pain can affect self-confidence and self-esteem due to limitations in physical abilities and appearance-related issues.

9. Everyday comfort: Basic activities like sitting at a desk, driving, or even eating can become uncomfortable due to back and neck pain.

10. Long-term effects: If not appropriately managed, unresolved back and neck discomfort can lead to chronic problems and more serious illnesses.

Given the far-reaching effects of back and neck discomfort, it's important to take a proactive approach to pain management, seek appropriate medical guidance, and adopt strategies to help relieve discomfort and improve overall health.

B. Essential Oils to Soothe Back and Neck Discomfort

Several essential oils are known for their potential to relieve back and neck pain. These oils can provide analgesic, anti-inflammatory, and muscle-relaxing properties to help relieve discomfort and promote relaxation. Here are some essential oils commonly used for this purpose:

1. Peppermint: Peppermint oil contains menthol, which has a cooling and analgesic effect. It can help relieve muscle tension and reduce pain. Mix a few drops of peppermint oil with carrier oil and apply it to the affected area for relief.

2. Lavender: Lavender oil is known for its calming and anti-inflammatory properties. It can help relax muscles and reduce pain and tension. Dilute lavender oil and apply it to the affected area or relax in a warm bath.

3. Eucalyptus: Eucalyptus oil contains compounds with anti-inflammatory and analgesic effects. It relieves muscle and joint pain. Mix eucalyptus oil with a carrier oil and massage it into the painful area.

4. Ginger: Ginger oil has warming properties that can help improve blood circulation and reduce muscle pain and inflammation. Mix ginger oil with a carrier oil and gently massage the painful area.

5. Marjoram: Marjoram oil is known for its muscle relaxant and analgesic properties. It can be used to relieve muscle spasms and tension. Dilute marjoram oil and massage it into the affected area.

6. Chamomile: Chamomile oil has anti-inflammatory and calming properties that can help relieve muscle pain and tension. Use chamomile oil in a hot compress or dilute it with a carrier oil for massage.

7. Rosemary: Rosemary oil has analgesic and anti-inflammatory properties that can help reduce pain and promote blood circulation. Mix rosemary oil with a carrier oil and use it in massage.

8. Black pepper: Black pepper oil contains warming compounds that can help relieve muscle stiffness and pain. Mix black pepper oil with carrier oil and apply it to the affected area.

When using essential oils to relieve back and neck pain, it's important to dilute them appropriately with a carrier oil before applying them to your skin. Also, do a patch test to ensure you have no adverse reactions to the oil. If you have any underlying health conditions or are taking medications, it is recommended that you consult a healthcare professional before using essential oils for pain relief.

Let's delve into the properties of essential oils commonly used to relieve back and neck pain:

1. Peppermint oil:

* Analgesic: Peppermint oil contains menthol, which has a cooling and numbing effect on the skin. It can help reduce pain by reducing pain signals and promoting a sense of relief.
* Anti-inflammatory: The anti-inflammatory properties of peppermint oil can help reduce inflammation in muscles and joints, helping to relieve pain.
* Muscle Relaxant: The muscle-relaxing properties of peppermint oil can help relieve muscle spasms and tension, which often lead to back and neck pain.

2. Lavender oil:

* Pain relief: Lavender oil has mild analgesic properties that can help relieve pain and discomfort by reducing pain signals.
* Anti-inflammatory: The anti-inflammatory properties of lavender can help reduce swelling and inflammation in the affected area, helping to relieve pain.
* Calming: The calming aroma of lavender oil also helps reduce stress

and tension, which can exacerbate muscle discomfort.

3. Eucalyptus oil:

* Analgesic: Eucalyptus oil contains compounds with analgesic properties, such as eucalyptol, which help numb and reduce pain sensations.
* Anti-inflammatory: Eucalyptus oil's anti-inflammatory properties can help reduce inflammation and relieve pain in sore muscles and joints.
* Enhance blood circulation: The warming effect of eucalyptus oil can improve blood circulation, aiding in healing and pain relief.

4. Ginger oil:

* Analgesic: Ginger oil contains gingerol, a compound with analgesic properties that can help relieve muscle and joint discomfort.
* Anti-inflammatory: Ginger oil's anti-inflammatory properties help reduce inflammation-related pain.
* Warming: The warming effect of ginger oil enhances blood flow to the affected area, which can help relieve pain and tension.

5. Marjoram Oil:

* Muscle relaxant: Marjoram oil is known for its muscle-relaxing properties, helping to relieve muscle spasms and tension that cause pain.
* Analgesics: Marjoram's analgesic properties can relieve pain and discomfort by attenuating pain signals.
* Anti-inflammatory: Its anti-inflammatory properties can help reduce inflammation and relieve pain and swelling.

6. Chamomile Oil:

* Anti-inflammatory: The anti-inflammatory properties of chamomile oil can help reduce inflammation and pain in muscles and joints.
* Muscle relaxant: Chamomile's muscle relaxant properties help relieve muscle tension and discomfort.
* Calming: The soothing aroma of chamomile promotes relaxation and can indirectly relieve pain caused by stress and tension.

7. Rosemary Oil:

* Analgesia: Rosemary oil contains compounds such as rosmarinic acid, which have analgesic properties and can relieve pain.

* Anti-inflammatory: Rosemary's anti-inflammatory properties can help reduce inflammation-related pain.
* Enhance blood circulation: The warming properties of rosemary oil improve blood circulation, helping with pain relief and healing.

8. Black pepper oil:

* Analgesia: Black pepper oil contains piperine, which can have an analgesic effect and reduce pain.
* Warming: Its warming effect enhances blood circulation and relieves muscle tension and soreness.
* Anti-inflammatory: The anti-inflammatory properties of black pepper oil help reduce pain and inflammation.

These essential oils can be used alone or mixed with a carrier oil for massage or other application methods. Their combined properties make them an effective natural choice for managing back and neck pain. However, it is important to remember that individual reactions to essential oils may vary, so if you have an underlying health condition or are taking medications, a patch test and consultation with a healthcare professional are recommended.

C. How to Use

Here's an overview of the different ways you can use essential oils to relieve back and neck pain:

1. Local application:

* Dilute your essential oil of choice in a carrier oil such as coconut, jojoba, or almond oil. A common dilution ratio is about 2 to 3% (10 to 15 drops of essential oil per 1 ounce of carrier oil).
* Gently massage the diluted essential oil into the affected area, focusing on the muscles and joints causing pain.
* This method allows the essential oils to penetrate the skin and provide topical relief.

2. Massage:

* Mix your choice of essential oils with a carrier oil to create a massage blend.
* Apply the mixture to your back and neck or ask a partner to help

massage.

    * Massage can help increase blood circulation, relax tense muscles, and provide the therapeutic properties of essential oils.

    3. Hot compress:

    * Add a few drops of essential oil of your choice to warm water.
    * Soak a clean cloth in water, wring it out, and apply a hot compress to the affected area.
    * This method combines the benefits of heat and aromatherapy to relax muscles and relieve pain.

    4. Bathing:

    * Add 5 to 10 drops of essential oil of your choice to a warm bath.
    * Swirl the water to disperse the oil evenly.
    * Soak in the bathtub for 15 to 20 minutes to allow the oil to penetrate and provide relaxation.

    5. Aromatherapy diffuser:

    * Use an aromatherapy diffuser to diffuse your favorite essential oils.
    * Inhaling aromatic molecules can have a calming and pain-relieving effect and contribute to overall relaxation.

    6. Inhalation:

    * Inhale directly from the bottle or place a few drops on a tissue or cotton ball and inhale deeply.
    * This method provides quick and effective immediate relief, especially while traveling.

    7. Ball mixing:

    * Add essential oils to a roller bottle and top with carrier oil to create a roll-on mixture.
    * Roll the mixture into the back of your neck and other tight areas.

    8. Acupoints:

    * Apply diluted essential oils to specific points on the body to relieve pain.

* Gently pressing these acupoints and essential oils can enhance the pain relief effect.

9. Hot/cold compress:

* Add a few drops of essential oil to hot or cold water, soak a cloth, and apply to the affected area.
* Alternating temperatures can help relax muscles and reduce inflammation.

Remember, it's important to patch-test diluted essential oils on a small area of your skin to check for any adverse reactions before applying it to a larger area. Additionally, if you have an underlying health condition or are taking medications, please consult a healthcare professional, especially if you are considering using essential oils for pain management.

Here's a breakdown of the benefits and considerations for each method of using essential oils to relieve back and neck pain:

1. Local application:

* Benefits: Targeted relief to specific areas of pain, allows dosage control, and can be easily incorporated into daily life.
* Caution: Some essential oils may cause skin irritation, so performing a patch test and using the appropriate dilution ratio is important.

2. Massage:

* Benefits: Combines the benefits of aromatherapy with physical contact to promote relaxation, enhance blood circulation, and help release muscle tension.
* Note: Requires someone to perform the massage and may not be suitable for people with sensitive or injured skin.

3. Hot compress:

* Benefits: Combines heat therapy with aromatherapy to achieve deep relaxation, improve blood flow, and relieve muscle soreness.
* Note: A warm water source is required, and the heat may not be suitable for certain conditions such as inflammation.

4. Bathing:

* Efficacy: Relax the whole body, and the water's warmth enhances the essential oils' effect, facilitating pain relief in multiple areas.
* Note: As the tub may be accessible, it may not be suitable for everyone, and the water temperature should be comfortable.

5. Aromatherapy Diffuser:

Benefits: Diffusing essential oils in the air provides long-lasting therapeutic benefits for relaxation and pain relief.
* Note: This method is more indirect and may not be as concentrated as a direct topical application.

6. Inhalation:

* Benefits: Fast and effective instant relief, perfect for use on the go.
* Note: Does not provide long-lasting results as applied topically or diffused.

7. Ball mixing:

* Advantages: Convenient and portable method, can be applied to the uncomfortable area accurately.
* Note: Roller bottles can leak or break if not handled properly.

8. Acupoints:

* Benefits: Combining aromatherapy with acupressure may enhance pain relief.
* Note: You must know the acupuncture points and their corresponding oils.

9. Hot/cold compress:

* Benefits: Provides the benefits of thermotherapy and aromatherapy, suitable for resolving pain and inflammation.
* Note: Requires hot or cold water; temperature preference may vary.

Each method has its advantages, and the choice depends on personal preference, available resources, and the severity of the pain. Listening to your body's reactions and adjusting your approach as needed is important. If you have an underlying health condition or concerns, it is recommended that you consult a healthcare professional before using essential oils for pain relief.

D. Create Soothing Blends and Massage Oils

Here are some personalized blends and massage oil recommendations using essential oils and carrier oils to help relieve back and neck pain:

Mint Cooling Relief Blend:

* 5 drops of peppermint essential oil
* 5 drops of eucalyptus essential oil
* 5 drops of lavender essential oil
* 2 tablespoons jojoba or coconut oil

Mix the essential oils with the carrier oil of your choice in a small glass bottle. Apply a small amount to the affected area and massage gently.

Soothing Lavender Massage Oil:

* 10 drops of lavender essential oil
* 5 drops of Roman Chamomile essential oil
* 2 tablespoons sweet almond oil or grapeseed oil

Mix essential oils with carrier oil and store them in dark glass bottles. Apply oil to the back and neck and massage gently.

Eucalyptus Soaking Bath:

* 8 drops of eucalyptus essential oil
* 6 drops of peppermint essential oil
* 4 drops of rosemary essential oil
* 1 cup Epsom salt

Mix essential oils with Epsom salt in a bowl. Add the mixture to a warm water bath and soak for 20 to 30 minutes to relax your muscles.

Hot compress mixture:

* 4 drops of ginger essential oil
* 4 drops of frankincense essential oil
* 4 drops of cypress essential oil

* 2 tablespoons jojoba or coconut oil

Mix essential oils with a carrier oil and apply a few drops as a warm compress. Apply the dressing to the affected area for soothing relief.

Remember to do a patch test before using any new mixture to make sure you're not sensitive to the oil. Additionally, the dilution ratio can be adjusted to your preference and skin sensitivity. If pain persists or worsens, consult a health care professional.

Proper dilution of essential oils is critical to ensure safety and avoid skin sensitization. Essential oils are highly concentrated, and applying directly to the skin without diluting them can cause irritation or adverse reactions. Diluting an essential oil in a carrier oil helps disperse the potency of the essential oil, making it safer to use.

Here are some general guidelines for dilution ratios:

1. Normal dilution (2%): This is the standard dilution for most adults. It involves adding approximately 12 drops of essential oil to 1 ounce (30 ml) of carrier oil.

2. Sensitive skin or facial use (1%): For more sensitive areas like the face, you can use a 1% dilution if you have sensitive skin. This will be approximately 6 drops of essential oil to 1 ounce of carrier oil.

3. Specific needs (3% or 5%): If you are dealing with a specific problem, such as acute pain, you may use a slightly higher dilution of 3% to 5%.

4. Children and the elderly (0.5% to 1%): For children, the elderly, or those with compromised immune systems, lower dilutions such as 0.5% to 1% are often recommended.

When choosing essential oils to relieve back and neck pain, consider the following factors:

* Types of pain: Different oils may be better suited for different types of pain. For example, analgesic oils like peppermint and wintergreen can provide cooling relief, while anti-inflammatory oils like eucalyptus and ginger can help relieve muscle tension.

* Personal preference: Choose an essential oil you like the scent of, as

aromatherapy can relieve pain. The scent of lavender may be soothing, while the uplifting scent of rosemary may help focus your mind during the massage.

* Symptoms: Think about the specific symptoms you are experiencing. If inflammation is a major issue, look for anti-inflammatory oils. If tension is a major problem, consider an oil with muscle-relaxing properties.

* Skin sensitivities: Some essential oils are more likely to cause skin sensitivities than others. Always do a patch test before using the new oil and dilute it more if you have sensitive skin.

Everyone's body is different, so what works for one person may not work for another. It's best to start with a lower dilution and gradually increase it if necessary. If you're unsure which oils to use or how to dilute them correctly, consult a qualified aromatherapist or healthcare professional.

E. Gentle Stretches and Exercises

Gentle stretches and exercises can help relieve back and neck discomfort. However, we must emphasize that if you are experiencing severe pain, it is important to consult a healthcare professional before attempting any exercise. Here are some general stretches and exercises you may find beneficial:

Neck discomfort:

1. Neck tilt:
Gently tilt your head to one side and bring your ears closer to your shoulders. Hold for 15 to 30 seconds. Repeat on the other side.

2. Neck rotation:
Turn your head to the side and look over your shoulder. Hold for 15 to 30 seconds. Repeat on the other side.

3. Chin fold:
Sit up straight and gently tuck your chin toward your chest. You should feel a stretch in the back of your neck.

Back discomfort:

1. Cat-Cow stretch:

Start on your hands and knees. As you exhale, arch your back upward (like a cat). Then, bring your belly toward the floor, lifting your head (like a cow) as you inhale. Repeat this movement slowly for a few rounds.

2. Child's posture:

Kneel on the floor and sit back on your heels. Extend your arms on the floor, bringing your chest toward the ground while keeping your hips over your heels.

3. Knee to chest stretch:

Lie on your back and bring one knee toward your chest while keeping the other leg straight. Gently hold your knees and feel the stretch in your lower back. Change legs.

4. Hamstring stretch:

Lie on your back and lift one leg, keeping it straight. Use your hands to pull the legs toward you gently. You should feel a stretch in the back of your legs.

Remember, these stretches should not cause pain. You should feel a slight stretch or mild discomfort but not severe pain. If any stretching worsens your discomfort, stop immediately. Incorporate these stretches into your daily routine gradually and consistently, and consider combining them with essential oil aromatherapy or topical application to enhance relaxation and relieve pain.

Stretching and strengthening play a vital role in promoting flexibility, relieving tension, and preventing future back and neck pain. Here are their contributions:

Stretch:

1. Flexibility: Regular stretching helps improve flexibility, which reduces stiffness and increases the range of motion of muscles and joints.

2. Relieve Tension: Stretching exercises help relax tight muscles and relieve tension and discomfort caused by knotted and stiff muscles.

3. Improve blood circulation: Stretching increases blood flow to mus-

cles, helping to reduce muscle soreness and promote healing.

4. Posture Improvement: Proper stretching can improve posture by targeting muscles that may have been shortened or tightened due to bad habits.

Reinforcement:

1. Muscle Support: Strengthening exercises target the muscles around the spine and neck to provide better support and stability to these areas.

2. Prevention: Strong muscles are less likely to develop strains and injuries. Strengthening helps prevent future pain and discomfort.

3. Posture improvement: Strong core muscles help improve posture and reduce stress on the back and neck.

4. Muscle balance: Strengthening exercise promotes muscle balance, which can help relieve imbalances that cause pain.

Combine stretching and strengthening:

The combination of stretching and strengthening is particularly effective:

1. Pre-strengthening stretches: Stretching before a strengthening workout helps warm up your muscles, making them more receptive to strengthening exercises.

2. Post-strengthening stretches: Post-strengthening stretches help lengthen and relax muscles that may have contracted during exercise.

3. Balance and flexibility: Building strength and flexibility creates a balanced and functional musculoskeletal system.

Remember, consistency is key. Gradually increase the intensity and duration of your stretching and strengthening routine. It's also important to listen to your body - don't push too hard or force movements that cause pain. If you have any existing medical conditions or concerns, please consult a healthcare professional or physical therapist before starting a new exercise regimen.

Integrating essential oils and aromatherapy into your stretching and strengthening routine can further enhance the experience. Oils such as peppermint, eucalyptus, and lavender can provide relaxation and focus during practice. Additionally, using essential oils during massage or diluted topical applications can help muscles recover and relax after exercise.

F. Posture and Ergonomics

Proper posture and ergonomics are crucial to preventing and managing back and neck pain. Here's why:

Correct posture:

1. Spinal alignment: Good posture aligns the spine with its natural curve, reducing stress on spinal structures and preventing strains.

2. Muscle balance: Correct posture ensures that the muscles effectively support the spine and maintain balance, reducing the risk of overuse or strain.

3. Prevention: Maintaining correct posture can help prevent muscle imbalances, joint problems, and chronic pain conditions caused by poor posture.

4. Reduce stress: Proper posture can reduce stress on ligaments, joints, and soft tissues, reducing discomfort and improving overall function.

Ergonomics:

1. Workplace comfort: Ergonomic adjustments to the workspace (such as chair height, keyboard position, and monitor position) support neutral body alignment and minimize stress during prolonged sitting.

2. Reduce strain injuries: Proper ergonomics reduce stress on muscles, tendons, and joints, helping to prevent repetitive strain injuries and discomfort.

3. Spine-health: Ergonomically designed furniture and equipment promote spinal health by minimizing awkward postures and maintaining proper alignment.

4. Efficiency: An ergonomic setup improves your efficiency and focus because you are less likely to feel discomfort that distracts you from your task.

Combine posture and ergonomics:

1. Awareness: Paying attention to your posture throughout the day, whether sitting, standing, or walking, is the first step to maintaining good alignment.

2. Ergonomic adjustments: Set up your workspace, including your desk, chair, and computer, to promote proper posture and reduce stress.

3. Frequent exercise: Avoid sitting or standing for long periods. Take breaks to stretch, change positions, and move around to prevent muscle stiffness.

4. Exercise: Regular physical activity, including stretching and strengthening exercises, supports good posture by maintaining muscle flexibility and balance.

5. Sleeping position: Maintain proper spinal alignment while sleeping using a supportive mattress and pillow that matches your preferred sleeping position.

6. Mindfulness: Practicing mindfulness of body alignment during daily activities helps reinforce good posture and ergonomics.

Incorporating essential oils into your daily routine can enhance your focus on posture and ergonomics. Oils like lavender, eucalyptus, and rosemary can provide refreshing scents that help you pay attention to your body's alignment. Using these oils in a diffuser in your workspace can create an environment that promotes focus and relaxation, supporting you in maintaining correct posture and ergonomics.

Here are tips and suggestions for improving posture during a variety of activities:

Sit:

1. Use a supportive chair: Choose a chair that provides adequate lumbar support and encourages neutral spine alignment.

2. Feet on the floor: Keep your feet flat on the floor or a footstool to maintain a comfortable and balanced sitting posture.

3. Knees and hips: Align your knees with your hips and maintain a 90-degree angle. Avoid crossing your legs for long periods.

4. Monitor position: Place your computer monitor at eye level to avoid straining your neck or leaning forward.

5. Keyboard and mouse: Hold the keyboard and mouse close to your body with your wrists in a neutral position.

Stand:

1. Weight distribution: Distribute your weight evenly between your feet to prevent excessive pressure on one side.

2. Exercise core muscles: Gently exercise core muscles to support the spine and maintain a more stable posture.

3. Shoulders back: Roll your shoulders back and down to avoid sagging or rounding your upper back.

4. Neutral spine: Maintain the spine's natural curve when standing. Avoid leaning forward or backward too much.

Promote:

1. Hip and knee bend: When lifting an object, squat down with your hips and knees instead of bending over.

2. Keep objects close: Keep objects close to your body when lifting to reduce pressure on your back.

3. Engage your core: Tighten your core muscles before lifting to stabilize your spine and protect your lower back.

4. Avoid twisting: Avoid twisting your body when lifting. Instead, turn your feet to face the direction you're moving.

5. Lift with legs: Use the strength of your leg muscles to lift instead of straining your back.

Additional tips:

1. Stretch breaks: Take short breaks to stretch and move around. Perform gentle neck, shoulder, and back stretching exercises.

2. Mindful awareness: Check your posture regularly during the day. Adjust as necessary to maintain proper alignment.

3. Postural exercises: Include exercises that strengthen core, back, and neck muscles to support better posture.

4. Use a mirror: Use a mirror to evaluate your posture and correct it if necessary.

5. Ergonomic accessories: Consider using lumbar pillows, ergonomic chairs, and posture reminder tools to support healthy alignment.

6. Posture reminders: Set reminders on your phone or computer to prompt you to check and adjust your posture throughout the day.

Remember, practicing good posture consistently is key to preventing discomfort and promoting overall health. Incorporating essential oils, such as those with an uplifting scent (like citrus) or a calming scent (like lavender), into your environment can help create a calming atmosphere and encourage mindful postures. Using these oils in a diffuser or inhaling them directly can remind you to pay attention to your body's alignment and make posture improvement a part of your daily routine.

G. Lifestyle Changes and Self-care

Here are some lifestyle changes and self-care practices that can support back and neck health:

1. Stress management:

Chronic stress can cause muscle tension and worsen back and neck discomfort. Incorporate stress-reduction techniques such as deep breathing, meditation, yoga, or mindfulness to help relax muscles and relieve tension.

2. Exercise regularly:

Engage in regular physical activity to strengthen the muscles that support your back and neck. Focus on exercises that improve core strength, flexibility, and posture, such as yoga, Pilates, and strength training.

3. Proper nutrition:

Maintain a balanced diet rich in essential nutrients, including vitamins and minerals that support bone health. Getting enough calcium, vitamin D, and magnesium can help strengthen bones and reduce the risk of spinal problems.

4. Hydration:

Staying hydrated helps with the health of your spinal discs and joints. Drink plenty of water throughout the day to keep your body hydrated.

5. Get enough rest:

Make sure you get enough sleep on a supportive mattress and pillow. Quality sleep allows your muscles to recover and supports overall health.

6. Ergonomic workspace:

Whether at home or in the office, set up your workspace ergonomically. Use an adjustable chair, proper keyboard and mouse placement, and a monitor at eye level to reduce stress on your back and neck.

7. To lift correctly:

Practice proper lifting techniques to prevent back and neck tension. Bend at your hips and knees, engage your core, and keep the object close to your body as you lift.

8. Maintain a healthy weight:

Being overweight can strain the spine and worsen back and neck pain. Maintain a healthy weight by eating a balanced diet and exercising regularly.

9. Stay active:

Avoid long periods of inactivity. Take breaks to move and stretch when sitting or standing for long periods.

10. Postural awareness:

Pay attention to your posture throughout the day. Practice sitting, standing, and moving with your back straight, shoulders relaxed, and neck in a neutral position.

11. Stretching program:

Incorporate regular stretching into your exercise routine to keep muscles flexible and prevent stiffness. Gentle neck and back stretches can help relieve tension.

12. Warm up before the activity:

Before engaging in physical activity or exercise, take a few minutes to warm up your muscles with light movements or stretches.

13. Consult a professional:

If you are experiencing chronic or severe back and neck pain, please consult a healthcare professional. They can provide personalized guidance, diagnose any potential problems, and recommend appropriate treatment or therapy.

Remember, a combination of these practices can help improve back and neck health and reduce the risk of discomfort. Essential oils can complement your self-care routine, helping to relax and provide a soothing atmosphere. However, if you experience persistent or worsening pain, it is important to seek medical care to address any underlying issues.

Essential oils promote relaxation, reduce stress, and support overall health through their aromatic and therapeutic properties. Here's how essential oils can help in these areas:

1. Aromatherapy and emotional wellbeing:

Inhaling essential oils directly impacts the limbic system, which is responsible for mood, memory, and emotions. The aromas of essential oils like lavender, chamomile, and bergamot have been shown to stimulate the release of neurotransmitters like serotonin and dopamine, promoting feelings of relaxation and well-being.

2. Stress reduction:

Certain essential oils, such as lavender, rose, and frankincense, has calming properties that can help reduce stress and anxiety. Inhaling these oils or using them in relaxation techniques can induce a state of relaxation, reduce cortisol levels (the stress hormone), and help combat stress's physical and emotional effects.

3. Improve sleep quality:

Lavender, chamomile, and cedarwood essential oils are known for their calming properties. Diffusing these oils or using them in your bedtime ritual can help create a relaxing environment, ease your mind, and improve the quality of your sleep.

4. Mood enhancement:

Citrus oils like orange, lemon, and grapefruit are known for their uplifting and uplifting scents. These oils can help improve mood and increase feelings of positivity. Inhaling or incorporating these oils into your environment is especially beneficial during times of stress or low energy.

5. Mindfulness and meditation:

Using essential oils in mindfulness practices and meditation can enhance the overall experience. Scents like sandalwood, patchouli, and vetiver are grounding and can help you achieve a more focused and focused state during meditation.

6. Relaxation techniques:

Essential oils can enhance various relaxation techniques, such as deep breathing, meditation, and progressive muscle relaxation. Inhaling calming oils during these exercises can deepen relaxation and enhance the effectiveness of stress-reducing techniques.

7. Calm the nervous system:

Certain essential oils have adaptogenic properties that can help balance the nervous system's response to stress. Oils like sage, bergamot, and Roman chamomile can promote relaxation while maintaining alertness.

8. Aromatherapy diffuser:

in your living or workspace to create a soothing atmosphere. Diffusers disperse oils into the air, allowing you to inhale their beneficial molecules. This method is particularly effective for relaxing and reducing stress.

9. Massage and bath:

Using essential oils in massage oil, bath salts, or bath oils can directly impact the mind and body. Massaging with diluted essential oils can relieve muscle tension and induce relaxation while adding essential oils to your bathtub can create a peaceful bathing experience.

10. Personalized wellness ritual:

Creating a routine involving essential oils to relax and reduce stress can help anchor positive habits and create a sense of routine in your daily life.

Keep in mind that individuals may react differently to essential oils, so it's essential to experiment and find the scent and technique that works best for you. Whether you choose to diffuse, inhale, apply topically, or incorporate essential oils into a variety of relaxation practices, they can be a powerful tool to promote relaxation, reduce stress, and support overall well-being.

After this chapter, we highlight the potential benefits of using natural remedies, such as essential oils, to relieve back and neck discomfort in men. By incorporating essential oils into their self-care routine and implementing lifestyle changes, men can relieve back and neck pain, improve posture, and enhance overall health. However, it is important to note that individual experiences may vary, and consultation with a healthcare professional is recommended for persistent or severe pain.

7.3 Solve Sports Injuries and Muscle Soreness

In this chapter, we'll explore the topic of addressing sports injuries and muscle soreness in men. We discuss common sports-related injuries and their impact on physical performance and guide on using natural remedies, including essential oils, to promote recovery, reduce pain, and support muscle health.

A. Understand Sports Injuries

Here is an overview of common sports injuries that men may experience:

1. Sprain: A sprain occurs when the ligaments that connect bones stretch or tear. Ligaments are tough, flexible tissues that stabilize joints. Sprains usually affect the ankles, wrists, and knees. A sudden movement, fall, or impact usually cause them.

2. Strain: A strain is an injury to a muscle or tendon, which is the tissue that connects muscle to bone. They can be caused by overstretching or overusing muscles. Strains typically occur in the hamstrings, quadriceps, and back muscles.

3. Muscle strain: A muscle strain, also known as a muscle tear, occurs when a muscle fiber is stretched beyond its limit, causing damage. This can occur during activities that require sudden, forceful movements. Muscle strains usually occur in the calf, groin, or hamstring muscles.

4. Tendinitis: Tendonitis is inflammation of tendons, which are the tissues that connect muscles to bones. It is often caused by repetitive motion or overuse of a specific joint. Common areas affected by tendonitis include the shoulders, elbows, and knees.

5. Shin splints: Shin splints are characterized by pain along the front or inner edge of the tibia (shin bone). They commonly occur in runners and athletes who engage in activities that involve repeated impact on the legs, such as jumping or running on hard surfaces.

6. Rotator cuff injury: The rotator cuff is a group of muscles and tendons that stabilize the shoulder joint. Rotator cuff injuries can cause pain, limited range of motion, and shoulder weakness. These injuries can be caused by repetitive overhead motion or direct impact.

7. Meniscus tear: The meniscus is the cartilage in the knee joint that acts as a shock absorber. Meniscal tears can occur during activities involving twisting or sudden changes in direction, such as basketball or football.

8. Achilles tendon injury: The Achilles tendon connects the calf muscle to the heel bone. Injuries to this tendon can range from mild inflammation (tendonitis) to complete tearing. Sudden bursts of activity, overuse, or lack

of proper warm-up can cause them.

9. Stress fractures: Stress fractures are tiny cracks in bones that often occur due to repeated impacts. They are common among athletes who engage in high-impact activities such as running or jumping.

10. Concussion: A concussion is a type of brain injury that can occur when a sudden blow to the head occurs or when the head is shaken violently. They are common in contact sports such as soccer and rugby.

It is important to note that proper warm-up, stretching, and use of appropriate protective equipment are critical to preventing sports injuries. If you experience a sports injury, rest, ice, compression, and elevation (RICE) can help immediately after the aftermath. However, seeking medical care is crucial for a proper diagnosis and treatment plan, especially for more serious injuries.

Proper warm-up, conditioning, and technique are important components of injury prevention in sports. Here are the reasons why each of these aspects is important:

1. Proper warm-up:

Warming up is essential before engaging in any physical activity as it prepares your body for more intense exercise. It helps increase blood flow to your muscles, making them more pliable and ready for action. A good warm-up should include light cardiovascular exercise (such as jogging or jumping jacks), followed by dynamic stretching. This combination helps improve flexibility, joint range of motion, and muscle coordination. Warming up gradually increases your heart rate and warms your muscles, reducing the risk of sudden strains and injuries.

2. Conditioning:

Regular physical conditioning is the key to strength, endurance, and overall health. By gradually increasing the intensity and duration of your workouts, you allow your muscles, tendons, and joints to adapt and become stronger. Conditioning also helps improve the body's ability to handle stress and reduces the risk of overuse injuries. Strength training and functional exercises can target specific muscle groups and enhance overall stability, reducing the chance of injury during exercise.

3. Correct technique:

Using correct techniques when performing exercises and physical activities can significantly reduce the risk of injury. Poor form and incorrect movement patterns can stress muscles, ligaments, and joints unnecessarily. Training with a qualified coach or instructor can help you learn and stay on track. For example, when lifting weights, using proper technique and not overloading the muscles is important to avoid strains and tears.

4. Progress:

Gradually increasing the intensity and difficulty of your workouts allows your body to adapt safely. Sudden increases in load or intensity can lead to injury. For example, it's important to increase the weight gradually in strength training rather than lifting heavy objects suddenly.

5. Rest and recovery:

Giving your body enough time to recover is crucial to preventing injury. Rest allows your muscles, tendons, and joints to repair and rebuild. Overtraining without adequate recovery can lead to fatigue, poor performance, and an increased risk of injury.

6. Listen to your body:

Pay attention to any pain, discomfort, or unusual sensations during exercise. Living with pain can exacerbate existing problems or cause new injuries. If you feel pain, stop the activity and assess the situation. It is wise to consult a medical professional if needed.

Remember, injury prevention is an ongoing process that involves consistency, proper planning, and mindfulness. Incorporating these principles into your fitness program can significantly reduce your risk of exercise-related injuries and allow you to enjoy a more active and fulfilling lifestyle.

B. Sports Injury Recovery Essential Oils

Essential oils can play a role in aiding recovery from sports injuries due to their potential analgesic, anti-inflammatory, and soothing properties. Here are some essential oils that are often considered beneficial in supporting recovery from sports injuries:

1. Eucalyptus: Eucalyptus oil is known for its refreshing fragrance and potential anti-inflammatory properties. It may help reduce muscle soreness and improve blood circulation. It is often used in massage mixtures or added to warm baths for relaxation.

2. Peppermint: Peppermint oil has a cooling feeling and contains menthol, which can temporarily relieve pain. It is often used topically in dilute form to soothe sore muscles and reduce discomfort.

3. Lavender: Lavender oil is known for its calming and relaxing properties. It may help reduce stress and anxiety associated with the injury, which may indirectly support the recovery process. Its mild analgesic properties may also provide some pain relief.

4. Helichrysum: Helichrysum oil is believed to have anti-inflammatory and analgesic properties. It is commonly used to manage bruises, sprains, and swelling. It's important to note that helichrysum oil is effective and usually requires proper dilution.

When using essential oils for sports injury recovery, you must keep the following points in mind:

* Dilution: Essential oils are highly concentrated and should be diluted in a carrier oil (such as coconut or jojoba) before applying to the skin. This helps prevent skin irritation.

* Patch test: Before applying any new essential oil to a larger area of skin, conduct a patch test by applying the diluted mixture to a small area and waiting 24 hours to check for any adverse reactions.

* How to use: Applying a dilute essential oil blend through gentle massage can help improve circulation and promote relaxation. You can also add a few drops of essential oil to a warm bath for a soothing soak.

* Consultation: If you have an existing medical condition, are taking medications, or are concerned about using essential oils due to allergies, it is wise to consult with a healthcare professional before using essential oils for injury recovery.

While essential oils can provide support, they should not replace proper medical treatment for serious injuries. If you have a severe or persistent injury, it is important to consult a healthcare provider for appropriate diagnosis and treatment. Additionally, consider working with a trained aromatherapist to ensure the safe and effective use of essential oils during recovery.

Let's delve into the properties of essential oils commonly used for sports injury recovery:

1. Eucalyptus:

* Analgesic: Eucalyptus oil contains compounds such as eucalyptol, which cools the skin and can temporarily relieve pain.
* Anti-inflammatory: Eucalyptus oil may have anti-inflammatory properties that can help reduce swelling and inflammation around injured muscles and joints.
* Circulation: Eucalyptus oil's uplifting fragrance and potential to improve blood circulation can boost blood flow to affected areas, which aids in the recovery process.

2. Mint:

* Analgesic: Peppermint oil contains menthol, which produces a cooling sensation and can temporarily numb the area, relieving pain and discomfort.
* Anti-inflammatory: The menthol in peppermint oil has anti-inflammatory properties that may help reduce inflammation and swelling.
* Muscle relaxant: The muscle-relaxing properties of peppermint oil can help relieve muscle tension and spasms commonly associated with sports injuries.

3. Lavender:

* Analgesic: The mild analgesic properties of lavender oil can relieve the pain and discomfort associated with sports injuries.
* Anti-inflammatory: The anti-inflammatory properties of lavender oil can help reduce inflammation and swelling around the injured area.
* Relaxation: The calming and relaxation-inducing properties of lavender oil can help manage stress and anxiety, which aids in the healing process.

4. Helichrysum:

* Anti-inflammatory: Helichrysum oil is known for its powerful anti-inflammatory properties, which can help reduce inflammation and pain.
* Healing: Helichrysum oil's potential to support tissue regeneration

and wound healing can help restore damaged muscles and joints.
* Pain relief: Helichrysum oil can relieve localized pain by numbing the area and reducing discomfort.

When using these essential oils for sports injury recovery, it's important to dilute them correctly and perform a patch test to make sure you don't have any adverse reactions. A dilute blend of essential oils through gentle massage can help relax muscles, reduce tension, and improve circulation. A combination of aromatherapy and topical application can provide physical and psychological benefits during recovery.

Remember, essential oils should be supplemented with proper medical care, especially for major injuries. If the injury is severe, persistent, or worsening, consult a healthcare professional for appropriate diagnosis and treatment.

C. How to Use

Let's explore various ways to use essential oils for sports injury recovery:

1. Local application:

Topical application involves applying a dilute mixture of essential oils directly to the affected area. This method provides localized relief and helps reduce pain, inflammation, and muscle tension. To use this method:
* Dilute the essential oil in a carrier oil (such as coconut oil, jojoba oil, or sweet almond oil) to the appropriate concentration (usually 1 to 3%).
* Gently massage the diluted mixture into the injured area using circular motions.
* Allow the oil to be absorbed into the skin. Avoid applying to broken skin or open wounds.

2. Massage:

Massage is a therapeutic technique that combines the benefits of essential oils with physical contact. Massage can help relax muscles, increase blood flow, and relieve pain. Using essential oils for massage:
* Dilute essential oils in a carrier oil.
* Rub the essential oil with your hands and heat the oil mixture slightly.
* Gently massage the oil into the injured area using long, sweeping

motions. Use appropriate pressure based on comfort.

* You can also combine gentle massage with stretching and range-of-motion exercises to improve flexibility.

3. Apply:

Dressing involves applying a cloth soaked in an essential oil solution to the injured area. This method can help relieve pain, reduce swelling, and provide targeted relief. Here's how to make and use the dressing:

* Add a few drops of essential oil to a warm or cold water bowl.
* Soak a clean cloth in the water-oil mixture, wring it out, and apply it to the injured area.
* Cover the dressing with a dry towel to retain heat or cold and to prevent oil stains.
* Leave the dressing in place for about 15 to 20 minutes. You can repeat this as many times a day as needed.

4. Warm water bath:

Soaking in a warm bath infused with essential oils can relieve overall relaxation and muscle tension. Add a few drops of your chosen essential oil to a carrier oil or bath salts before adding to the bath water. Mix well to disperse the oil.

5. Cooling gel or cream:

You can make a cooling gel or cream by combining essential oils with aloe vera gel or unscented lotion. Apply this mixture to the affected area for a cooling sensation that helps reduce inflammation.

Essential oils are potent, and proper dilution is crucial to prevent skin irritation. If the injury is severe or does not improve, consult a healthcare professional for appropriate treatment. Always conduct a patch test before using new essential oils and discontinue use if you experience any adverse reactions.

Each method of using essential oils for sports injury recovery has its benefits and considerations, and its effectiveness can vary based on the nature of the injury and personal preference. Here's a breakdown of the benefits and considerations for each method:

Topical application:

* Benefits: Topical application provides direct and targeted relief to injured areas. It allows essential oils to penetrate the skin and reach affected tissues. This method suits localized pain, muscle tension, and joint discomfort.

* Precautions: Ensure proper dilution to prevent skin irritation. A patch test is recommended, especially if this is your first time using essential oils. Avoid using this method on broken or sensitive skin.

Massage:

* Benefits: Massage combines the therapeutic benefits of essential oils with physical contact. It enhances relaxation, improves blood circulation, and reduces muscle tension. It's also great for promoting flexibility and range of motion.

* Note: Choose a carrier oil appropriate for your skin type. Use appropriate pressure when massaging and avoid putting too much pressure on injured or sensitive areas. If you are new to massage techniques, consider seeking help from a trained massage therapist.

Apply:

* Benefits: Dressings are great for providing targeted relief and reducing inflammation. The warmth or coolness of the dressing can help reduce pain and swelling.

* Note: Make sure the water-oil mixture is at a comfortable temperature before applying the dressing. Monitor the skin for any adverse reactions during and after dressing application.

Warm bath:

* Benefits: A warm bath infused with essential oils relaxes the entire body and relieves muscle tension. It's a convenient way to relax overall and promote a sense of well-being.

* Note: Essential oils can be diluted in a carrier oil or unscented bath product before adding to the bath water. Ensure the water temperature is comfortable, and avoid using hot water, especially for injuries involving inflammation.

Cooling gel or cream:

* Benefits: Cooling gel or cream can provide a soothing and cooling sensation to the injured area, which can help relieve pain and reduce inflammation.

* Precautions: Make sure to apply cooling gel or cream lightly to avoid additional discomfort. Avoid contact with eyes, mouth, and sensitive areas.

Overall, the effectiveness of these methods depends on the specific injury, the essential oil used, and personal response. Listening to your body and adjusting your approach as needed is crucial. Consult a medical professional if the injury is severe or does not improve. Additionally, always follow safety guidelines, including proper dilution and patch testing, to ensure a safe and beneficial experience.

D. Create Healing Blends and Massage Oils

Here are some recipes and suggestions for creating personalized blends and massage oils to aid sports injury recovery:

Muscle Soothing Massage Oil:

* 10 drops of eucalyptus essential oil
* 10 drops of peppermint essential oil
* 10 drops of lavender essential oil
* 2 tablespoons carrier oil (such as jojoba, sweet almond, or coconut oil)

Mix essential oils with a carrier oil in a dark glass bottle. Shake and mix well. Use this massage oil to gently massage the affected area to relieve muscle tension and promote blood circulation.

Joint Soothing Blend:

* 15 drops of helichrysum essential oil
* 10 drops of frankincense essential oil
* 5 drops of ginger essential oil
* 2 tablespoons carrier oil

Mix essential oils with a carrier oil in a glass bottle. Shake to mix. Apply this mixture to joints to provide soothing relief and support joint movement.

Cooling compress mixture:

* 10 drops of peppermint essential oil

* 5 drops of eucalyptus essential oil
* 5 drops of lavender essential oil
* 2 cups cold or warm water

Mix the essential oils in water and soak a clean cloth or towel in the mixture. Wring out excess liquid and apply the dressing to the affected area for about 10 to 15 minutes. This can help reduce inflammation and provide a cooling sensation.

Relaxing bath:

* 10 drops of lavender essential oil
* 5 drops of chamomile essential oil
* 5 drops of cedarwood essential oil
* 1/2 cup Epsom salt

Mix essential oils with Epsom salt in a bowl. Add the mixture to a warm water bath and soak for about 20 minutes. This can help relax muscles and provide overall relaxation.

Remember to patch-test any new mixture or oil before using it on a larger area of skin. Also, adjust the number of drops according to your preference and sensitivity. If you have any existing medical conditions or are taking medications, please consult a healthcare professional before using essential oils for sports injury recovery.

Proper dilution ratios and selecting the right essential oil for specific injuries and symptoms are critical to ensuring safety and effectiveness. Here are some guidelines to help you make an informed choice:

Dilution ratio:

* Adults: A general guideline is to use a 2% dilution, which means adding approximately 12 drops of essential oil per 1 ounce (30 ml) of carrier oil. This ratio is suitable for most situations, including sports injury recovery. You can adjust the dilution to your personal needs, but no more than a 5% dilution (30 drops of essential oil per 1 ounce of carrier oil) is recommended for topical use.

Choose essential oils:

* Eucalyptus: Known for its analgesic and anti-inflammatory proper-

ties, eucalyptus helps relieve muscle and joint pain.

* Peppermint: Contains menthol, which provides a cooling sensation and helps relieve pain and inflammation.

* Lavender: Known for its calming and anti-inflammatory effects, lavender is great for promoting relaxation and aiding healing.

* Helichrysum: Has strong anti-inflammatory and analgesic properties and can be used on bruises, sprains, and muscle soreness.

* Frankincense: Contains anti-inflammatory compounds that help reduce inflammation and support tissue repair.

* Ginger: Known for its warming properties, ginger essential oil can help relieve muscle pain and soreness.

* Chamomile: Has anti-inflammatory properties to help soothe skin irritations.

* Cedarwood: Has a grounding effect that promotes relaxation and aids recovery.

Injury-specific guidance:

* Muscle strain: Peppermint, eucalyptus, and lavender are good choices. They provide a cooling sensation, help reduce inflammation, and relieve muscle discomfort.

* Joint pain: Helichrysum and frankincense are effective for joint pain. They can help reduce inflammation and support joint health.

* Bruises: Helichrysum and lavender are often recommended for their ability to help reduce bruising and promote healing.

* Tendinitis: Eucalyptus and ginger can help relieve the pain and inflammation associated with tendonitis.

Remember, essential oils are effective; a little goes a long way. Be sure to dilute them appropriately in carrier oil before applying them to your skin. Conduct a patch test before using a new oil or mixing it on a larger skin area. If you have any underlying health conditions or are taking medications, please consult a healthcare professional before using essential oils for injury recovery. It's also a good practice to keep track of the oils you use and their effects to help you tailor your approach over time.

E. Rest and Recovery

Rest, proper nutrition, and hydration play key roles in supporting recovery from sports injuries. Here's why each of these factors is essential:

Rest:

Rest is essential for the body to repair and heal. When you are injured, your body needs time to recover, rebuild damaged tissue, and reduce inflammation. Overexertion or continued strenuous activity can worsen the injury and delay healing. Give your body the necessary time to heal and rest and recover.

Proper nutrition:

Nutrition is the foundation of recovery. Nutrient-rich foods provide essential building blocks for tissue repair and healing. Essential nutrients include:

* Protein: required for tissue repair and muscle recovery. Sources include lean meats, poultry, fish, beans, lentils, nuts and seeds.

* Vitamins and Minerals: Vitamins like vitamin C and minerals like zinc and magnesium are essential for collagen production, wound healing, and immune function. Include a variety of fruits, vegetables, whole grains, and nuts in your diet.

*Omega3 fatty acids: These anti-inflammatory fats support healing and reduce inflammation. Found in fatty fish (such as salmon and mackerel), flax seeds, chia seeds, and walnuts.

* Antioxidants: Found in colorful fruits and vegetables, antioxidants help fight oxidative stress and promote healing.

Hydration:

Proper hydration is essential for a variety of body functions, including tissue repair and fluid balance. Water supports the transport of nutrients and oxygen to cells and helps remove waste products. Staying hydrated can also help relieve muscle spasms and maintain joint lubrication.

Balanced diet:

A balanced diet rich in whole foods provides essential nutrients for recovery. Prioritize lean protein, complex carbohydrates, healthy fats, and a variety of vitamins and minerals.

Anti-inflammatory foods:

Include foods with anti-inflammatory properties such as turmeric, ginger, berries, green leafy vegetables, and green tea. These can help reduce inflammation and support healing.

Lean protein:

Protein is essential for muscle repair. Include sources such as lean meats, fish, poultry, eggs, dairy products, legumes, and plant-based proteins.

Complex carbohydrates:

Carbohydrates provide energy for healing and recovery. Choose whole grains like brown rice, quinoa, oats, and whole wheat.

Healthy fats:

Omega-3 fatty acids found in fatty fish, flax seeds, chia seeds, and walnuts have anti-inflammatory properties.

Hydration:

Drink water regularly to stay hydrated. Dehydration hinders the body's ability to heal.

Replenish:

After consulting with a health care professional, you may consider certain supplements that support healing, such as collagen, vitamin C, and omega-3 fatty acids.

Consult a professional:

If you are dealing with a serious sports injury, it is recommended that you work with a healthcare provider or sports nutritionist who can provide personalized recommendations based on your needs, type of injury, and overall health.

Essential oils can promote relaxation, reduce inflammation, and support the body's natural healing process. Here are how essential oils can help with these aspects of sports injury recovery:

Promote relaxation:

Recovering from a sports injury often involves physical discomfort and emotional stress. Essential oils like lavender, chamomile, and frankincense have calming and soothing properties. When inhaled or used in aromatherapy, these oils can help relieve stress, anxiety, and tension. By promoting relaxation, essential oils contribute to a more positive mindset, which improves overall healing.

Reduce inflammation:

Inflammation is a natural response to injury, but excessive or prolonged inflammation can hinder healing. Many essential oils have anti-inflammatory properties. Oils such as eucalyptus, peppermint, and ginger contain compounds that can help reduce inflammation when applied topically or used in massage. These oils may help reduce swelling, redness, and discomfort associated with inflammation.

Supports the natural healing process:

The body has innate healing mechanisms that repair damaged tissue and restore function. Certain essential oils, such as helichrysum, lavender, and tea tree, contain compounds that can support these natural healing processes. For example, helichrysum has skin-regenerating properties that can aid in wound healing, while tea tree oil has antibacterial properties that can help prevent infection in minor cuts and scrapes.

Massage and topical application:

One effective way to harness the benefits of essential oils is through massage or topical application. Diluted essential oils can be applied to the affected area and gently massaged into the skin. This helps improve blood circulation, reduce muscle tension, and promote the absorption of the beneficial compounds in the oil.

Hot compress:

A hot compress infused with essential oils can help relieve pain and relax you. For example, adding lavender oil to a hot compress can soothe sore muscles and enhance relaxation.

Aromatherapy and inhalation:

Inhaling essential oils through a diffuser or inhalation stick can have a calming effect on the nervous system. Aromatherapy using oils like lavender, bergamot, or sage can help reduce stress and promote relaxation.

Custom blends:

Creating a personalized essential oil blend based on your specific needs and symptoms can provide targeted support. For example, a blend of lavender and chamomile may help relax, while a blend of peppermint and eucalyptus may address localized inflammation.

Precaution:

While essential oils can be beneficial, using them safely is important. Be sure to dilute essential oils appropriately before applying them to your skin and perform a patch test to check for allergies or sensitivities. If you are pregnant, nursing, have an underlying health condition or are taking medications, please consult a healthcare professional before using essential oils.

Personal changes:

It's worth noting that individual reactions to essential oils may vary. What works for one person may have a different effect on another. It's a good idea to start with a small amount of oil and see how your body reacts.

Overall approach:

Essential oils should be considered part of a holistic approach to sports injury recovery. They can complement other strategies such as rest, proper nutrition, physical therapy, and medication. If you have a serious injury or chronic illness, consult a healthcare professional for guidance on how to incorporate essential oils safely and effectively into your recovery plan.

F. Rehabilitation and Physical Therapy

Incorporating essential oils into sports injury rehabilitation and physical therapy procedures can provide various benefits and contribute to a more effective and comprehensive recovery process. Here are some advantages of using essential oils in these situations:

1. Pain relief: Many essential oils have analgesic properties that can help relieve pain associated with sports injuries. Oils such as peppermint, eucalyptus, and lavender can be used topically or massaged to relieve localized

pain and reduce discomfort during rehabilitation exercises.

2. Muscle Relaxation: Essential oils like chamomile, sage, and marjoram have muscle-relaxing properties. Applying these oils to tight or sore muscles as part of a massage or stretching routine can help relax muscle fibers and reduce muscle spasms, promoting better flexibility and range of motion.

3. Improve blood circulation: Certain essential oils, including ginger, black pepper, and cypress, have properties that can improve blood circulation. Enhanced circulation can help speed healing by delivering oxygen and nutrients to injured tissue and removing waste products.

4. Reduce inflammation: Essential oils with anti-inflammatory properties, such as frankincense, helichrysum, and turmeric, can help reduce inflammation that often accompanies sports injuries. Applying these oils topically or using them in aromatherapy can help manage swelling and discomfort.

5. Relax and reduce stress: Recovering from a sports injury can be mentally and emotionally taxing. Essential oils like lavender, bergamot, and cedarwood have calming properties that can help reduce stress and anxiety. Incorporating these oils into relaxation techniques, such as deep breathing or meditation, can support overall health during the recovery process.

6. Enhance focus and motivation: Essential oils like rosemary, lemon, and peppermint have uplifting and uplifting scents that enhance focus and mental clarity. Using these oils during rehabilitative exercises or physical therapy may help improve focus and motivation.

7. Aromatherapy for mental and emotional support: The recovery process can be physically demanding and emotionally challenging. Essential oil aromatherapy can create a positive and supportive environment. Inhaling calming and soothing oils during treatment can promote feelings of relaxation and emotional balance.

8. Personalized approach: Essential oils can be tailored to individual needs and preferences. Creating a customized blend based on specific symptoms and goals allows for a personalized approach to recovery.

9. Non-invasive and natural: Essential oils are derived from plants and provide a natural, non-invasive way to support the body's healing process. They can be integrated into recovery procedures without interfering with other medical treatments.

10. Holistic therapy: Incorporating essential oils into rehabilitation and physical therapy routines requires a holistic approach to recovery. By addressing the physical, spiritual, and emotional aspects of healing, essential oils contribute to a holistic and comprehensive recovery process.

A word of caution: While essential oils can provide many benefits, it's crucial to use them safely and consult a healthcare professional, especially if you have an existing medical condition, allergies, or sensitivities. Always conduct a patch test before applying essential oils to larger areas and ensure proper dilution for topical use.

Partnering: If you are working with a physical therapist or rehabilitation professional, consider discussing incorporating essential oils into your treatment plan. Collaboration between healthcare providers and aromatherapists can lead to an integrated and holistic approach to recovery.

Supplementation techniques combined with the use of essential oils can significantly aid the recovery process from sports injuries. These techniques focus on improving flexibility, strength, and circulation, enhancing overall healing, and minimizing the risk of future injury. Here are some complementary technologies to consider:

1. Stretching: Incorporating dynamic and static stretching into your recovery routine can help improve flexibility and range of motion. Stretching helps prevent muscle imbalances, reduce muscle tension, and enhance overall mobility. Essential oils with muscle-relaxing properties, such as lavender, chamomile, and marjoram, can be used to increase their effectiveness before stretching.

2. Strengthening exercises: Targeted strengthening exercises performed under the guidance of a physical therapist can help rebuild muscle strength and stability in the affected area. Strengthening exercises promote proper alignment and support joint health. Essential oils can be used before and after exercise to warm up muscles and aid recovery.

3. Foam rolling: Foam rolling, or auto myofascial release, involves using a foam roller to apply pressure to tight or sore muscles. This technique can help release muscle knots, improve blood circulation, and relieve muscle tension. Applying essential oils before foam rolling can enhance the relaxing and soothing effects of the practice.

4. Cross-training: Engaging in low-impact activities such as swimming, biking, or yoga can help maintain fitness levels while minimizing stress on the injured area. Essential oils can be used during these activities to promote relaxation and mental focus.

5. Active recovery: Perform light exercise and activity on your rest days to promote blood flow and prevent stiffness. Essential oils with analgesic and anti-inflammatory properties can provide support during an active recovery process.

6. Hydration and nutrition: Staying properly hydrated and eating a balanced, nutrient-rich diet can aid the body's recovery process. Drinking water, eating anti-inflammatory foods, and getting enough protein can support tissue repair and reduce inflammation.

7. Rest and sleep: Adequate rest and quality sleep are critical to recovery. Essential oils known for their calming properties, such as lavender and chamomile, can be diffused in your bedroom to promote relaxation and improve sleep quality.

8. Mind-body exercises: Techniques like meditation, deep breathing, and mindfulness can help reduce stress and increase mental clarity. Essential oils with soothing scents can enhance the relaxing benefits of these practices.

9. Support equipment: Wearing appropriate support equipment, such as braces, dressings, or supportive shoes, can help prevent further injury and provide comfort during the recovery process.

10. Consult a healthcare professional: Always consult with your healthcare provider, physical therapist, or rehabilitation specialist before incorporating supplemental techniques into your recovery plan. They can guide the most appropriate techniques based on your specific injury, condition, and recovery goals.

Combining these supplementary techniques with the use of essential oils creates a comprehensive and holistic approach to recovery that promotes optimal healing and a faster return to physical activity.

G. Precautions and Injury Prevention

Preventing sports injuries requires a proactive approach that includes proper preparation, understanding your body's signals, and incorporating smart habits into your daily life. Here are some preventive measures to help reduce the risk of sports injuries:

1. Warm-up: Always start your workout or exercise session with a dynamic warm-up. Perform light cardiovascular activity and dynamic stretches to increase blood flow to your muscles, improve flexibility, and prepare your body for more intense exercise.

2. Proper technique: Make sure you use proper form and technique in your workouts and physical activities. Improper form can stress muscles and joints unnecessarily, increasing the risk of injury. Ask a coach or trainer for guidance if you're unsure about your form.

3. Gradually increase your workouts' intensity, duration, and complexity over time. Sudden changes in training load can lead to overuse injuries.

4. Cool down: After your workout, cool down with gentle static stretches to help relax muscles and prevent stiffness. Cooling also helps remove waste products from the muscles and reduces the risk of post-exercise soreness.

5. Hydration: Maintain proper hydration before, during, and after exercise. Dehydration can impair muscle function and increase the risk of cramps and injury.

6. Balanced nutrition: A balanced diet provides the nutrients needed for muscle repair, recovery, and overall health. Includes a blend of carbohydrates, proteins, healthy fats, vitamins, and minerals.

7. The right shoes: Wear the right shoes for your activity to provide proper support, cushioning, and stability. Ill-fitting shoes can lead to various types of injuries.

8. Rest and Recovery: Allow adequate rest and recovery time between strenuous exercise or exercise sessions. Overtraining can lead to fatigue, weakened immune function, and increased risk of injury.

9. Cross-training: Cross-training to prevent overuse injuries. Alternating between different types of activities can give specific muscle groups a break while still staying fit.

10. Protective Equipment: Wear appropriate protective equipment such as helmets, pads, goggles, or braces, depending on the sport or activity. This gear reduces the impact of bumps and falls.

11. Listen to your body: Listen to your body's signals. If you experience pain, discomfort, or fatigue during exercise, stop and assess the situation. Living with pain can lead to more serious injuries.

12. Stretching and flexibility: Regularly perform flexibility and stretching exercises to keep your muscles and joints mobile. Flexible muscles are less likely to be affected by strains and strains.

13. Strength training: Include strength training in your daily routine to build muscle strength and stability. Strong muscles provide better support for joints and prevent injuries.

14. Warm-up and cool-down routine: Develop a consistent warm-up and cool-down routine specific to your activity. A consistent routine can help prepare your body for activity and aid recovery afterward.

15. Professional guidance: Consult with an athletic trainer, fitness trainer, or physiotherapist to design a comprehensive training program that considers your fitness level, goals, and any existing conditions.

Following these precautions can significantly reduce your risk of sports injuries and allow you to enjoy a safer, more fulfilling sports and exercise experience.

Essential oils can play a supportive role in promoting muscle flexibility, reducing muscle tension, and preventing overuse injuries. Here's how they can be beneficial:

1. Muscle relaxation: Many essential oils, such as lavender, chamomile, and eucalyptus, have natural muscle relaxation properties. When used in massage or aromatherapy, these oils can help relax tense muscles, reduce muscle stiffness, and promote flexibility.

2. Massage: Essential oils can be diluted with a carrier oil and used for massage. The massage action combined with the aromatherapeutic effects of essential oils can help improve blood circulation to muscles, relieve tension, and increase flexibility.

3. Warm-up ritual: Incorporate essential oils into your warm-up routine. Applying a diluted mixture of warm oils, such as ginger and black pepper, before a workout can help increase blood flow to your muscles and improve flexibility.

4. Stretching aid: Apply a dilute essential oil mixture before stretching. The soothing aroma and potential muscle-relaxing effects of essential oils may make stretching and holding postures easier.

5. Post-workout recovery: Essential oils like peppermint and eucalyptus have cooling properties that can be soothing after strenuous exercise. A dilute mixture applied to areas of tension or fatigue can promote relaxation and relieve muscle discomfort.

6. Self-care rituals: Incorporate essential oils into your self-care routine. Add them to your bath, use them during a self-massage, or practice gentle yoga or stretching while diffusing a calming oil like lavender or bergamot.

7. Focus before exercise: Aromatherapy can help establish a focused mindset before exercise. Inhaling energizing oils like citrus or rosemary can provide mental clarity and help you perform your workouts with better form and awareness.

8. Mind-body connection: Essential oils can enhance the mind-body connection, allowing you to be more aware of your body's signals during exercise. This increased awareness can help you avoid overexertion and prevent overuse injuries.

9. Reduce stress: High-stress levels can lead to muscle tension and reduced flexibility. Essential oils with stress-relieving properties, such as lavender or sage, can help calm the mind and indirectly aid muscle relaxation.

10. Regular aromatherapy practice: Incorporating regular aromatherapy sessions, whether by diffusion, inhalation, or diluted topical application, can support overall relaxation and help maintain flexibility over time.

11. Incorporate breathing techniques: Combining deep breathing techniques with aromatherapy can enhance relaxation and oxygenation of muscles, promote flexibility, and reduce the risk of strain injuries.

Remember, while essential oils can supplement muscle flexibility efforts, they should not replace a proper warm-up, cool-down, and stretching routine. If you have any underlying health conditions or wish to use essential oils as part of a fitness regimen, please consult a fitness professional or health-care provider.

These points cannot be overstated when using essential oils for sports injury recovery or other therapeutic purposes. Staying safe and seeking professional guidance when needed are critical steps in enjoying essential oils' benefits while minimizing potential risks.

1. Proper dilution: Essential oils are potent and concentrated substances. Proper dilution of them in a carrier oil can help reduce the risk of skin irritation and sensitization. To ensure safe use, follow the recommended dilution ratio, usually around 2 to 3% for adults.

2. Patch test: Always perform a patch test before applying any new essential oil to a larger area of skin. Apply a small amount of diluted to a small skin area and wait 24 hours to check for any adverse reactions or allergies.

3. Medical consultation: If you are dealing with a serious or ongoing injury, you must consult a medical professional or healthcare provider before using essential oils. They can guide whether essential oils are appropriate for your specific condition and how to integrate them into your overall treatment plan.

4. Knowledge of contraindications: Essential oils may have contra-indications, especially if you have an existing medical condition, are taking medications, or are pregnant / nursing. Some oils may not be suitable or may interact with medications. In this situation, the advice of a healthcare provider is crucial.

5. Professional aromatherapist: If you are new to using essential oils or are dealing with a complex injury, seeking the guidance of a certified aro-matherapist can provide personalized advice and ensure you are using the correct essential oils and techniques.

6. Listen to your body: Pay attention to how your body reacts to essential oils. If you experience discomfort, irritation, or worsening symptoms, discontinue use immediately.

7. Serious injuries: For serious injuries, fractures, or illnesses that require medical attention, essential oils should be used as a complementary approach rather than as a standalone treatment. Consultation with a healthcare

professional is crucial.

8. Ongoing problems: If you are dealing with chronic or ongoing problems, consider a holistic approach that includes medical treatment, physical therapy, and lifestyle modifications in addition to essential oils.

Remember, essential oils can provide supportive benefits but should not replace professional medical care when needed. Combining medical expertise and informed essential oil use contributes to a comprehensive approach to recovery and wellness.

After this chapter, we highlight the potential benefits of using natural remedies, such as essential oils, to address sports injuries and muscle soreness in men. By incorporating essential oils into their recovery routine, men can experience pain relief, enhanced healing, and improved physical function. However, it is important to note that individual experiences may vary, and consultation with a healthcare professional or sports therapist is recommended for proper diagnosis and treatment of sports injuries.

Chapter 8

Men's Health Problems at Various Stages

Men have health problems that are different from women at every stage of their lives, which can be collectively referred to as "andrology" in medical terms. In this chapter, we will discuss how to use essential oils to regulate, prevent, or assist in treating problems faced by men at every stage of their lives, and provide some DIY essential oil methods.

There are female and male animals and female and male humans. There is never a complete and reasonable understanding of the concept of male. The concept of the male should be: " Male Heart " - majestic spirit; " Male " - rough and Strong; " Male Body " - tough, tenacious, and erect. Mind, sex, and body are both independent and interdependent, thus constructing a complete boy's life.

In the vast world, yin and yang blend, and plants and animals survive and benefit each other. It is precisely because of the harmonious coexistence of animals and plants in nature that a splendid world exists. As the understanding of nature continues to deepen, the dazzling aromatherapy of traditional Chinese medicine gradually emerges. This treatment spreads quickly like a scent filled with the fragrance of love. Aromatherapy is a great natural remedy.

Its main magic weapon is the essential oil extracted from the seeds, flowers, fruits, leaves, stems, and roots of plants. Since the advent of therapeutic-grade essential oils in modern times, it has the characteristics of harmlessness, innocence, and effectiveness. It also has the characteristics of high permeability, high synergy, and high volatility. It can safely act on all aspects of the human body to prevent disease. The purpose of prevention and prevention of existing diseases. During practice, fruitful results have been achieved.

The male reproductive system is mainly composed of the pituitary gland in the brain, the ejaculation center in the lumbar spine, the adrenal glands in the endocrine system, and the testicles in the hormone system. Only when these neuroendocrine organs and genitals cooperate and coordinate can they better function in both sexes. role in reproduction. Special attention should be paid to a characteristic of the male system, that is, the ejaculation and urinary system share an anterior urethra, which increases the complexity of the male reproductive system. This article focuses on the results of applying traditional Chinese aromatherapy (natural therapy) to the male reproductive system. Preliminary success.

Men's diseases mainly refer to male erectile dysfunction, ejaculation dysfunction, male infertility, male genital diseases, prostate diseases, etc.

The male reproductive system consists of internal genitalia and external genitalia. The internal genitals consist of gonads (testes), deferens ducts (epididymis, vas deferens, ejaculatory ducts, and urethra), and accessory glands (seminal vesicles, prostate, bulbourethral glands). External genitalia include the scrotum and penis.

The testicles are in the scrotum, about 3cm × 3cm in size, and hard in texture. They are mainly used for reproductive and sexual functions. The testicular seminiferous tubules produce primary sperm, which mature in the coiled epididymal duct and enter the seminal vesicle for later use. During sexual intercourse, it is mixed with prostatic fluid and seminal vesicle fluid to form semen, which is excreted from the body through the urethra.

The nutrition of the testicles is supplied by the testicular artery, which originates from the abdominal aorta, which shows the importance of the testicle as an organ. The spermatic vein returns to the general circulation. Because the left spermatic vein is at a right angle, the resistance to its return to the renal vein is greater. Long-term standing or excessive participation in sports such as basketball, volleyball, long-distance running, etc., will lead to left varicocele, resulting in malnutrition of the testicles and epididymis on the blood supply side and poor sperm development, ultimately leading to male infertility.

The prostate is the largest organ that produces semen. Its fluid mainly provides a variety of enzymes, is alkaline, and is the protagonist of liquefied semen. Once the semen enters the female reproductive tract, it neutralizes the acidic vaginal fluid so that the sperm can swim upstream to achieve pregnancy. When sexual life is excessive, the human body is malnourished, and the prostate is inflamed by bacterial (rare), biochemical, and physical factors, the composition of the prostatic fluid will change, causing reproductive dysfunction.

Although the male urethra is not prone to exogenous lower urinary tract bacterial infections if the foreskin is too long, phimosis and the hygiene of the external genitalia are not paid attention to, urinary tract infections (including bacterial and viral) can easily occur.

8.1 Phimosis and Excessive Foreskin in Children

Phimosis and foreskin in children refer to the phenomenon of phimosis or foreskin in boys.

Under normal circumstances, most boys are born with phimosis. As they age, the foreskin will gradually relax, and the foreskin can turn up to expose the glans. After the age of 3, the foreskin will loosen on its own and can be partially turned up, but generally cannot be completely turned up to expose the coronal sulcus. If it still cannot be turned up by puberty, it is called pathological phimosis.

Phimosis and prepuce are common worldwide.

The World Health Organization estimates that approximately 130 million men worldwide suffer from phimosis.

In Africa and Asia, the prevalence of phimosis is higher, about 50%-80%.

In Europe and North America, the prevalence of phimosis is approximately 10%-20%.

In recent years, circumcision has become increasingly popular around the world.

In the United States, Canada, Australia, and other countries, the neonatal circumcision rate is as high as 80%-90%.

In countries such as Europe and Asia, the rate of circumcision is also gradually increasing.

A. What Is Phimosis and Foreskin in Children?

Phimosis refers to the narrowing of the foreskin opening or the adhesion between the foreskin and the glans penis, which prevents the foreskin from turning up and the external urethral opening and glans penis from being exposed.

Paraphimosis refers to a person whose foreskin is long and completely covers the glans penis and external urethral opening, but the foreskin opening is large and can naturally turn up to above the coronal sulcus.

B. Clinical Manifestations of Phimosis and Foreskin in Children

Phimosis or foreskin is congenital in children. When children start normal metabolism and secretion after birth, phimosis or foreskin will have a certain impact on urination. After urination, there is often a little residual urine in the foreskin cavity. Coupled with the accumulated sebum secretions and epithelial desquamation, massive smegma, which is a petri dish for bacterial reproduction, will gradually form. If you do not pay attention to local hygiene, it can easily lead to balanitis, urinary tract infection, and penile cancer.

Dangers of excessive foreskin and phimosis:

- Excessive foreskin and phimosis can easily harbor dirt, lead to the accumulation of smegma, breed bacteria, and cause diseases such as foreshitis, balanitis, and urinary tract infection.

- Phimosis may also affect penile development, resulting in a short penis.

- Foreskin and phimosis are one of the important transmission routes of sexually transmitted diseases, which can increase the risk of contracting sexually transmitted diseases such as AIDS and syphilis.

There are two main treatments for prepuce and phimosis:

- Conservative treatment: suitable for patients with excessive foreskin and no obvious symptoms such as foreshitis or balanitis. Prevent infection mainly by keeping the area clean and hygienic and washing the foreskin and glans regularly.

- Surgical treatment: Suitable for patients with phimosis, redundant foreskin, and obvious symptoms such as foreshitis and balanitis. The most common surgical method is circumcision, which involves removing part or all of the foreskin. Circumcision is a safe and effective treatment that can effectively prevent the health risks of foreskin and phimosis.

Suggestion:
- Parents should check their children's foreskin regularly. If they find phimosis or excessive foreskin, they should consult a doctor promptly.

- For children with redundant foreskin and phimosis, attention should be paid to keeping the local area clean and hygienic and regular cleaning of the foreskin and glans to prevent infection.

- Children with symptoms such as posthitis and balanitis should seek medical treatment in time.

C. How to Take Care of Phimosis and Foreskin in Children with Essential Oils

For children with phimosis that cannot be turned up, surgical treatment can be considered within 2 years of age. Children's phimosis can also be turned up on its own. With the help of adults, it can be turned up a little every day. At the same time, diluted tea tree and frankincense essential oils can be applied to the local area to reduce inflammation and relieve pain, repair damaged cells, and relieve discomfort. Certain essential oils have anti-inflammatory, antibacterial, analgesic, and other effects, and may be helpful for symptoms such as posthitis and balanitis. Parents should choose to use them after consulting doctors and aromatherapists.

D. Aroma Application Guidelines

1. Recommended oils: tea tree, frankincense, marjoram.

2. Usage: 1 to 2 drops each of frankincense and tea tree essential oils, diluted with coconut oil 1: (3 to 10), apply on the foreskin, twice a day, a course of treatment every 3 days. It activates blood circulation and removes blood stasis, enhances the elasticity of the foreskin, facilitates foreskin inversion, and shortens foreskin inversion time, and relieves foreskin pain (micro-tears of the foreskin) caused by excessive foreskin inversion every day. You can also add 1 drop of marjoram and dilute it with coconut oil for external application, which can soothe muscle tissue.

8.2 Glans Ulcer

Glans ulcers are common worldwide.

• The World Health Organization estimates that approximately 500 million people worldwide are infected with the herpes simplex virus every year, and some of these patients will develop glans ulcers.

• Sexually transmitted diseases such as syphilis and chancroid are also common causes of glans ulcers.

In recent years, the incidence of glans ulcers has been on the rise. This may be related to factors such as changes in sexual lifestyle and the prevalence of sexually transmitted diseases such as AIDS.

A. What Is Glans Ulcer

Glans ulcers are ulcerative lesions that occur on the glans penis and can be caused by a variety of causes, including:

• Infection: The most common pathogen is herpes simplex virus (HSV), followed by Treponema pallidum, Chancroid, Candida, etc.

• Inflammation: such as balanitis, balanitis circumscripta plasma-cellularis wait.

- Autoimmune diseases: such as Behçet's disease, Behçet Disease, etc.

- Drugs: such as certain antibiotics, chemotherapy drugs, etc.

- Tumors: such as penile cancer, glans cancer, etc.

B. Clinical Manifestations of Glans Ulcer

Due to allergies (common to sulfonamide drugs) or unclean sex, the glans surface of the penis may blister or even become infected and rupture. It manifests as pain and excessive mucus secretion, and some patients may also experience pruritus.

- Local redness, swelling, pain, erosion, ulcers, etc., appear on the glans penis.

- There may be exudation and scab on the surface of the ulcer.

- Some patients may be accompanied by systemic symptoms such as fever and lymphadenopathy.

Treatment of glans ulcers should be based on the specific cause.

- Infectious glans ulcer: Treatment should be directed to the causative agent. For example, herpes simplex virus infection can be treated with antiviral drugs and syphilis infection can be treated with antibiotics.

- Inflammatory glans ulcers: can be treated with anti-inflammatory drugs.

- Autoimmune glans ulcer: It can be treated with glucocorticoids, immunosuppressants, and other drugs.

- Drug-induced glans ulcer: Suspicious drugs should be discontinued.

- Tumor glans ulcer: should be treated surgically.

Suggestion:

- Pay attention to sexual hygiene and avoid infectious diseases.

- Regular physical examination, early detection, and early treatment.

- If a glans ulcer occurs, you should seek medical treatment promptly for a clear diagnosis and standardized treatment.

C. How to Take Care of Glans Ulcers with Essential Oils

Since ulcers are caused by allergies and infections, anti-allergy and anti-infection treatments are key. The skin of the glans is a sensitive area. Choose frankincense, cypress, tea tree, and other blood-activating channels to achieve the purpose of leaking poisons. Tea tree fights infection and promote healing; lavender is the main essential oil for treating skin problems, and adding peppermint essential oil can speed up dirt removal and wound healing. Please do it under the guidance of a doctor or aromatherapist.

D. Aroma Application Guidelines

1. Recommended oils: frankincense, cypress, lavender, peppermint.

2. Method: 1 drop each of frankincense, cypress, and tea tree, diluted 1:1 with coconut oil, and apply directly to the skin on the back of the penis, 1cm away from the coronal sulcus. In addition, you can use salt-warmed water (normal saline is better) to clean the ulcer 3 to 4 times a day, and then use 10 drops of coconut oil, 1 drop of lavender, and 1 drop of peppermint to clean the glans.

It is worth noting that during the treatment process, the foreskin should always be kept upturned to the coronal sulcus. If it is often dislocated, anti-allergic tape can be used to fix it. If the clothes you are wearing affect the wound, you can also use sterilized gauze, add 1 drop of lavender and 1 drop of peppermint essential oil, and fix it on the pubic symphysis to prevent the glans from being rubbed by clothes and hindering wound healing.

8.3 Pyllosthrosis

Pyllosthrosis disease is uncommon worldwide.

- There are currently no precise epidemiological data.

- The disease may be related to race, region, and other factors.

In recent years, the incidence of Pyllosthrosis disease has been on the rise. This may be related to the increased incidence of autoimmune diseases, sexually transmitted diseases, etc.

A. What is Pyllosthrosis Disease

The presence of plaque-like hardness in the cavernous body of the penis is called Pyllosthrosis disease. Pyllosthrosis disease is a chronic inflammatory disease that occurs in the tunica albuginea of the penis and can cause symptoms such as induration, pain, and curvature of the penis.

Cause:

The exact cause of Pyllosthrosis disease is unknown, but it may be related to the following factors:
Autoimmune diseases: such as Behçet's disease. etc.
Infections: such as syphilis, gonorrhea, etc.
Trauma: such as injury to the corpus cavernosum of the penis.

B. Clinical Manifestations of Pyllosthrosis

The penis is composed of two corpora cavernosa, corpora cavernosa (containing the urethra) and the glans. In common cases of colds and tooth-aches, sexual intercourse causes plaque-like nodules to form in part of the cavernous sinus within the cavernous body, which manifests as penile erection and bending pain, affecting sexual life. The main clinical manifestations of Pyllosthrosis disease include:

- The tunica albuginea of the penis appears indurated, with a hard texture and unclear boundaries.

- Penile pain can be spontaneous or painful during erection.

- A curvature of the penis can cause difficulty in sexual intercourse.

C. How to use Essential Oils to Take Care of Penile Stiffness

Because Pyllosthrosis disease is the degeneration of the cavernous sinus in the cavernous body, the cavernous body is congested, and the blood return function is blocked. It is difficult for general drugs to enter the sinus, making treatment difficult. Physiotherapy-grade essential oils have high penetration, effectiveness, and synergy. features, it is a good choice. Frankincense and myrrh can be used to promote blood circulation and remove blood stasis, helichrysum can be used to stop bleeding and remove blood stasis to regenerate vascular endothelium, and tea tree can be used to reduce inflammation and relieve pain. Please do it under the guidance of a doctor or aromatherapist.

D. Aroma Application Guidelines

1. Recommended oils: frankincense, myrrh, helichrysum, tea tree, angelica.

2. How to use: 1 drop each of frankincense, myrrh, and tea tree, dilute with coconut oil 1: 5, apply on the penis skin centered on the "nodule," 1-2cm above and below, 3 times a day, at night The effect will be better if you apply it again before clinical use. You can also add 1-2 drops of Perfect Repair to the smear formula at the same time. If conditions permit, you can add 1 drop of Helichrysum to the smear formula 3 days after nodules are discovered. There is no need to use it again after 3 days. Patients should note that if they seek medical treatment late, they should consult a senior aromatherapist or andrologist.

8.4 Testicular Hydrocele

Testicular hydrocele is common worldwide.

- According to statistics, about 15% of men will develop testicular hydrocele in their lifetime.

- The disease is more common in children, with about 1% of boys born with testicular hydrocele.

In recent years, the incidence of testicular hydrocele has increased. This may be related to factors such as the increased incidence of male infertility and scrotal trauma.

Suggestion:

- Pay attention to personal hygiene and avoid infectious diseases.

- Avoid scrotal trauma.

- Regular physical examination, early detection, and early treatment.

- If symptoms such as scrotal enlargement and pain occur, you should seek medical treatment promptly for a clear diagnosis and standardized treatment.

A. What Is the Testicular Hydrocele

The normal testicular tunica vaginalis has a small amount of fluid to protect the testicles. If there is too much fluid in the tunica vaginalis, a scrotal mass will appear, which is called testicular hydrocele. It can be divided into two types: congenital and acquired.

Congenital testicular hydrocele:Congenital testicular hydrocele is caused by failure of the peritoneal sheath to close, causing peritoneal fluid to flow into the testicular vaginal cavity.

Acquired testicular hydrocele:

Acquired testicular hydrocele can be caused by:

- Inflammation: such as orchitis, epididymitis, etc.

- Trauma: such as scrotal trauma, etc.

- Tumors: such as testicular tumors, spermatic cord tumors, etc.

- Congestion: such as varicose veins, etc.

B. Clinical Manifestations of Testicular Hydrocele

When the secretory fluid of the secretory layer of the testicular vaginal membrane is greater than the absorbed fluid of the vaginal absorptive layer due to inflammation or acute injury, more and more fluid will accumulate in the vaginal sac, and the scrotum will become larger, and larger. The main clinical manifestations of testicular hydrocele include:

- The scrotum is enlarged and may appear as a cystic mass.

- A feeling of swelling in the scrotum, which may be accompanied by pain.

- Testicular palpation may reveal a smooth, cystic mass.

C. How Essential Oils Regulate Testicular Hydrocele

Inflammation, trauma, and reflux blockage are the causes. Promoting blood circulation and removing blood stasis, aromatic dampness, and anti-inflammation is the key. Frankincense, myrrh, tea tree, and cypress can be used. Please do it under the guidance of a doctor or aromatherapist.

D. Aroma Application Guidelines

1. Recommended oils: Frankincense, Cypress, Myrrh, Tea Tree, DDR (an essential oil blend).

2. How to use: 1 drop each of frankincense, myrrh, and cypress, diluted with coconut oil 1:10, apply directly to the scrotal skin of the affected side, 3-4 times a day. When the "lump" does not shrink significantly after 3-4 days, you can use an injection needle under the guidance of a professional doctor to suck out the fluid (often fluid that is larger than a fist) to reduce the blood supply and reabsorption of the "lump" that compresses the surrounding tissue.

You can get twice the result with half the effort. You can also apply the above compound essential oil to the groin of the affected thigh to strengthen the circulation of the veins and promote the disappearance of the lump.

8.5 Epididymitis

Epididymitis is common worldwide.

- According to statistics, about 10% of men will develop epididymitis in their lifetime.

- The disease is more common in teenagers and men of childbearing age.

In recent years, the incidence of epididymitis has been on the rise. This may be related to factors such as the increased incidence of sexually transmitted diseases and unclean sexual life.

Suggestion:
- Pay attention to personal hygiene and avoid infectious diseases.

- Use condoms correctly to prevent sexually transmitted diseases.

- Avoid strenuous exercise.

- Regular physical examination, early detection, and early treatment.

- If symptoms such as scrotal pain and swelling occur, you should seek medical treatment promptly for a clear diagnosis and standardized treatment.

A. What is an Epididymitis

Epididymitis is often caused by infection of adjacent organs, leading to retrograde invasion of the epididymis by viruses such as streptococci and staphylococci. It is often secondary to infection of the urethra, prostate, or seminal vesicles. Epididymitis is inflammation of the epididymis, the male reproductive organ located behind and above the testicles. The epididymis is responsible for storing and transporting sperm.

Cause:

The most common cause of epididymitis is a bacterial infection, usually sexually transmitted. Other causes include:

- Nonspecific urinary tract infection

- Tuberculosis

- Viral infection

- Trauma

B. Clinical Manifestations of Epididymitis

Clinically, the common symptoms include enlargement of the epididymis on the affected side with obvious tenderness, pain in the scrotum with or without a sinking feeling, and referred pain in the lower abdomen and groin, which is aggravated when standing or walking. If the acute phase is not completely cured, it will turn into chronic epididymitis. At this time, the epididymis often enlarges and hardens to varying degrees, with mild tenderness, and the ipsilateral vas deferens may become thicker. The main clinical manifestations of epididymitis include:

- Scrotal pain, which can be severe and usually affects one side.

- Swelling of the scrotum

- Epididymis is tender to palpation

- Fever

- Frequent urination

- Urgency to urinate

• Dysuria

C. How Essential Oils Help Epididymitis

Bacterial retrograde infection is an important cause of epididymitis. If the inflammation does not subside for a long time, it will cause swelling and induration of the epididymis. Promoting blood circulation and removing blood stasis, clearing heat, and detoxifying are the keys to treatment. Frankincense, myrrh, cypress, tea tree, lemon, etc. can be used. Please do it under the guidance of a doctor or aromatherapist.

D. Aroma Application Guidelines

1. Recommended oils: frankincense, cypress, myrrh, tea tree, lemon, DDR (an essential oil blend).

2. How to use:

(1) Oral administration: 4 drops of lemon, 2 drops of tea tree, 2 drops of DDR, drop into about 250ml of warm water and drink once every 4 hours. You can usually drink more warm water to promote metabolism.

(2) Apply 1 drop each of frankincense, myrrh, and cypress, diluted with coconut oil 1:10, and apply directly to the scrotal skin of the affected side 3-4 times a day. You can also apply the above compound essential oil to the groin of the affected thigh to strengthen the circulation of the veins and promote the disappearance of the lump.

8.6 Varicocele

Varicocele is also common worldwide.

• According to statistics, about 15% of men will develop varicocele.

• The disease is more common in teenagers and men of childbearing age.

In recent years, the incidence of varicocele has increased. This may be related to factors such as the increased incidence of male infertility and sedentary life.

Suggestion:

- Pay attention to personal hygiene and avoid infectious diseases.

- Avoid sitting for long periods and exercise appropriately.

- Regular physical examination, early detection, and early treatment.

- If symptoms such as scrotal swelling and pain occur, you should seek medical treatment promptly for a clear diagnosis and standardized treatment.

Varicocele is a common disease in men and can lead to male infertility. Therefore, men should pay attention to the prevention and early treatment of varicocele.

A. What is the Varicocele?

Varicocele is a vascular disease, which refers to the abnormal expansion, elongation, and tortuosity of the pampiform venous plexus in the spermatic cord, which can lead to pain and discomfort and progressive testicular hypofunction. It is one of the common causes of male infertility. The spermatic vein is a vein located in the scrotum that carries blood to the testicles.

Cause: The exact cause of varicocele is unknown, but it may be related to the following factors:

- Increased abdominal pressure: such as chronic constipation, prostatic hyperplasia, etc.

- Valvular dysplasia: leading to venous blood return disorder.

- Genetic factors: People with a family history are at increased risk.

B. Clinical Manifestations of Varicocele

Due to long-term standing fatigue, the valve function in the veins is damaged and disordered, and the blood reflux is incomplete and refluxes into the lower veins. The venous volume is forced to expand and twist, forming a palpable earthworm-shaped and mass-like structure in the scrotum and a varicose spermatic cord. Due to overexertion of the veins, scrotal pain, discomfort, and sinking sensation may occur. In addition, the function of excreting waste and toxins is reduced, which may cause malnutrition of the testicles and epididymis on the affected side, affecting male fertility. The main clinical manifestations of varicocele include:

- Scrotal swelling

- scrotal pain

- Palpable vermiform mass in scrotum

- Symptoms worsen when standing

- Symptoms reduce with bed rest

C. How Essential Oils Help Varicocele

If you suffer from varicocele, it is recommended to go to the hospital for examination. For patients with varicocele of third degree or above, surgical treatment is recommended as the first choice. The disease will recur after surgery, and aromatherapy can be used to prevent it. Those with less than two degrees may consider aromatherapy. Frankincense and cypress essential oils can be used to activate blood circulation, improve blood circulation, and slow down varicose veins. Please do it under the guidance of a doctor or aromatherapist.

D. Aroma Application Guidelines

1. Recommended oils: frankincense, cypress, etc.

2. Usage: 2 drops of each of frankincense and cypress, diluted with coconut oil 1:5, apply directly to the inner thigh of the left side. It can also be used on the scrotum and lower abdomen on the same side at the same

time. Generally, once every 4 hours within a week and once a week after that. three times. At the same time, it is recommended to change the exercise to swimming or push-ups once every 3 days. The intensity of exercise should be stopped when you feel slightly tired. If you can take a cold bath before going to bed, dry, and rub the red skin after the bath, the effect will be better.

8.7 Male Urinary Tract Infection

Male urinary tract infections are common worldwide.

- According to statistics, about 50% of men will develop a urinary tract infection in their lifetime.

- Male urinary tract infections are more common in adolescents and men of childbearing age.

In recent years, the incidence of male urinary tract infections has been on the rise. This may be related to factors such as the increased incidence of sexually transmitted diseases, unclean sex, urinary tract obstruction, etc.

Suggestion:
- Pay attention to personal hygiene and avoid infectious diseases.

- Use condoms correctly to prevent sexually transmitted diseases.

- Drink plenty of water to keep your urinary tract clear.

- Regular physical examination, early detection, and early treatment.

- If symptoms such as frequent urination, urgent urination, and painful urination occur, you should seek medical treatment promptly for a clear diagnosis and standardized treatment.

Male urinary tract infection is a common disease in men and can affect men's sexual life and fertility. Therefore, men should pay attention to the prevention and early treatment of male urinary tract infections.

A. What Is a Male Urinary Tract Infection

A male urinary tract infection is an infection that occurs in the male urethra and can be caused by a variety of reasons, including:

- Bacterial infection: The most common pathogen is Escherichia coli, and other pathogenic bacteria include Neisseria gonorrhoeae, Chlamydia trachomatis, Mycoplasma, etc.

- Non-bacterial infections: such as Candida, viruses, etc.

- Urinary tract obstruction: such as prostatic hyperplasia, urethral stricture, etc.

- Other factors: such as sexual life, trauma, etc.

B. Clinical Manifestations of Male Urinary Tract Infection

Urethral tingling and pus discharge can be seen. Delay in seeking treatment can lead to infection, causing symptoms of frequent urination, painful urination, urgency, or even fever. If the fever exceeds 39°C, you should go to the hospital; although there is urethral discharge but no fever, you can receive aromatherapy first.

C. How Essential Oils Help Male Urinary Tract Infection

Traditional Chinese medicine believes that stranguria syndrome is caused by dampness poisoning. Clinically, essential oils that can clear away heat, detoxify, and promote dampness, such as tea tree, lemon, etc., should be used. Please do it under the guidance of a doctor or aromatherapist.

D. Aroma Application Guidelines

1. Recommended oils: lemon, tea tree, eucalyptus, Onguard (an essential oil mixture), etc.

2. Instructions:
(1) Oral administration: 4 to 6 drops of lemon essential oil, drop into warm water and drink once every 4 hours; in severe cases, use 4 drops of lemon and 2 to 4 drops of tea tree essential oil, drop into a glass with 250 ml of

warm water and then drink 500ml of warm water to promote the excretion of toxins after 10 minutes.

(2) Application: Topically apply 1 to 2 drops each of tea tree, eucalyptus, and Onguard essential oils directly on the outer surface of the urethra and the skin on the ventral side of the penis (sensitive bodies can dilute it with coconut oil 1:1). If you have frequent urination, for bladder irritation symptoms such as urgent urination and painful urination, you can apply it on the lower abdomen and bladder area once every 4 hours, and three times a day after the symptoms improve.

8.8 Prostatitis

Prostatitis is common worldwide.

- According to statistics, about 30% of men will develop prostatitis in their lifetime.

- Prostatitis is more common in teenagers and men of childbearing age.

In recent years, the incidence of prostatitis has been on the rise. This may be related to factors such as the increased incidence of sexually transmitted diseases and sedentary life.

Suggestion:
- Pay attention to personal hygiene and avoid infectious diseases.

- Avoid sitting for long periods and exercise appropriately.

- Maintain good sexual habits.

- Regular physical examination, early detection, and early treatment.

- If symptoms such as frequent urination, urgent urination, and painful urination occur, you should seek medical treatment promptly for a clear diagnosis and standardized treatment.

Prostatitis is a common disease in men that can affect their sexual life and fertility. Therefore, men should pay attention to the prevention and early treatment of prostatitis.

A. What is Prostatitis

Prostatitis is an acute and chronic inflammation of the prostate caused by prostate-specific and non-specific infections, with urethral irritation symptoms and chronic pelvic pain as the main clinical manifestations. Most cases are chronic aseptic, and acute bacterial prostatitis is rare. Due to the unique capsule barrier of the prostate, infection, and inflammation are generally less likely to occur. Only when there is a decrease in the body's resistance, excessive fatigue, irregular sexual life, too much (including masturbation), too little or long-term abstinence, excessive addiction to tobacco, alcohol, spicy food, and having sex when you have a cold or are unwell can cause prostate cancer. Long-term chronic blood stasis and reduced resistance provide opportunities for pathogenic bodies to become infected.

B. Clinical Manifestations of Prostatitis

Prostatitis belongs to the categories of urinary turbidity, hot stranguria, and strain in traditional Chinese medicine. Its onset is related to dampness and heat in the liver meridian, liver qi stagnation, inability to do what one wants, blood stasis blocking the collaterals, excessive sexual exertion, kidney yin damage, etc. Acute prostatitis refers to acute inflammation caused by prostate-specific bacterial infection, which mainly manifests as urinary urgency, frequent urination, dysuria, rectal and perineal pain, and often an aversion to cold and fever. Chronic prostatitis has many clinical manifestations. This is because the prostate is in the pelvic cavity and is affected by many sympathetic and parasympathetic hormones. There are three common categories:

1. The clinical manifestations of the neurotic type include insomnia, abdominal discomfort, frequent urination, poor urination, poor sexual function, or even disorder. Once the illness lasts for a long time and the correct treatment is not obtained, people often believe that chronic prostatitis is the disease. If the disease is incurable, it will cause mental disorders, often painful urination, especially symptoms of abdominal discomfort, perineal prolapse, abnormal urination and defecation, and other symptoms of autonomic nervous system dysfunction.

2. The inflammatory type is characterized by frequent urination, urgen-

cy, less abdominal discomfort, and less painful urination. It is mostly caused by sexual intercourse after drinking, colds, chronic gingivitis, and pharyngitis treatment. It can also be caused by too much or too little sexual intercourse. Mostly non-bacterial inflammation. Inflammation causes the prostate to swell and the prostate sympathetic nerves to become overly sensitive, leading to dysfunction of the opening and closing of the posterior urethral muscles at the bladder neck opening.

3. No morning erection or weak erection characterizes kidney deficiency type. Even if it is done reluctantly, it is prone to backache, dizziness, dizziness, premature ejaculation, listlessness after intercourse, or general weakness and lack of energy. It is also accompanied by lumbosacral soreness and lower abdominal discomfort. Frequent urination or even dribbling of urine.

C. How Essential Oils Help Chronic Prostatitis

Due to the existence of the prostate "capsule barrier," it is difficult for drugs to enter the prostate, which directly affects the therapeutic effect. Some high-quality plant essential oils have small molecular weight, strong lipophilicity, and strong permeability and can reach the hospital directly through the envelope. In addition, plant essential oils are excellent in antibacterial, antiviral, immune regulation, antioxidant repair, cell repair, and mood regulation. Performance. We have observed for many years that prostatitis can achieve the desired results as long as the diagnosis is clear and the oil is used appropriately. In addition, it should be noted that the symptoms caused by chronic prostatitis are not very clear clinically, which requires clinical aromatherapists to handle them appropriately, and the expected results can also be achieved. Please do it under the guidance of a doctor or aromatherapist.

D. Aroma Application Guidelines

(1) Neurotic type

1. Recommended Oils: wild orange, Balance (a blend of essential oils), Digestzen (a blend of essential oils), Zendocrine (a blend of essential oils), DDR (a blend of essential oils), lavender, vetiver, cedarwood, etc.

2. Instructions:
(1) Inhalation: Inhale wild orange essential oil, 3 to 4 times a day.
(2) Aromatherapy: For insomnia, fatigue, etc., you can add 2 drops

of each of lavender, vetiver, and cedar. Drop it into an aromatherapy diffuser before going to bed to enhance the effect of soothing your mood.

(3) Application: Apply the Balance essential oil to the Baihui point on the top of the head, 3 to 4 times a day, and apply it to the Yongquan point on the soles of the feet at night. If patients have discomfort in the lower abdomen and perineum, they can apply the Digestzen essential oil to soothe the liver and regulate qi on the lower abdomen and coccyx, 3 times a day, 1 to 2 drops each time, and apply it to the soles of the feet at night.

(4) Oral administration: If you have symptoms of poor erectile function or erectile dysfunction, you can take 4 drops of Zendocrine and DDR and pour it into an empty capsule, 1 capsule each time, 2 times a day. Or take 1 to 2 capsules of Zendocrine capsules and DDR capsules directly, twice a day. A course of treatment is 3 months, and it can be used every other day after taking effect.

(2) Inflammatory type

1. Recommended oils: DDR (an essential oil blend), lemon, lavender, peppermint, yarrow, tea tree, Digestzen (an essential oil blend), and other essential oils.

2. Instructions:

a. Oral administration: 6 to 8 drops of DDR essential oil, put into a capsule and taken, 1 capsule each time, 3 times a day. You can also take 1 to 2 drops each of lemon, lavender, peppermint, and tea tree into an empty capsule, 1 capsule each time, 3 times a day, with warm water. If you have lower abdominal discomfort, you can also use 2 drops each of Digestzen and Yarrow and add them to warm water for drinking.

b. Application: If you have lower abdominal discomfort, you can also use 2 drops each of Digestzen and yarrow essential oil, diluted with coconut oil 1: (1-3), and apply it locally.

It is worth noting that please do not resume sexual life immediately after the above symptoms disappear. You should decide based on your physical condition.

(3) Kidney deficiency type

1. Recommended oils: Zendocrine (an essential oil blend), clary sage, yarrow, cypress, DDR (an essential oil blend), and other essential oils.

2. Instructions:

a. Oral administration

Take 2 drops each of Zendocrine, clary sage, and yarrow, and pour into an empty capsule, 1 capsule each time, 3 times a day.

If the illness lasts for a long time and does not heal, taking the LLV (a supplement kit) 2 times a day, 2 capsules each time, on an empty stomach is recommended.

b. Application: If you have pain in the lumbosacral area, you can use 2 drops each of Zendocrine, clary sage, cypress, and DDR essential oil, diluted with coconut oil 1: (1-3), and apply it locally.

8.9 Prostatic Hyperplasia

Prostatic hyperplasia is common worldwide.

- According to statistics, about 50% of men over 50 years old suffer from prostatic hyperplasia, and the prevalence rate among men over 80 years old can reach 90%.

- Prostatic hyperplasia is more common in developed countries.

In recent years, the incidence of prostatic hyperplasia has been on the rise. This may be related to factors such as men's extended life span and changes in dietary structure.

Suggestion:

- Pay attention to personal hygiene and avoid infectious diseases.

- Maintain a healthy lifestyle and avoid sitting for long periods.

- Regular physical examination, early detection, and early treatment.

- If symptoms such as frequent urination, urgent urination, and painful urination occur, you should seek medical treatment promptly for a clear diagnosis and standardized treatment.

If you have symptoms of prostatic hyperplasia, please seek medical treatment promptly for a clear diagnosis and standardized treatment.

A. What is Prostatic Hyperplasia

Prostatic hyperplasia, also known as benign prostatic hyperplasia (BPH), refers to the enlargement and enlargement of the prostate than normal. Prostatic hyperplasia is a common disease among middle-aged and elderly men. The prostate is located at the mouth of the bladder neck. Its size is 4cm × 3cm × 2cm. It is shaped like a chestnut and contains the prostate urethra. Therefore, irregular prostate hyperplasia can compress the urethra or affect urination due to irregular contraction of the bladder neck, or prostate capsule.

B. Clinical Manifestations of Prostatic Hyperplasia

Once urination obstruction, frequent urination, weak urination, increased nocturia, B-ultrasound examination shows that the prostate is larger than 4cm×3cm×2cm, the residual urine in the bladder is less than 80mL, and there are plaques and irregular shadows in the prostate, it can be considered as prostatic hyperplasia with inflammation, treatment is necessary. The main clinical manifestations of prostatic hyperplasia include:

- Symptoms of urinary tract irritation: frequent urination, urgency, painful urination, and increased nocturia

- Difficulty urinating: hesitant urination, thin urine stream, incomplete urination

- In severe cases, urinary retention may occur.

C. How Essential Oils Regulate Prostate Hyperplasia

Cell repair compound, kidney-nourishing liver compound essential oil can be used to improve the contractility of the bladder and regulate the opening and closing of the bladder neck. Essential oils from large trees such as cinnamon and fir can also be used. Please do it under the guidance of a doctor or aromatherapist.

D. Aroma Application Guidelines

1. Recommended oils: Juniper Berry, Frankincense, DDR (an essential oil blend), Cedarwood, Digestzen (an essential oil blend), Zendocrine (an essential oil blend), etc.

2. Instructions:

(1) 2 drops each of DDR and Zendocrine essential oils, diluted with coconut oil 1:3, apply to the perineum, lumbosacral area, and soles of the feet before going to bed. A course of treatment is 3 months. For long-term prostatic hyperplasia, it is recommended to add frankincense essential oil for care. 2 drops each of the above essential oils plus frankincense, 1 to 2 courses a year, with a stage of 3 years.

(2) For those with symptoms of prostatitis, such as pain in the lower abdomen and lumbosacral region, add 1 to 2 drops each of Digestzen, frankincense, juniper berry, and cedarwood, and apply it locally with coconut oil 1:1 as a base.

8.10 Sexual Dysfunction

Sexual dysfunction is common worldwide.

- According to statistics, about 50% of men will experience sexual dysfunction during their lifetime.

- Sexual dysfunction is more common in middle-aged and older men.

In recent years, the incidence of sexual dysfunction has been on the rise. This may be related to factors such as the accelerated pace of life, increased stress, and poor lifestyle.

Suggestion:

- Maintain a healthy lifestyle and avoid sitting for long periods.

- Quit smoking and drinking and avoid excessive drinking.

- Maintain a good mental state and avoid anxiety and depression.

- Regular physical examination, early detection, and early treatment.

- If sexual dysfunction occurs, you should seek medical treatment promptly for a clear diagnosis and standardized treatment.

A. What Is Sexual Dysfunction

Male sexual function and sexual satisfaction are incompetent, often manifested by sexual desire disorder, impotence, premature ejaculation, spermatorrhea, no ejaculation, and retrograde ejaculation. Sexual behavior is not only an instinctive reaction but also a physiological activity based on mental and psychological activities. Therefore, male sexual dysfunction is partly caused by systemic diseases, reproductive system diseases, and organic diseases. Most patients have sexual psychological dysfunction and organ dysfunction. Rarely caused by disease (such as paraplegia due to spinal cord trauma). Without a correct view of sex, sexual dysfunction will occur, and sexual dysfunction must be treated by both men and women.

B. Clinical Manifestations of Sexual Dysfunction

1. Weak erection: For severe impotence, it is necessary to understand whether the cause is emotional or due to chronic prostatitis. If it is psychological, the clinical manifestation is that it does not stand up when it needs to stand up and does not wilt when it needs to wilt. You can use essential oils to regulate your mood.

2. Premature ejaculation: refers to the discharge of semen outside the female reproductive tract during sexual intercourse. The main reason is that the ejaculation threshold is too low or there is a lack of self-discipline in self-regulating excitability.

3. Anejaculation: refers to a condition in which sexual intercourse lasts for a long time without ejaculation, and the penis shrinks without ejaculation afterward. The reason is that ejaculation stasis increases, or semen volume is insufficient (insufficient gunpowder), and the failure to ejaculate. In severe cases, it can lead to hyperactivity of yang.

4. Hyperactivity: The penis is often lifted without impotence, which can last for a few hours or more than 24 hours. As the so-called "male heart" is impure, it violates lust and caution, the yang energy is floating on the penis, and the penis cannot be lifted, or it may be due to the penis. The entrance of the cavernous sinus in the cavernous body should be closed or not, and the outlet should be open or not. The imbalance of closing and opening causes this.

5. Azoospermia: Azoospermia is the absence of sperm in the semen.

Azoospermia caused by congenital small testicles, such as prostatitis, spermatic corditis, etc., can also lead to azoospermia. Azoospermia caused by vas deferens obstruction has normal testicular size.

6. Infertility: Male infertility refers to a couple living together for more than 1 year without taking any contraceptive measures, and the woman is infertile due to the man's factors. Any factor that affects sperm production, maturation, ejaculation, capacitation, or fertilization can lead to male infertility. Common causes of male infertility include primary infertility and secondary infertility. Primary cases are mostly related to Y chromosome defects, abnormal testicular development, congenital absence of vas deferens, etc. Secondary cases are more common in male varicocele, chronic prostatitis, and abnormal sperm development caused by testicular dysfunction.

C. How Essential Oils Regulate Sexual Dysfunction

Different methods are used to target different causes, pathogenesis, and clinical manifestations of sexual dysfunction. For example, infertility due to abnormal sperm development is mainly related to malnutrition. In addition to dietary factors, physical factors, and excretion factors, improving the nutritional status of the human body also requires the application of essential oils that support fertility and improve sperm quality, such as juniper berry, Geranium, jasmine, rose, clary sage, etc. Please do it under the guidance of a doctor or aromatherapist.

D. Aroma Application Guidelines

(1) Weak erection and severe impotence

1. Recommended oils: Ylang-Ylang, Clary Sage, Cedarwood, Balance Blend (an essential oil blend), Cinnamon, Rose, Hawaiian Sandalwood, DDR Blend (an essential oil blend), Zendocrine Blend (an essential oil blend) and other essential oils.

2. Instructions:
a. Aromatherapy: If psychological factors cause it, choose 2 to 3 essential oils such as ylang-ylang, clary sage, cedar, rose, etc., take 2 drops of each, and add it to the aroma diffuser for aromatherapy.
b. Topical apply: Use Balance compound essential oil and apply it on Baihui and Yongquan points before sex; if necessary, you can use 2 to 3 types of ylang-ylang, clary sage, cedarwood, cinnamon, etc., 1 to 2 drops of each,

dilute coconut oil 1:3 and apply it to the roots of the thighs; and for woman can also apply rose essential oil at the same time. The application time needs to be adjusted by both parties, usually 1 to 2 hours before intercourse.

c. Oral administration: If it is caused by chronic prostatitis, you can use DDR compound and Zendocrine compound essential oil, pour 2 to 3 drops of each into a capsule, and take 1 to 2 capsules each time, twice a day in the morning and evening.

(2) Premature ejaculation

1. Recommended oils: Zendocrine (an essential oil blend), Balance (an essential oil blend), Clary Sage, Rose, Jasmine, Ylang-Ylang.

2. Instructions for use: 4 drops each of Zendocrine, clary sage, and ylang-ylang, 2 drops of jasmine, diluted with coconut oil 1:3, apply to Guanyuan point, Qihai point, perineum, inner thigh, or Apply 2 drops of lavender and 2 drops of Balance on the soles of the man's feet. The woman should use 2 drops of rose and ylang-ylang essential oils before intercourse. Inhale and apply on the Guanyuan point, Qihai point, perineum, etc., to enhance sexual interest. It is usually pleasant. Happy essential oils can be applied to enhance satisfaction for both parties.

(3) Anejaculation

1. Recommended oils: Ylang-Ylang, Schisandra chinensis, Zendocrine (an essential oil blend), Balance (an essential oil blend), and Cinnamon.

2. Instructions:
a. Oral administration: Take Schisandra chinensis and Yuanqi compound 3 times a day, add 2 drops each time into a glass of 250ml warm water and drink, and then drink 500ml of warm water after 5-15 minutes to facilitate the metabolism of essential oils. Add a total of 4-6 drops of lemon essential oil and take it together for better results.

b. Apply 1-2 times each of balancing compound essential oil, juniper berry, and vitality compound, diluted with coconut oil 1:5, and apply to the ejaculation center of lumbar vertebra 4-5, twice a day, and once before going to bed. For better results, you can use Vitality Complex, Clary Sage, and Perfect Repair Complex, 1-2 drops each, diluted 1:5 with coconut oil, and apply it to the base camp (testicles, scrotum) to promote spermatogenesis and fluid transfer.

It is worth noting that aromatherapy should be used for 1-2 weeks before sexual intercourse. After success, the subrhythm will still be maintained for more than 1 month. Afterward, the patient can adjust the rhythm by himself depending on his health status. If necessary, consult a senior aromatherapist or urologist to avoid future troubles.

(4) Hyperactivity

1. Recommended Oils: Balance (an essential oil blend), Angelica Sinensis, Frankincense, DDR (an essential oil blend), Zendocrine (an essential oil blend), Helichrysum, Cypress.

2. Instructions:
a. Apply: Use 1 drop each of Balance, Frankincense, Helichrysum, and DDR, diluted 1:5 with coconut oil, and apply it to the raised penis body, perineum, and root of the corpus cavernosum, once every 4 hours. If the penis body is weak, you can reduce the number of applications. It is better to add 1 drop of Angelica sinensis to the application compound to achieve faster and better results.
b. Orally: 2 drops of DDR, 1 drop of frankincense, drop into a glass with warm water, 2 times a day. If possible, add 4 drops of lemon, 1 drop of peppermint, and 1 drop of lavender, 4 times daily for better results.
If you encounter special circumstances, such as after surgery, please consult a professional nurse or andrologist to use oil to prevent sequelae.

(5) Azoospermia

Obstructive azoospermia should first exclude azoospermia caused by congenital microorchidism. Physical examination: The testicles on both sides were normal in size, the structure of the epididymis and spermatic cord were normal, and there was no varicocele. Ultrasound: If the size of the bladder and prostate is normal, but the seminal vesicles are full and enlarged, and there is no sperm in the semen examination, it can be diagnosed as obstructive azoospermia.

1. Recommended oils: rose, frankincense, clary sage, angelica, DDR (an essential oil blend), Zendocrine (an essential oil blend) essential oils.

2. Instructions:
a. External application: Take 1 drop of each of the above essential oils, dilute 1:10 with coconut oil, and apply directly to the scrotum and groin on both sides. It is recommended to apply it in categories, massage, and massage appropriately according to the direction of sperm movement in physiological

anatomy, twice a day, and once before going to bed for better results.

b. Oral administration: Take 1 drop of each of the above essential oils into a capsule three times a day, one capsule at a time, and drink plenty of water.

c. Semen testing once a month.

(6) Infertility

Primary infertility generally cannot be cured. For secondary infertility, treatment mainly focuses on the cause. This article mainly focuses on abnormal sperm development caused by abnormal testicular function.

1. Recommended oils: rose, ylang-ylang, clary sage, Zendocrine (an essential oil mixture), and other essential oils.

2. Instructions:

a. External application: Take 2 drops of the above essential oils, dilute it 1:1 with coconut oil, and apply it on the lower abdomen, inner thighs, and lumbosacral area.

b. Oral administration: Take 2 drops of each of the above essential oils into a capsule, 1 capsule each time, 2 times a day, morning and evening.

In this chapter, we analyze the health problems faced by men in various periods and propose countermeasures for using plant essential oils for conditioning. Various application methods are taught; please consult a doctor or aromatherapist before using it.

Chapter 9

Integrating Essential Oils into

Men's Lifestyles

W e guide safely incorporating essential oils into a man's lifestyle. We cover selecting and using essential oils, blending techniques, and application methods and provide DIY projects and recipes.

9.1 Hybrid Technology and Application Methods

In this chapter, we'll explore the art of blending essential oils and various application methods for optimal results and enjoyment. We discuss the principles of blending and the importance of synergy and provide practical guidance on creating blends and applying essential oils to maximize their therapeutic benefits.

A. Understand the Mixing Principles of Essential Oils

Synergy in the context of essential oils refers to the combined effect of different essential oils that work together to enhance their individual properties and create a more powerful and balanced therapeutic effect. When essential oils are strategically blended, their chemical components can interact with each other, amplifying their benefits and creating a unique and harmonious aromatic profile.

Here are the synergies with essential oils:

1. Complementary properties: Different essential oils have different chemical compositions, and each has its own set of therapeutic properties. By combining oils with complementary properties, you can target multiple problems at the same time. For example, mixing an oil with antibacterial properties and an oil with anti-inflammatory properties can address infection and inflammation.

2. Enhance aroma: Combining oils with pleasant aromas can create more complex and appealing scents. This is particularly beneficial in aromatherapy, where the aroma of a mixture can have a positive impact on mood and mood.

3. Balance effects: Some oils can be very potent on their own, and mixing them with milder oils can help balance their effects and reduce the risk of adverse reactions, such as skin sensitivity.

4. Broad spectrum of action: Synergistic blends can have a wider range of action than single oils. This is particularly useful when dealing with multifaceted issues or promoting overall well-being.

5. Unique therapeutic properties: The combined chemical composition of different oils can produce therapeutic properties that are not present in any single oil. This allows for a more nuanced and versatile approach to solving a variety of problems.

6. Personalized solutions: By blending essential oils, you can customize the blend to meet your specific needs or preferences. This makes aromatherapy a highly customizable practice.

When creating a synergistic blend, it is important to consider the following factors:

* Chemical compatibility: The chemical makeup of some essential oils may not interact well with other essential oils. Research the chemical composition of the oil you use to ensure compatibility.

*Treatment goals: Determine your desired results. Is your goal for relaxation, energy, immune support, or pain relief? Choose an oil that meets these goals.

* Aroma: Consider the aroma you want to achieve. Some oils have strong, uplifting scents, while others are more calming. Mixing oils with complementary aromas creates a more pleasant and balanced scent.

* Ratios: Try different mixing ratios to find the right balance of oils. Start with a small amount of each oil and adjust as needed.

*Skin sensitivity: Keep in mind that some oils can be skin irritants, especially when used undiluted. Thinning with a carrier oil is crucial, especially when mixing multiple oils.

Synergy is a fundamental concept in aromatherapy, allowing for the creative and effective use of essential oils to address a wide range of physical, emotional, and spiritual issues.

When creating effective and safe blends, it is crucial to choose essential oils with complementary aromas, therapeutic properties, and safety profiles. Here are some things to keep in mind:

1. Aroma compatibility:

* Choose essential oils with a harmonious blend of aromas to create a pleasant scent. The balanced and comprehensive aroma enhances the overall experience.
* Some oils have a strong dominant scent, while others are more subtle. Consider the scent intensity of each oil and how they interact with each other.

2. Therapeutic properties:

*Determine your desired treatment goals. Is your goal to relax, uplift, soothe, or uplift? Choose an oil with properties that match your intentions.
* Research the specific healing properties of each oil. For example, if you're looking for a pain reliever, choose an oil with analgesic and anti-inflammatory properties.

3. Security configuration file:

* Assess the safety of each oil. Some oils are generally safe for most people, while others have specific precautions, contraindications, or age restrictions.
* Consider the possibility of skin irritation, photosensitivity, and other adverse reactions. Always follow recommended dilution guidelines and perform a patch test.

4. Chemical composition:

* Research the chemical composition of each oil. Certain chemical families (such as monoterpenes, sesquiterpenes, esters, etc.) have specific therapeutic properties.
* Look for oils with complementary chemical profiles for synergistic effects.

5. Balance strength:

* If using a strong oil, balance it with a milder oil to avoid overpowering the fragrance or effects of the mixture.
* Milder oils can also act as carriers for stronger oils, helping to distribute their properties more evenly.

6. Personal preference:

* Your personal preference and sensory response play an important role in choosing an oil. Some scents resonate more personally, so choose oils that you find attractive and comforting.

7. Intent and application:

* Consider the context in which you will use the mix. Is it for relaxation, mood enhancement, respiratory support, or skincare? Tailor your oil selection to your specific application.
* Choose an oil appropriate for the intended method of use, whether topically, inhaled, or diffused.

8. Mixing ratio:

* Experiment with different mixing ratios to find the right balance of aroma and therapeutic effect.
* Start with a small amount of strongly scented oil and gradually add

other essential oils while evaluating the aroma.

9. Research and resources:

* Use reputable aromatherapy references, books, and online resources to learn about the properties and aromas of different oils.
* Please consult an experienced aromatherapist or essential oil expert for guidance.

Remember, essential oil blending is both an art and a science. It involves creativity, intuition, and a deep understanding of the oils you are using. It's also good practice to keep detailed records of the mixtures you create, noting the oils used, their proportions, and the effects observed. This can help you improve your blending skills over time and develop your signature blend based on your needs and preferences.

B. Basic Mixing Techniques

Introducing basic blending techniques such as the top, middle, and base notes system can greatly improve your ability to create a balanced and harmonious blend of essential oils. This technique is based on the concept of layering oils with different volatilities to create depth and longevity in the aroma of the blend. Here's how it works:

1. Top notes:

* The top notes are the most volatile and evaporate quickly. They provide the initial aroma, which is often bright, uplifting, and refreshing.
* Common top-note oils include citrus oils such as lemon, lime, and bergamot, and herbal oils such as peppermint and eucalyptus.
* When creating a blend, start with a small portion of the top notes. They add a lively and uplifting quality to the aroma.

2. Middle notes:

* The middles have a moderate evaporation rate and are the heart of the blend. They balance the aroma between the top and base notes.
*Middle notes are usually floral and slightly sweet, contributing to the overall body of the blend.
* Essential oils such as lavender, geranium, and chamomile are often used as middle notes.

3. Basic notes:

* Base notes are minimally volatile, providing depth, richness, and staying power to blends.
* They have a grounding effect that helps anchor lighter tops and middles.
* Wood oils such as cedar, sandalwood, and patchouli are often used as base notes.

4. Mixing ratio:

* To create a balanced mix, follow proportions that align with the top, mid, and base systems. A common ratio is about 30% top notes, 50% mid-range, and 20% base notes.
* However, these ratios can be adjusted to your preference and the specific effect you want.

5. Layering and testing:

* Start by selecting essential oils for each note category. Layer them one by one, starting with the base notes, then the middle and top notes.
* Mix a small amount of oil and evaluate the aroma. Keep adjusting the ratio until you reach the desired balance.

6. Mixed synergies:

* The synergy of essential oils from different note categories creates a multi-dimensional aroma that evolves.
* When mixed properly, different notes transition seamlessly, providing a complete and complex olfactory experience.

7. Personalization:

* Top, mid, and base systems provide a structured framework, but don't hesitate to experiment and adjust the proportions to suit your preferences and intentions.
* Personalization is the key to creating a blend that resonates with you and provides the desired therapeutic benefits.

The system of top, middle, and base notes is a fundamental technique in aromatherapy, allowing you to create blends with depth, complexity, and harmonious aroma profiles. With experience, you'll develop an intuitive understanding of how different oils interact and can adjust this technique to suit your unique blending style.

Here are some examples of essential oils for each note category (top, middle, and base notes) and their characteristics:

Top notes:

Top notes are usually light and fresh and evaporate quickly. They provide the initial aroma, which is often uplifting and uplifting. Some examples include:

1. Lemon: Energetic and cheerful, lemon oil is commonly used for its fresh and welcoming scent.
2. Peppermint: Peppermint oil is rich in menthol, is invigorating, and is known for its cooling and refreshing aroma.
3. Bergamot: Bergamot oil has a citrusy and uplifting aroma and is known for its calming and balancing qualities.
4. Eucalyptus: Camphor oil has clear properties and is often used to promote a feeling of rejuvenation.

Middle notes:

The mid-note oil is balanced and comprehensive, providing body to the blend. They generally have a moderate evaporation rate and contribute to the core of the aroma. Examples include:

1. Lavender: Floral and calming, lavender oil is widely used for its soothing and relaxing properties.
2. Geranium: Rose-colored and harmonizing, geranium oil is known for its balancing and calming effects.
3. Chamomile: Sweet and herbal, chamomile oil is often used for its mild, comforting scent.
4. Rosemary: Herbal and energizing, rosemary oil is valued for its stimulating and uplifting properties.

Base notes:

The base oil is deep, grounding, and slow to evaporate. They provide stability and longevity to the mix, creating a solid foundation. Examples include:

1. Cedar: Woody and warm, cedar oil is often used for its calming and grounding properties.

2. Sandalwood: Earthy and exotic, sandalwood oil is prized for its meditative and relaxing qualities.

3. Patchouli: Rich and musky, patchouli oil is known for its aphrodisiac and calming properties.

4. Vetiver: Woody and smoky vetiver oils are used for their calming and stabilizing effects.

Keep in mind that these are just a few examples; many other essential oils fall into each note category. The beauty of aromatherapy is the wide variety of essential oils, each with its own unique scent and therapeutic benefits. When blending, consider the characteristics of each note and how they work together to create a balanced and harmonious aromatic experience.

C. Create a Personalized Blend

Creating a personalized essential oil blend can be an enjoyable and rewarding process. Here's a step-by-step guide to help you create a blend for a specific purpose:

Step 1: Determine your intent

Determine the purpose of the mix. Is it for relaxation, concentration, breathing support, or some other goal? This intention will guide your oil selection.

Step 2: Choose essential oils

Choose essential oils that match your intentions. Consider oils from different fragrance categories to create a balanced and harmonious scent. For example, for relaxation, you might choose lavender (middle note), bergamot (top note), and cedar wood (base note).

Step 3: Research properties

Research the properties of each selected oil. Learn about their aroma, therapeutic benefits, and potential preventative measures.

Step 4: Choose a carrier Oil

Choose a carrier oil to dilute your essential oils. Common carrier oils include jojoba oil, sweet almond oil, and coconut oil. This step is critical for safe topical application.

Step 5: Calculate the dilution ratio

Calculate the dilution rate based on your intended use and the age of the person using the mixture. A common dilution ratio for adults is 2 to 3% (12 to 18 drops of essential oil per ounce of carrier oil). For children or sensitive individuals, use a lower dilution ratio.

Step 6: Create your mixture

Use a dropper to measure selected essential oils and add them to a container of your choice. Start with the fundamental note, then the middle and top notes. Keep track of total droplets to ensure you stay within the recommended dilution ratio.

Step 7: Mix and test

Gently mix the essential oil and carrier oil by rolling the container between your palms. Do a patch test on a small area of skin to check for any adverse reactions. Wait 24 hours to ensure there is no sensitivity.

Step 8: Adjust as needed

If the aroma or effect of the mixture isn't what you want, you can adjust the proportions of essential oils or add different oils to achieve the desired effect.

Step 9: Label your mixture

Label your mixture with purpose, ingredients, and dilution ratios. This ensures that you can recreate it in the future and use it safely.

Step 10: Enjoy your blend

Use your personalized blend as needed, apply it to pulse points, use it in a diffuser, or add it to a warm bath. Observe its effect and adjust as necessary.

Keep in mind that blending essential oils is an art form, and it may take a few tries to create the perfect blend that resonates with you. Pay attention to how each oil makes you feel and be open to experimentation. Enjoy the journey of creating unique scents to support your health.

Experimentation is a key aspect of creating personalized essential oil blends. Everyone may have different preferences and reactions to different oils, so it's important to try different combinations and adjust. Here's why it's crucial to experiment, take notes, and adjust your ratios:

1. Personal Reaction: Everyone's body chemistry is unique, so an oil that works for one person may not have the same effect on another. Experimenting allows you to find something that resonates with you.

2. Aroma Preferences: Aroma is subjective, and what may be pleasant to one person may be off-putting to another. By trying different blends, you can discover the scents you find most appealing and comforting.

3. Targeted effects: Essential oils have a range of therapeutic properties, and some may be better than others for certain purposes. Experimentation can help you determine which oils are most effective in achieving your desired results.

4. Adjust the proportions: If the mixture is not providing the desired effect, you can adjust the proportions of essential oils. Increasing or decreasing the amount of a specific oil can change the overall aroma and therapeutic effect.

5. Take notes: Keeping a journal of your experiments is invaluable. Note the oils you used, their proportions, your impression of the scent, and any effects you experienced. This record will help you track your progress and optimize your mix over time.

6. Incremental Change: Sometimes, small changes can make a big difference. Adjusting the ratio of one oil in the blend can result in a more balanced aroma or more dramatic therapeutic effects.

7. Safety Precautions: Experiments should always be performed safely. Follow the recommended dilution ratios and perform a patch test to avoid adverse reactions. If you are trying a new oil, start with a lower dilution and work your way up if necessary.

8. Creativity and Expression: Creating mixes is a creative process. Think of it as making your aromatic masterpiece. Experimentation allows you to express your unique preferences and create something that works for you.

9. Learn and grow: The more you experiment with essential oils, the more you understand their properties and interactions. This knowledge will enable you to create effective blends to meet your specific needs.

Remember, patience is key when trying essential oils. The mixture may take time to fully develop its aroma, and its therapeutic effects may be more pronounced with continued use. Be open to the journey of discovery and enjoy the process of creating blends that support your health.

D. How to Use

Let's explore the different ways to apply essential oils:

1. Local application:

* Dilution: Essential oils are effective and should be diluted with a carrier oil (such as jojoba, coconut, or almond oil) before applying to the skin. This helps prevent skin sensitivity and allows for safer use.
*Pulse points: Apply diluted essential oil to pulse points such as your wrists, temples, and behind your ears. Blood vessels in these areas are close to the surface of the skin, which enhances absorption.
*Massage: Add essential oils to massage oil for a relaxing experience. Massage also helps with the absorption and distribution of oils.
* Targeted areas: Apply to specific areas of concern, such as muscle soreness or joints, to promote comfort and relaxation.
* Bath: Add a few drops of essential oil to a warm bath. Mix the oil with an emulsifier, such as a carrier oil or bath salts, to disperse them evenly in the water.

2. Inhalation:

* Direct inhalation: Inhale the aroma directly from the bottle. This is quick and convenient for a burst of scent.
* Hand inhalation: Place a few drops of essential oil in your hands, rub them together, and cover your nose with a cup. Take a deep breath.
* Steam inhalation: Add a few drops of oil to a bowl of hot water. Cover your head with a towel, lean against the bowl, and inhale the steam. This can

relieve congestion and breathing problems.

*Personal inhaler: Use a personal inhaler stick or inhaler necklace for on-the-go aromatherapy. They allow you to inhale the oil discreetly.

3. Diffuse:

* Ultrasonic diffusers: These devices combine essential oils with water to create a fine mist that disperses in the air. They are perfect for creating a pleasant atmosphere and aromatherapy.

* Mist diffusers: These diffusers break down essential oils into tiny particles, delivering a strong concentration of aroma. They require no water and are ideal for larger spaces.

* Passive diffusion: Place a few drops of essential oil on a cotton ball, paper towel, or fabric. The aroma will naturally diffuse into the air.

* Reed diffuser: Place a reed stick in a container of diluted essential oil. The oil flows up the reeds, releasing the aroma into the room.

Each application method has its advantages and considerations. For example, topical application is great for targeted effects, inhalation provides a quick and effective mood boost, and diffusion is great for creating an inviting ambiance in a room. Always follow recommended dilution ratios, use oils safely, and be aware of your body's reactions. Enjoy the versatility of essential oils as you explore these different application methods.

Let's dive deeper into the benefits, considerations, and suitability of each essential oil application method for different situations and expected results:

Topical application:

* Benefits: Targeted relief of specific problems such as muscle tension, skin problems, and localized discomfort. Provides a sensory experience through skin absorption.

*Note: Always dilute to avoid skin irritation. Perform a patch test to check sensitivity. Avoid use near sensitive areas such as eyes and mucous membranes.

* Suitability: Ideal for pain relief, skincare, relaxation, and supporting emotional well-being.

Inhalation:

* Benefits: Rapid effects on mood and mood. Can quickly solve breath-

ing problems. Directly enters the limbic system, affecting mood and memory.

*Caution: With some oils, inhaling directly from the bottle can be strong. Care should be taken when inhaling steam to avoid burns.

* Suitability: Great for stress relief, respiratory support, emotional balance, and mental clarity.

Diffuse:

* Benefits: Creates a pleasant atmosphere with sustained release of fragrance. Great for larger spaces. Supports relaxation, mindfulness, or respiratory health, depending on the oil used.

*Note: Some diffusers require water, which can dilute the fragrance. Mist diffusers may be too strong for sensitive people.

* Applicability: Suitable for enhancing the atmosphere, promoting sleep and concentration, and creating a warm environment.

Massage:

* BENEFITS: Combines the therapeutic benefits of touch with aromatherapy. Promotes relaxation, relieves muscle tension, and enhances emotional well-being.

* Note: Always dilute essential oil before using for massage. Choose the right carrier oil based on your skin type.

* Suitability: Effective for relaxation, muscle relief, stress reduction, and overall health.

Bath:

* Benefits: Provides relaxation, promotes detoxification, and may relieve muscle soreness. Experience essential oils all over your body.

*Note: Essential oils should be dispersed using emulsifiers to prevent skin irritation. Be careful not to slip into the tub.

* Suitability: Ideal for relaxation, muscle relief, and supporting skin health.

Personal inhalers and hand inhalers:

* Advantages: Portable and discreet. Can be used anywhere for a quick boost of mood or respiratory support.

*Note: Personal inhalers need to be refilled occasionally. Hand inhalation requires reapplication as the odor subsides.

* Suitability: Great for relieving stress, mental concentration, and

breathing issues on the go.

Keep in mind that the suitability of each method depends on your personal preferences, circumstances, and desired results. You can also combine methods for a more comprehensive effect. Always be aware of any allergies or sensitivities you may have and adjust accordingly.

E. Local Application Technology

Here is a guide to safe and effective topical application techniques for using essential oils:

Mmassage:

1. Dilute: Always dilute essential oils with a carrier oil before applying to skin. A typical dilution ratio is 2 to 3 drops of essential oil per teaspoon (5 ml) of carrier oil for adults.
2. Mix: Mix the essential oil of your choice with a carrier oil, such as sweet almond, jojoba, coconut, or grapeseed oil. You can mix them in a small bottle or the palm of your hand.
3. How to use: Gently massage the oil blend into the skin in the desired area. Use long, sweeping movements to relax, or use concentrated techniques to relax your muscles.

Apply:

1. Dilute: Dilute the essential oil as mentioned before, then add a few drops of the mixture to warm or cold water.
2. Soaking: Soak a clean cloth or towel in the water-oil mixture, wring it out, and apply it to the affected area.
3. Relaxation: Leave the dressing on for 15 to 20 minutes. This method is great for relieving pain, soothing sore muscles, and reducing inflammation.

Spot healing:

1. Dilute: Dilute the essential oil as described above. For spot healing, you can use higher concentrations of essential oils, but dilution is still essential.
2. How to use: Apply a small amount of the diluted mixture to specific areas of concern, such as blemishes or muscle soreness.
3. Cover: If needed, you can cover the area with a bandage or cloth to

prevent the oil from evaporating too quickly.

Topical application tips:

* Always do a patch test on a small area of skin before applying new essential oils to a larger area.
* Use gentle circular motions when massaging to avoid friction and irritation.
* Consider carrier oil absorption rate. Light oils, such as fractionated coconut oil, are absorbed quickly, while heavy oils, such as castor oil, are absorbed more slowly.
* Avoid applying essential oils to broken or irritated skin.
* Be careful on sensitive areas such as the face, neck, and genital area. Use milder oils and lower dilutions.
* Keep oil away from eyes, mucous membranes, and areas of the body with thin skin.
* If you are pregnant, nursing, or have a medical condition, consult a qualified healthcare professional before using essential oils topically.

Remember, everyone's skin is different, so it's important to monitor your skin's reactions and adjust your practices accordingly.

Below is a more detailed discussion of appropriate dilution ratios, areas of application, and considerations for sensitive skin or specific concerns:

Dilution ratio:

The dilution ratio ensures the essential oil is safe and effective for use on the skin. For general topical application, it is generally recommended that adults dilute 2 to 3 drops of essential oil per teaspoon (5 ml) of carrier oil. However, this ratio can be adjusted based on individual sensitivity, the specific oil used, and the purpose of the mixture.

Application areas:

Essential oils can be applied to various parts of the body, depending on the desired effect. Here are some common application areas:

1. Pulse points: Apply to areas with good blood supply, such as wrists, temples, and behind ears for quick absorption.
2. Chest and Back: For respiratory support, you can massage the essential oil blend into your chest and upper back.

3. Abdomen: To support digestive comfort, apply diluted oil to the abdomen in a clockwise direction.

4. Feet: The pores on the soles of the feet are larger and are effective areas for absorbing and diffusing oils.

5. Topic: Apply directly to areas of concern, such as temples where you have a headache or muscle soreness.

Precautions for sensitive skin:

If you have sensitive skin, take extra precautions:

1. Lower dilutions: Start with a lower dilution ratio (1% dilution, or about 1 drop of essential oil per teaspoon of carrier oil) and gradually increase if there are no adverse reactions.

2. Patch test: Always perform a patch test by applying a small amount of the diluted mixture to a small area of skin, such as the inside of your forearm. Wait 24 hours to check for any adverse reactions.

3. Mild essential oils: When trying a new oil for the first time, use a mild essential oil like lavender, chamomile, or frankincense.

4. Carrier oil choice: Choose a mild carrier oil such as sweet almond, jojoba, or fractionated coconut oil.

Specific focus and areas:

Different problems may require a tailored approach:

1. Facial application: Due to sensitive skin, use extra caution on the face. Always use well-diluted oil and avoid the eye area.

2. Children and the elderly: Children and the elderly have more delicate skin. For these groups, use a very mild oil and a lower dilution.

3. Pregnancy and breastfeeding: Consult a qualified health care professional before using essential oils during pregnancy or breastfeeding. Certain oils should be avoided, especially in the first trimester.

4. Photosensitive oils: Some oils can increase skin sensitivity to sunlight. These include citrus oils like lemon and bergamot. Avoid sun exposure after applying these oils topically.

Remember, essential oils are potent and should be used with caution. If you feel any discomfort or adverse reactions, please stop using it immediately. Always listen to your body and adjust your practice accordingly.

F. Inhalation Method

Inhalation is a direct and effective way to experience the therapeutic properties of essential oils. It offers a variety of benefits and can be a powerful solution to physical and emotional problems. Here is a detailed discussion of the benefits of inhalation:

1. Fast-acting: Inhalation accesses the aromatic compounds in essential oils almost immediately. When you inhale, these volatile molecules go directly to olfactory receptors in the nose and then to the brain, where they can have rapid effects on mood, mood, and even physiological processes.

2. Respiratory support: Inhalation is particularly effective for respiratory problems. Essential oils with decongestant, expectorant, and antibacterial properties can be inhaled to relieve congestion, coughs, and sinus discomfort.

3. Emotional balance: Inhaling certain essential oils can affect the limbic system, which is responsible for mood and memory. Calming oils like lavender, chamomile, and frankincense can help reduce stress, and anxiety and promote relaxation.

4. Cognitive benefits: Inhaling oils with cognitive-enhancing properties, such as rosemary and peppermint, can improve concentration, concentration, and mental clarity. These oils stimulate the brain and increase alertness.

5. Immune support: Some essential oils have immune-boosting properties. Inhaling these oils can help support the immune system and provide protection against pathogens.

6. Mood enhancement: Scents can trigger specific emotional responses. Inhaling uplifting oils like citrus oils (such as lemon and orange) can improve your mood and boost energy levels.

7. Non-invasive: Inhalation is non-invasive and does not require direct contact with the skin, making it a convenient option for people with sensitive skin or who do not like to apply oil topically.

8. Versatility: Inhalation adapts to a variety of situations. You can use a personal inhaler, diffuse the oil around your room, or even inhale it directly from the bottle.

Inhalation method:

There are several methods of inhalation:

1. Direct inhalation: Inhale directly from the bottle or rub a drop of oil between your palms and cover your nose and mouth with your hands.

2. Steam inhalation: Add a few drops of essential oil to a bowl of hot water, place your face on the bowl, cover your head with a towel, and inhale deeply.

3. Diffuse: Use an essential oil diffuser to disperse aromatic molecules into the air to create a pleasant, therapeutic atmosphere.

4. Personal inhaler: You can carry an inhaler with an essential oil-infused wick with you to enjoy the benefits throughout the day.

Inhalation is generally safe for most people, but remember to use caution if you have a respiratory condition like asthma or allergies. Also, make sure the room is well-ventilated when diffusing oils. Always follow recommended inhalation guidelines and be aware of your body's reactions.

Let's dive into these inhalation techniques using essential oils:

1. Direct inhalation:

Direct inhalation involves inhaling the aroma of essential oil directly from the bottle or into your hands. This method is quick and convenient and can be used anywhere. The specific operation method is as follows:

* Open the bottle of desired essential oil.
* Hold the bottle about an inch or so away from your nose.
* Inhale deeply through your nose, breathing slowly and steadily.
* Exhale slowly through your mouth.
* Repeat for a few breaths or as needed to relax or give a quick energy boost.

2. Steam inhalation:

Steam inhalation involves adding a few drops of essential oil to hot water and inhaling the steam. This method is particularly effective for respiratory problems. The specific operation method is as follows:

* Boil a pot of water and pour it into a heatproof bowl.
* Add 3~5 drops of essential oil of your choice (e.g., eucalyptus, tea tree, peppermint) to hot water.
* Place your face about 8 to 12 inches above the bowl and drape a towel over your head to create a tent.
* Close your eyes and inhale the steam deeply through your nose for about 5 to 10 minutes.
* If the steam feels too strong, take a break.

3. Diffuse:

Diffusing essential oils is a popular and effective way to enjoy their scent throughout a room. Essential oil diffusers disperse tiny droplets of oil into the air, creating a pleasant and healing environment. The specific operation method is as follows:

* Fill the diffuser with water up to the filling line.
* Add 5 to 10 drops of your chosen essential oil or blend with the water.
* Turn on the diffuser according to the instructions.
* Let the scent fill the room and inhale deeply as you perform activities.

4. Personal inhaler:

Personal inhalers are compact, portable devices that you can take with you to enjoy the benefits of essential oils on the go. Here's how to use them:

* Open the personal inhaler and insert the cotton wick or pad.
* Add 5 to 15 drops of essential oil of your choice or mix into wick.
* Close the inhaler tightly.
* Hold the inhaler close to your nose and inhale deeply through your nostrils.
* You can use your inhaler on the go while traveling or at work.

Each of these inhalation techniques has unique benefits and can be chosen based on your preference and situation. Remember, essential oils are potent, so start with fewer drops and adjust to your comfort level. If you experience any adverse reactions or discomfort, discontinue use and seek guidance from a healthcare professional.

G. Diffuse

Diffusing essential oils is a popular and effective method of ambient aromatherapy that offers many benefits for mood enhancement and overall health. Here are some of the main advantages:

1. Aromatherapy enjoyment: Diffusing essential oils allows you to enjoy the natural and pleasant aroma of various plant extracts. Scent can create a pleasant and inviting atmosphere in your living space.

2. Mood-enhancing: Different essential oils have specific aromatic characteristics that can influence mood and mood. For example, lavender is known for its calming properties, while citrus oils like lemon and orange can uplift and energize.

3. Stress relief: Certain essential oils, such as lavender, chamomile, and frankincense, have stress-relieving properties. Diffusing these oils can help create a soothing environment and reduce feelings of stress and anxiety.

4. Improves sleep: Lavender, cedarwood, and bergamot are known for promoting relaxation and better sleep. Diffusing these oils before bed can create a calming bedtime routine and improve sleep quality.

5. Increases focus: Essential oils like rosemary, peppermint, and eucalyptus have uplifting scents that can enhance mental clarity and focus. Diffusing these oils in your workspace or study area can increase productivity.

6. Air purification: Many essential oils have natural antibacterial properties. When diffused, they can help clean the air by reducing airborne pathogens and promoting a healthier indoor environment.

7. Benefits of aromatherapy: Diffusing essential oils allows you to experience the therapeutic benefits of aromatherapy. Inhaling aromatic molecules directly affects your limbic system, which is involved in mood, memory, and more.

8. Energy boost: Citrus oils such as lemon, grapefruit, and orange are known for their uplifting and energizing qualities. Diffusing these oils can provide a natural boost of energy and vitality.

9. Enhance the ambiance: The aroma of essential oils can create a unique and inviting atmosphere in your home. You can customize your scent

to suit different occasions or times of day.

10. Holistic health: Diffusing essential oils supports overall health by not only addressing physical health but also emotional and spiritual aspects. Fragrance can create a feeling of balance and harmony.

To experience the benefits of diffusing essential oils, invest in a high-quality essential oil diffuser. Follow the manufacturer's instructions for your specific diffuser model. Start with a small amount (usually 3 to 5 drops) of the essential oil of your choice, or mix and adjust based on the size of the room and your preference. Remember, essential oils are potent, so moderation is key. It is generally recommended to diffuse for 30 to 60 minutes at a time, with breaks between sessions.

Always consider safety guidelines, especially if you have pets or young children at home. Consult a resource, reputable source, or aromatherapy professional to choose the right essential oils to enhance your desired mood and ensure a safe and enjoyable experience.

Choosing the right diffuser, choosing the right oil, and determining the best time to diffuse are important steps in ensuring a safe and effective aromatherapy experience. Here are guides to help you in every aspect:

Choose the right diffuser:

1. Ultrasonic diffusers: These diffusers use ultrasonic vibrations to disperse a fine mist of water and essential oils into the air. They often come with LED lights to add to the ambiance. They are great for maintaining the therapeutic properties of the oil.

2. Nebulizer diffuser: Nebulizers release pure essential oils directly into the air in the form of tiny droplets. They require no water and provide a richer aroma. They are best for larger spaces and areas where you want a strong scent quickly.

3. Evaporative diffusers: These diffusers use fans or natural airflow to diffuse oils. They usually involve placing a few drops of essential oil on a mat or surface, with a fan dispersing the aroma. They are simple and cost-effective.

Choose a diffuser oil:

1. Single oils: Choose essential oils based on your desired mood or

purpose. For relaxation, lavender, chamomile, and bergamot are excellent choices. For energy and focus, consider peppermint, rosemary, or citrus oils.

2. Blends: Many essential oil companies offer pre-made blends designed for specific purposes such as relaxation, energy, or immune support. These save you time and effort in creating your blends.

Best time to diffuse fragrance:

1. Start slowly: When you are new to diffusing, start with a shorter diffusing time, about 15 to 30 minutes. This allows you to gauge how your body reacts to the aroma.

2. Avoid prolonged use: While aromatherapy can be beneficial, it is generally recommended not to diffuse oils for hours on end. Resting between diffuse sessions is important.

3. Customize to your needs: Depending on the size of the room and your sensitivity to scents, you may need to adjust the number of drops of essential oil and the diffusion time. Some oils are more effective, so you may need fewer drops.

4. Diffuse your oil before bed: If you diffuse your oil before bed, start about 30 minutes before you plan to go to bed and stop diffusing just before bed. This allows the scent to fill the room without overwhelming your senses while you sleep.

5. Open a window: If your room is getting stuffy or you've been diffusing for a while, consider opening a window to freshen the air and prevent sensory overload.

Remember, less is more when it comes to essential oils. Start with a conservative number of drops (usually 3 to 5 drops) and adjust based on your preference and room size. Always follow the manufacturer's instructions for your specific diffuser model.

Finally, if you have pets or specific health conditions, research the safety of essential oils based on your situation, as some essential oils may be harmful to animals or individuals with certain sensitivities. If you are unsure, consult a qualified aromatherapist or healthcare professional before diffusing essential oils.

H. Enhance Daily Life Application

Incorporating essential oils into your daily life can enhance your overall health and support your specific goals. Here are some ways to seamlessly integrate essential oils into your daily life:

1. Morning routine:

* Wake up refreshed: Diffuse, uplifting essential oils like citrus (e.g., lemon, orange) boost your mood and energy as you start your day.
* Shower Aromatherapy: Apply a drop or two of your favorite essential oil to the shower floor before you step in. The steam will dissipate the aroma for a spa-like experience.

2. Working or studying time:

* Focus and productivity: Inhale focus-enhancing oils like rosemary or peppermint directly from a personal inhaler, or use a diffuser, where oils are known for their cognitive support properties.
* Tabletop diffuser: Use a small tabletop diffuser filled with oils like eucalyptus or bergamot to maintain a clean and positive environment.

3. Lunch break:

* Stress relief: Keep a roll-on mixture of calming oils in your bag or on your desk. Apply to wrists and temples during your lunch break to relax.

4. Afternoon slump:

* Energy boost: Inhale revitalizing oils like peppermint or wild orange to help combat the afternoon slump and restore focus.

5. Exercise or Yoga:

* Pre-workout energizing cream: Apply a diluted blend of energizing oils before exercise to add extra energy.
* Post-workout recovery: Use a soothing oil like lavender or chamomile in your post-workout massage oil to relax your muscles.

6. Evening liquidation:

* Aromatherapy bath: Add a few drops of a relaxing oil, such as laven-

der or cedarwood, to your bath water for a calming soak before bed.

* Bedtime ritual: As you relax, diffuse a sleep-inducing oil like chamomile or sandalwood in your bedroom.

7. Before going to bed:

* Nighttime Routine: Apply a relaxing essential oil blend to the soles of your feet or pulse points before bed to promote a restful night.

8. Mindfulness practice:

* Meditation: Use the calming oil blend in a diffuser or directly on your wrist to enhance your meditation practice.
* Breathe deeply: Inhale soothing oils while practicing deep breathing exercises to enhance relaxation.

Remember, essential oils are highly concentrated, so a little goes a long way. Dilution is key, especially when applying them topically. Always conduct a patch test and consider personal sensitivities and health conditions before applying new oil to your skin. If you are pregnant, nursing, or have specific health conditions, please consult a healthcare professional or aromatherapist before incorporating essential oils into your daily life.

Finally, keep a small essential oil kit with you that contains your favorite blends and single oils so you can easily access them throughout the day. Try different oils and procedures to find the one that works best for you and supports the results you want.

Here's a more detailed breakdown of how to incorporate essential oils into different daily routines:

Morning routine:

* Wake-up diffuser: Start your day right with an essential oil diffuser. Oils like citrus (like lemon, orange, or grapefruit) are uplifting and can lift your mood.
*Personal inhaler: Keep a personal inhaler containing an energy blend (such as peppermint and rosemary) next to your bed. Take a deep breath and build up as soon as you wake up.
* Revitalizing shower: Add a few drops of stimulating oil (e.g., eucalyptus, peppermint) to the corner of the shower and wake up with an aroma.

Exercise or exercise class:

* Pre-workout energizing cream: Apply a dilute blend of essential oils like peppermint, eucalyptus, and bergamot to your pulse points before exercise to invigorate your mind.
* Cooling massage: Create a post-workout massage oil using soothing essential oils like lavender, chamomile, and frankincense to help relax muscles and relieve tension.

Work or study environment:

* Desktop diffuser: Use a compact diffuser with oils like rosemary, lemon, or cedarwood in your workspace to increase focus and productivity.
* Inhalation breaks: Carry a personal inhaler filled with a focus-enhancing essential oil blend for a quick inhalation during study or work breaks.

Lunch break or stress relief:

* Roll-on blend: Prepare a roll-on blend with calming oils like lavender, bergamot, and sage. Apply to wrists or temples at rest to relieve stress.

Light evening:

* Aromatherapy bath: Add a few drops of a soothing oil like lavender, ylang-ylang, or chamomile to your evening bath to relax your body and mind.
* Bedrooms diffuse: Diffuse calming blends like lavender and cedarwood in your bedroom to create a peaceful atmosphere before bed.

Bedtime ritual:

* Inhale before bed: Use an essential oil pillow spray or inhale a calming oil like chamomile or frankincense before bed to signal sleep.
* Foot massage: Apply a sleep-inducing essential oil blend to the soles of your feet or spine for a relaxing bedtime ritual.

Remember, essential oils are versatile so that you can tailor your use to your preferences and needs. Dilution is essential, especially for topical application. Always patch-test new oils and be aware of potential sensitivities. Also, please consider your medical condition and seek advice from a healthcare professional if you have concerns, especially during pregnancy or when taking medications.

Incorporating essential oils into these routines can help you take advantage of their benefits throughout your day.

After this chapter, we highlight the art and science of blending essential oils and the various application methods that can be used to obtain optimal results. By understanding the principles of blending, trying different essential oils, and applying them through appropriate methods, men can harness the full potential of essential oils to boost their health. Prioritizing safety, following guidelines, and personalizing the mixture to personal preferences and needs are critical. With knowledge and creativity, essential oils can enhance daily life and contribute to a more balanced and enjoyable lifestyle.

9.2 DIY Projects and Recipes for Men

In this chapter, we'll explore exciting do-it-yourself (DIY) projects and recipes specifically for men. We provide step-by-step instructions, ingredient lists, and tips for making homemade products using essential oils. These items range from beauty and personal care items to home fragrances and wellness treatments, allowing men to customize their self-care routines and enhance their overall wellness.

A. DIY Beard Oil

Here's a simple recipe for nourishing and conditioning beard oil using essential oils and carrier oils:

Element:

* 1 oz (30 ml) jojoba oil
* 0.5 oz (15 ml) argan oil
* 0.5 oz (15 ml) sweet almond oil
* 5 drops of cedarwood essential oil
* 3 drops of sandalwood essential oil
* 2 drops of bergamot essential oil
* 2 drops of frankincense essential oil

Guide:

1. Choose a clean, dry glass bottle with a dropper cap to store your beard oil.

2. Mix the carrier oils (jojoba, argan, and sweet almond) in a glass bottle. These carrier oils provide nutrients and moisture to your beard and skin underneath.

3. Add the essential oil to the carrier oil mixture drop by drop. Cedarwood, sandalwood, bergamot, and frankincense were chosen for their conditioning, soothing and aromatic properties.

4. Close the bottle tightly and shake gently to mix the oil thoroughly.

5. Let the mixture sit for a few hours or overnight to allow the scents to meld together.

Instructions:

1. After showering or cleaning your face, dry your beard with a clean towel.

2. Put a few drops of beard oil into your palms and rub your hands together to distribute the oil evenly.

3. Gently massage the oil into your beard, making sure to reach the skin underneath.

4. Use a beard comb or brush to distribute oil throughout your beard for even coverage.

5. Enjoy the conditioning and aromatherapy benefits of beard oil!

This beard oil formula not only helps condition and soften your beard, but it also provides a pleasant masculine scent. Adjust essential oil drops to your personal preference. Always conduct a patch test before using a new mixture to ensure no adverse reactions. Consider consulting a healthcare professional before using essential oils if you have sensitive skin or specific health concerns.

Beard oil is a multi-purpose beauty product that offers a range of benefits to promote healthy facial hair and achieve a groomed appearance. Here are some of the main advantages:

1. Moisturize and condition: The primary function of beard oil is to moisturize and condition beard hair and the skin underneath. The natural oils

in beard oil, such as jojoba, argan, and sweet almond, help prevent dryness and itchiness in the beard area. Well-moisturized hair is less prone to breakage and split ends.

2. Softens and Tames: Beard oil softens coarse beard hair, making it more manageable and easier to comb. This is especially beneficial for those with longer beards that tend to get tangled easily.

3. Soothes Itchy Skin: Many men experience itching and discomfort when their beard grows. Beard oil helps relieve this itchiness by moisturizing the skin underneath and reducing irritation.

4. Promotes healthy beard growth: The carrier oil used in beard oil is rich in vitamins, minerals, and fatty acids that nourish the hair follicles and promote healthy beard growth. Well-nourished hair follicles are more likely to produce strong, thick hair.

5. Enhances shine: Beard oil adds a subtle shine to your beard, making it look healthy and groomed. This can make your beard look smoother and more attractive.

6. Prevent beard dandruff: Similar to dandruff, "beard dandruff" refers to flakes of skin that can accumulate under your beard. Applying beard oil regularly will help keep your skin moisturized and reduce the likelihood of flaking.

7. Provides a Subtle Fragrance: Beard oil often contains essential oils that provide a pleasant and subtle fragrance. This can be used as a natural alternative to cologne or perfume.

8. Supports skin health: Beard oil isn't just for your hair; it also benefits the skin underneath. Healthy skin is essential for healthy hair growth. The moisturizing and anti-inflammatory properties of certain carrier oils and essential oils contribute to overall skin health.

9. Enhanced grooming: Applying beard oil makes grooming more enjoyable and efficient. It helps prevent tangles and makes the process of combing or brushing your beard smoother.

10. Boosts Confidence: A well-groomed beard enhances your appearance and confidence. Regular use of beard oil helps maintain a groomed and polished appearance.

To fully enjoy these benefits, choosing a high-quality beard oil with natural ingredients and no synthetic additives is essential. When applying beard oil, start with a small amount and increase as needed, focusing on evenly distributing it throughout your beard and massaging it into your skin. When choosing a beard oil, consider your skin type and any allergies you may have. As with any grooming product, do a patch test on new beard oils to ensure they don't cause adverse reactions.

B. Natural Aftershave balm

Here's a simple recipe for a soothing and hydrating aftershave balm using essential oils, aloe vera, and natural ingredients:

Soothing Aftershave Balm Recipe:

Element:

* 1/4 cup aloe vera gel
* 2 tablespoons jojoba oil (or other carrier oil of your choice)
* 1 tablespoon shea butter
* 1 teaspoon beeswax pellets
* 5~7 drops of lavender essential oil
* 3~5 drops of cedar essential oil
* 2~3 drops of chamomile essential oil (optional, for extra soothing)
* Small glass or metal container for balm

Guide:

1. Prepare your workspace: Make sure all your equipment and containers are clean and sanitized.

2. Double boiler method: Melt the shea butter and beeswax granules over low heat in a double boiler. If you don't have a double boiler, you can create one by placing a heatproof bowl over a pot of simmering water.

3. Add the carrier oil: Once the shea butter and beeswax are melted, remove the mixture from the heat and stir in the jojoba oil. Jojoba oil is a great choice because of its moisturizing and non-greasy properties.

4. Cool and add aloe vera: Let the mixture cool slightly, but not so-

lidify. Add aloe vera gel and stir gently or stir to combine. Aloe vera provides soothing and moisturizing benefits to the skin.

5. Add essential oils: Add essential oil drops once the mixture is thoroughly blended. Lavender, cedarwood, and chamomile are great choices for skin-calming and aromatic properties. Adjust the number of drops to your liking.

6. Mix and store: Mix ingredients thoroughly. Pour the mixture into a clean, airtight glass or metal container. Allow the container to cool and set completely before sealing it.

7. How to use: Paint your skin dry with a clean towel after shaving. Take a small amount of aftershave balm and gently massage onto your face and neck. The balm will help soothe irritation, moisturize the skin, and provide a subtle fragrance.

8. Storage: Store aftershave balm in a cool, dry place. Keep it away from direct sunlight and extreme temperatures to maintain its quality.

This homemade aftershave balm is customizable, so feel free to adjust the essential oil blend to your liking. Always do a patch test before applying the balm to larger areas of your skin, especially if you have sensitive skin or are prone to allergies.

Remember, a little goes a long way, so start with a small amount and increase as needed. This balm can also be given as a gift to a friend or loved one who loves natural beauty products.

Using a natural aftershave balm provides several benefits of calming and protecting your skin after shaving. Here are some benefits:

1. Soothes irritation: Shaving can cause skin irritation, redness, and micro-cuts. Natural aftershave balms formulated with ingredients like aloe vera and essential oils can help soothe these irritations and provide relief.

2. Moisturize: Many natural aftershave balms contain moisturizing ingredients like shea butter, jojoba oil, and aloe vera. These ingredients help replenish lost moisture, keeping skin hydrated and preventing dryness or tightness.

3. Reduce inflammation: Essential oils like lavender, chamomile, and

cedarwood have anti-inflammatory properties that help reduce inflammation and redness caused by shaving.

4. Antibacterial benefits: Some essential oils, such as tea tree and lavender, have natural antibacterial properties. Applying these oils to your aftershave balm can help prevent infections and promote overall skin health.

5. Aromatherapy: Aftershave balms often contain essential oils to create a pleasant aroma. Aromatherapy can positively impact your mood, making the post-shave experience more enjoyable and relaxing.

6. Protect natural aftershave balm, which forms a protective barrier on the skin, protecting it from environmental pollutants and harsh elements. This barrier also prevents chafing and discomfort.

7. Non-greasy formula: Natural aftershave balms are usually formulated to be non-greasy and can be quickly absorbed into the skin. This means you get the benefits of no heavy or oily residue.

8. Nourishing ingredients: Natural ingredients like shea butter and carrier oils provide essential nutrients to the skin, promoting skin health and helping to maintain its natural balance.

9. Gentle and safe: Natural aftershave balms are typically free of harsh chemicals, synthetic fragrances, and artificial additives, reducing the risk of adverse reactions and sensitivity.

10. Promotes healing: Ingredients with healing properties, like aloe vera and essential oils, can help the skin recover faster from small scratches or cuts.

Overall, using a natural aftershave balm can help provide a more comfortable post-shave experience while supporting the health and well-being of your skin. Choosing a balm that suits your skin type and preferences is important to maximize the benefits.

C. Vitality Body Scrub

Here's a recipe for an invigorating and rejuvenating body scrub that uses essential oils, exfoliating ingredients, and nourishing oils:

Revitalizing Citrus Body Scrub

Element:

* 1 cup granulated sugar (or salt for coarser scrubs)
* 1/4 cup carrier oil (such as sweet almond, jojoba, or coconut oil)
* 10~15 drops of refreshing essential oil (such as citrus oils such as lemon, grapefruit, or orange, and a little peppermint)
* The peel of a citrus fruit (such as lemon, orange, or grapefruit)
* 1 teaspoon vitamin E oil (optional, for added skin nutrition)
* 1 teaspoon natural honey (optional for extra hydration)
* Sealable glass jar for easy storage

Guide:

1. In a mixing bowl, combine granulated sugar (or salt) with the carrier oil of your choice. Mix well to form a paste consistency.

2. 10 to 15 drops of refreshing essential oil to the mixture. You can customize the blend by using a combination of citrus oils and a dash of mint. Adjust the number of drops according to your preference for scent intensity.

3. Add the zest of citrus fruit (lemon, orange, or grapefruit) to the mixture. The leather flavor adds a refreshing fragrance and natural color.

4. Add 1 teaspoon of vitamin E oil to the mixture if desired. Vitamin E oil is known for its skin-nourishing properties and can help extend the shelf life of your scrub.

5. Optional: Add 1 teaspoon of natural honey to the mixture for added moisture. Honey is soothing and moisturizing to the skin.

6. Stir all ingredients thoroughly until well-mixed.

7. Transfer the scrub to an airtight glass jar for storage. Make sure the jar is clean and dry before filling it with scrub.

Instructions:

1. Scoop a small amount of body scrub into your hands in the shower or bath.

2. Gently massage the scrub into damp skin using circular motions. Focus on areas that could benefit from exfoliation, such as your elbows, knees, and feet.

3. Leave the scrub on the skin for a few minutes to allow oils and nutrients to penetrate.

4. Rinse off the scrub thoroughly with warm water.

5. Pat dry skin and enjoy the revitalizing and hydrating benefits of the scrub.

NOTE: Essential oils are potent, so start with a few drops and adjust to your preference. Before using the scrub all over your body, do a patch test on a small area of skin to ensure you don't have any adverse reactions. If you have sensitive skin or any allergies, consult a healthcare professional before using new skin care products.

This homemade body scrub will leave your skin feeling soft, smooth, and rejuvenated, thanks to the exfoliating action of sugar (or salt) and the moisturizing properties of carrier oil and honey. The refreshing scent of citrus essential oil provides a refreshing boost to your senses.

Exfoliation is a skincare practice that involves removing dead skin cells from the skin's surface. It offers a range of benefits for smooth, revitalized, and healthy skin. Here are some of the key benefits of exfoliation:

1. Remove dead skin cells: The outermost layer of the skin is composed of dead skin cells, which can make the skin look dull and rough. Exfoliation helps slog off these dead cells, revealing fresher, more radiant skin.

2. Enhance skin texture: Regular exfoliation helps eliminate uneven patches and rough areas, leaving skin with a smooth texture. This results in a soft and touchable complexion.

3. Unclog pores: Exfoliation helps remove dirt, oil, and debris from your pores, preventing them from clogging. Cleaned pores are less likely to cause blackheads, whiteheads, and acne breakouts.

4. Improve skin tone: Exfoliation can help improve the appearance of uneven skin tone, hyperpigmentation, and sunspots by promoting the turnover of new skin cells and fading dark spots.

5. Promote blood circulation: The physical action of exfoliation stimulates blood flow to the skin's surface, promoting a healthy complexion and natural glow.

6. Enhance skin care product penetration: By removing the barrier of dead skin cells, exfoliation allows skin care products, such as moisturizers and serums, to penetrate more effectively and deliver their benefits to the deeper layers of the skin.

7. Boosts collagen production: Regular exfoliation can boost collagen production, a protein that supports skin firmness and elasticity.

8. Prevent ingrown hairs: Exfoliation can help prevent ingrown hairs by keeping hair follicles clean and reducing the likelihood of hair becoming trapped beneath the skin's surface.

9. Revitalize dull skin: Exfoliation can instantly revive dull skin, leaving it fresh and rejuvenated.

10. Prevent acne: Exfoliation can help prevent the buildup of excess oil and dead skin cells that can lead to breakouts for those prone to acne.

It is important to note that exfoliation should be done in moderation and using the correct technique. Excessive exfoliation or the use of harsh exfoliants can lead to skin irritation, sensitivity, and disruption of the skin's natural barrier. Choosing the right exfoliation method for your skin type and incorporating it into your skincare routine can help achieve healthier, smoother, more vibrant skin.

D. DIY Room Spray

Here's a simple recipe for a refreshingly scented room spray using essential oils and natural ingredients:

Refreshing Citrus Room Spray

Element:

* 1/2 cup distilled water
* 1/2 cup witch hazel or vodka (as a preservative)

* 15 to 20 drops of citrus essential oil (such as lemon, orange, grapefruit, or bergamot)

* 5 drops of peppermint essential oil (brings a cooling and energizing scent)

* 5 drops of lavender essential oil (soothing)

Guide:

1. Combine distilled water and witch hazel or vodka in a glass or plastic spray bottle. The alcohol content in witch hazel or vodka helps preserve the spray and extend its shelf life.

2. Add essential oil drops into the mixture. You can adjust the number of drops based on your preference for scent intensity.

3. Close the spray bottle tightly and shake well to combine all ingredients.

4. Before using room spray, shake gently to ensure essential oils are fully dispersed in the liquid.

5. Before using it in a larger space, test the spray on a small, inconspicuous area to ensure you are not sensitive to any ingredients.

6. To use, spray the room into the air to instantly refresh your space with the uplifting and uplifting scent of citrus and mint.

NOTE: Since this room spray contains water, storing it in a cool, dark place is best to prevent bacterial growth. Shake well before each use to ensure even distribution of essential oils.

Feel free to customize the essential oil blend to your liking. You can create other variations using different essential oils (such as eucalyptus and lavender) or a combination of floral and woody scents. This DIY room spray not only adds a pleasant scent to your surroundings but also provides a natural and chemical-free way to enjoy the benefits of essential oils.

Using a homemade room spray with a masculine scent can provide several advantages for refreshing your living space:

1. Personalized scent: Creating your room spray allows you to customize the scent to your liking. You can choose essential oils that evoke masculine

aromas, such as woody, earthy, or spicy scents, making your living space feel more customized and cozier.

2. Natural and chemical-free: Homemade room sprays are often made from natural ingredients, including essential oils, water, or alcohol. This means you can avoid the synthetic fragrances and chemicals commonly found in commercial air fresheners, which is better for your health and the environment.

3. Aromatherapy benefits: Many essential oils used in masculine scents have aromatherapy benefits. For example, woody scents like cedarwood promote relaxation and grounding, while citrus oils like bergamot can uplift and energize. So, in addition to freshening the air, your room spray can boost your overall health.

4. Cost-effectiveness: Making your room spray may be more cost-effective in the long run than purchasing commercial products. A small bottle of essential oil can go a long way, allowing you to make multiple batches of room spray.

5. Easy to make: DIY room sprays are easy to make with just a few ingredients and minimal equipment. You don't need to be a DIY expert to create a custom scent that suits your preferences.

6. Impression of cleanliness: A well-scented room can give the impression of being clean and tidy. Use a masculine room spray to help create a welcoming atmosphere for you and your guests.

7. Flexibility: With a homemade room spray, you can switch scents based on the season, mood, or occasion. You can try different essential oil combinations to find the one that resonates best with you.

8. Thoughtful and thought-provoking: Carefully selected masculine scents can be thought-provoking and evoke specific memories or emotions. Whether you use an earthy scent that evokes the outdoors or a warm, spicy scent that provides a sense of comfort, your room spray can help create the overall ambiance of your living space.

9. Conversation starter: When guests enter your home and are greeted by a pleasant and unique scent, it can be a conversation starter and a way to leave a lasting impression.

10. Cultivate a cozy space: The right scent helps create a cozy and

inviting atmosphere. Homemade room spray can help you create a cozy and inviting environment.

Remember, scent preference is personal, so feel free to experiment with different essential oils and ratios until you find the masculine scent that resonates best with you and complements your living space.

E. Muscle Soothing Ointment

Here is a recipe for a soothing and soothing muscle salve using essential oils, carrier oils, and herbal ingredients:

Soothing Muscle Ointment

Element:

* 1/4 cup carrier oil (such as coconut, olive, or sweet almond oil)
* 1 tablespoon beeswax granules (for setting the ointment)
* 10 drops of eucalyptus essential oil
* 10 drops of peppermint essential oil
* 8 drops of lavender essential oil
* 6 drops of rosemary essential oil
* 1 tablespoon arnica oil (infused carrier oil)
* 1 tablespoon calendula oil (infused with carrier oil)
* Optional: 1 teaspoon of vitamin E oil (increases skin nutrition)

Guide:

1. Melt beeswax pellets over low heat in a double boiler or heat-safe glass bowl.

2. Once the beeswax has melted, add a carrier oil (such as coconut oil) and stir well until completely combined.

3. Remove the mixture from the heat, let it cool slightly, then add the essential oils and other herbal oils (arnica and calendula).

4. Add eucalyptus, peppermint, lavender, and rosemary essential oils to the mixture. Stir well to ensure even distribution.

5. If you use vitamin E oil, add it to the mixture and stir again.

6. Carefully pour the mixture into clean and sterilized containers, such as small jars or glass jars.

7. Allow mixture to cool and set completely before sealing the container.

8. When using, massage a small amount of muscle ointment on the affected area. The warmth of your skin will help melt the ointment and promote absorption.

Notes:

* Arnica and calendula oils are known for their soothing properties. You can make an infused oil by placing dried arnica and calendula petals in a carrier oil (such as olive oil) and letting it sit in a cool, dark place for a few weeks before filtering.

*This ointment is for external use only. Avoid applying to broken or irritated skin.

* Before using the ointment on a larger area, do a patch test to ensure you don't have any adverse reactions.

* Store the ointment in a cool, dark place to extend its shelf life.

* Feel free to adjust the amount of essential oil according to your preference and desired potency.

This homemade muscle salve provides natural relief for sore and tired muscles. The combination of essential oils and herbal ingredients provides a soothing and comforting experience for muscle discomfort.

Homemade muscle salve can provide a variety of benefits for relieving soreness and discomfort and promoting relaxation:

1. Natural pain relief: Essential oils such as eucalyptus, peppermint, lavender, and rosemary used in the ointment have analgesic and anti-inflammatory properties. They can help relieve muscle soreness, tension, and discomfort when used topically.

2. Improves blood circulation: Peppermint and rosemary essential oils

have vasodilatory properties, which can help improve blood circulation when applied to the skin. This can help relieve muscle stiffness and promote the delivery of nutrients to the muscles.

3. Relaxation: Lavender essential oil is known for its calming and relaxing effects. When applied to the skin, it can help soothe the mind and body, promoting a feeling of relaxation and ease.

4. Anti-inflammatory support: Arnica and calendula-infused oils are known for their anti-inflammatory properties. These oils can help reduce inflammation in muscles and joints, helping to provide overall relief.

5. Moisturizing: The carrier oil used in the salve, such as coconut oil or almond oil, provides moisture to the skin. This prevents dryness and ensures that skin remains soft and supple.

6. Topical application: Ointments allow for targeted application to specific areas of discomfort. This is especially beneficial for sore muscles, neck or shoulder tension, or any local discomfort.

7. Aromatherapy benefits: Besides physical effects, essential oils also provide aromatherapy benefits. Inhaling the soothing scents of eucalyptus, peppermint, and lavender can help relax the mind and provide relief.

8. DIY and personalized: Making your muscle salve allows you to control the ingredients, customize the scent to your liking, and adjust the potency of the essential oils. This personalization enhances the overall experience and effectiveness of the ointment.

9. Non-invasive and natural: Homemade muscle salve offers a non-invasive and natural way to relieve discomfort. They may be a preferable option for people looking for alternatives to over-the-counter ointments and medications.

10. Preventive care: Regular use of muscle ointments can also help prevent muscle soreness and tension. Massaging the ointment into your muscles before or after physical activity can support muscle recovery and reduce the risk of post-exercise discomfort.

Everyone's body reacts differently, so it's important to do a patch test and see how your skin reacts to the ointment before using it more widely. If you have any underlying medical conditions or concerns, it is recommended that you consult a healthcare professional before using any new products, including homemade products.

F. DIY Natural Cologne

Creating a personalized and natural cologne using essential oils and alcohol-free ingredients is a great way to have a unique scent that suits your preferences. Here's a simple recipe to get you started:

Element:

* Carrier oil (such as jojoba, fractionated coconut, or sweet almond): 2 tablespoons
* Essential oils (a combination of your favorite scents; see below for suggestions): 20 to 30 drops total
*Glass roller bottle (10ml or 15ml)

Essential oil combination:

Choose essential oils based on your preferred scent. Here are some suggestions:

1. Wood and soil:
* Cedarwood: 7 drops
* Sandalwood: 7 drops
* Vetiver: 5 drops
* Bergamot: 5 drops (a touch of freshness)

2. Citrus and spices:
* Sweet orange: 7 drops
* Cardamom: 5 drops
* Frankincense: 5 drops
* Ginger: 5 drops

3. Herbal and fresh:
* Lavender: 7 drops
* Rosemary: 6 drops
* Mint: 5 drops
* Eucalyptus: 5 drops

Guide:

1. Choose your preferred size (10ml or 15ml) glass roller bottle.

2. Using a small funnel, pour the carrier oil into a roller bottle. The carrier oil will serve as the base of the cologne and help dilute the essential oils.

3. Add desired essential oil drops to carrier oil. You can use a single essential oil or a combination of oils to create your desired scent profile.

4. Close the roller bottle securely and gently roll between your palms to mix the carrier and essential oils.

5. Let the cologne sit for a few hours or overnight before use. This allows the essential oils to blend and create their fragrance.

6. To use, apply cologne to pulse points (wrists, neck, and behind ears). Gently roll the roller ball onto the skin and gently tap the area with your finger to apply cologne.

Note: Always conduct a patch test before using cologne on a larger area of skin, especially if you have sensitive skin or allergies. If you experience any irritation, discontinue use.

Skill:

* Feel free to adjust the number of drops of essential oil to achieve your desired scent level. Some essential oils are more potent than others so that you may need fewer drops for a stronger scent.

* The scent of a cologne may evolve as the essential oils are blended and matured. It's normal for the scent to change slightly after a few days.

*Remember that natural colognes made with essential oils tend to have a softer, more subtle scent than commercial alcohol-based colognes. You may need to reapply cologne throughout the day to maintain the scent.

Creating your natural cologne is a fun and creative process that allows you to have a unique scent that reflects your personality. Enjoy trying different essential oil combinations to find the perfect fragrance for you.

Using a homemade cologne made with essential oils offers a range of advantages, especially compared to the synthetic fragrances found in many commercial colognes. Here are some reasons why using homemade cologne and essential oils may be a good choice:

1. Natural ingredients: Homemade cologne is made from natural ingredients, primarily essential oils and carrier oils. This means you avoid the synthetic chemicals and potentially harmful additives often found in commer-

cial fragrances. Using natural ingredients reduces the risk of skin sensitivity and allergic reactions.

2. Unique scent: One of the most significant advantages of making your cologne is creating a unique scent based on your preferences. Essential oils come in various scents, from floral and herbal to spicy and woody. You can mix and match essential oils to create a signature, truly your own scent.

3. Customization: You have complete control over the ingredients and proportions with homemade cologne. This allows you to adjust the intensity and balance of the fragrance to your liking. You can try different essential oil combinations until you find the perfect scent that suits your personality and style.

4. Therapeutic benefits: Essential oils provide a pleasant aroma and various therapeutic benefits. Many essential oils have aromatherapy properties that can lift your mood, reduce stress, and even promote relaxation. For example, lavender and chamomile are known for their calming effects, while citrus oils like bergamot and sweet orange can provide an energizing boost.

5. Longevity: Natural colognes made with essential oils may have a softer, more subtle scent than synthetic fragrances, but they can still have decent longevity when applied to pulse points. You can easily reapply your homemade cologne throughout the day to maintain your desired scent.

6. Environmental considerations: Making your cologne reduces your need for synthetic fragrances, often involving environmentally harmful production processes. By using natural ingredients, you are making a more environmentally friendly choice.

7. Avoid overpowering smells: Many commercial colognes can be overpowering due to their high concentration of synthetic fragrances. Homemade colognes made with essential oils tend to have more subtle and refined scents, making them suitable for various occasions without overpowering those around them.

8. Sense of accomplishment: Making your cologne can be a rewarding experience. It allows you to use your creativity, learn about the properties of different essential oils, and take pride in using the products you make.

In summary, using homemade cologne containing essential oils offers a range of benefits, from creating a unique and appealing scent to avoiding synthetic chemicals and enjoying potential therapeutic benefits. It's a great way to express your personality while embracing natural and holistic fragrances.

G. Calming Pillow Spray

Using essential oils to create a calming pillow spray is a great way to promote relaxation and improve the quality of your sleep. Here's a simple recipe for a soothing pillow spray:

Element:

* 2 ounces (60 ml) of distilled water
* 1/2 oz (15 ml) witch hazel or vodka (as a dispersant for the essential oil)
* 10 ~ 15 drops of lavender essential oil
* 5 drops of chamomile essential oil (optional)
* 5 drops of bergamot essential oil (optional)

Guide:

1. Sterilize a 2 oz (60 ml) spray bottle to ensure cleanliness.

2. Combine distilled water and witch hazel or vodka in a small glass or stainless-steel bowl. Witch hazel and vodka help disperse the essential oils, and mix them thoroughly in the water.

3. Drop the essential oil into the water mixture. Because of its calming effect, you can use 10 to 15 drops of lavender essential oil. If desired, add 5 drops of Chamomile Essential Oil for extra relaxation and 5 drops of Bergamot Essential Oil for an uplifting scent.

4. Gently stir the mixture to ensure the essential oils are fully dispersed in the liquid.

5. Carefully pour the mixture into a spray bottle using a small funnel. When installing the nozzle, leave a little space at the top to avoid spillage.

6. Seal the spray bottle tightly with the nozzle.

7. Shake the bottle well before each use to ensure essential oils are

evenly distributed in the mixture.

8. When using, gently rub pillows and bedding before going to bed. Let the mist settle before lying down.

NOTE: Always conduct a patch test before using any new essential oil on your skin or bedding. If you experience any adverse reactions, discontinue use. It's also a good idea to consult a healthcare professional before using essential oils if you have any medical conditions or concerns.

This calming pillow spray creates a calming environment, supports relaxation, and encourages a good night's sleep. Lavender, chamomile, and bergamot are all known for their soothing properties, which can help you relax and unwind after a long day.

Use an essential oil-infused pillow spray to promote relaxation and restful sleep and create a peaceful environment in your bedroom:

1. Promotes relaxation: Essential oils like lavender, chamomile, and bergamot are known for their calming and soothing properties. When you spray these oils on your pillows and bedding, their scent can help you relax and reduce stress and tension.

2. Improve sleep quality: The calming scent of essential oils can help signal your body that it's time to relax and prepare for bed. Inhaling these scents while lying down can create a peaceful environment that supports uninterrupted sleep and better sleep quality.

3. Reduce anxiety: Many essential oils have been studied for their potential to reduce anxiety and promote a sense of tranquility. The act of using a pillow spray and inhaling these oils can have a positive impact on your overall emotional state, helping you feel more at ease.

4. Helps relieve stress: Stress can be a major disruptor of sleep. Essential oils in pillow spray can help lower stress levels and promote relaxation, making it easier to transition into a calmer state before bed.

5. Create a sleep ritual: Incorporating a pillow spray into your nightly routine can serve as a relaxation ritual, signaling your body that it's time to wind down. Over time, this consistent practice can help regulate your mind and body for better sleep.

6. Refresh your bedding: Besides aromatherapy benefits, pillow spray can also help refresh your bedding between washes. This helps create a more inviting and comfortable sleeping environment.

7. Nourishes the senses: Smell is closely linked to memory and emotion. Using a pillow spray with a pleasant scent can create a positive sensory connection with sleep, making you more likely to look forward to your bedtime.

8. Improve sleeping environment: Fragrance can transform a space. Spraying a soothing mist on pillows and around your bedroom can help create a cozy, peaceful atmosphere that supports relaxation and sleep.

9. Encourage mindfulness: Using pillow spray encourages mindfulness and present-moment awareness. As you spray the mist and inhale the scent, you can take a moment to focus on your breathing and release the stress of the day.

10. Supports overall health: Quality sleep is vital to overall health and well-being. By promoting restful sleep and relaxation, pillow spray can boost your physical, mental, and emotional health.

Remember that individuals may react differently to scents, so it's best to choose a scent that resonates with you. Additionally, practicing good sleep hygiene and maintaining a consistent sleep schedule can further enhance the relaxation and sleep support benefits of using pillow spray.

H. DIY Shampoo and Body Wash

Here are recipes for homemade shampoo and body wash using essential oils and natural cleansers:

Homemade Lavender Mint Shampoo and Body Wash

Element:

* 1 cup liquid castile soap (unscented or your preferred scent)
* 2 tablespoons vegetable glycerin
* 10 ~ 15 drops of lavender essential oil
* 5 ~ 10 drops of peppermint essential oil
* 2 teaspoons jojoba oil (optional, to add moisture)

* 1 teaspoon vitamin E oil (optional, as a natural preservative)
* Distilled water (to adjust consistency)
* BPA-free plastic or glass container with a pump

Guide:

1. Combine liquid Castile soap and vegetable glycerin in a mixing bowl. Mix well.

2. Add lavender and peppermint essential oils to the mixture. Adjust the number of drops according to your scent preference; fewer drops will produce a milder scent, while more drops will provide a stronger scent.

3. If using jojoba oil and vitamin E oil, add them to the mixture and stir until everything is well combined.

4. Gradually add distilled water to the mixture while stirring. Add water until the desired consistency is reached. Shampoo and body wash should be easy to pour but not too watery.

5. Carefully transfer the mixture to a clean, empty, BPA-free plastic or glass container and pump.

6. Label the container with the product name and date of preparation.

7. To use, pump a small amount of shampoo and shower gel onto your hands or towel, then rub it into a lather and clean your hair and body. Rinse thoroughly with water.

Note: As with any homemade product, it is recommended to patch-test a small area of skin before using shampoo and body wash all over your body to make sure you don't have any adverse reactions. Consult a dermatologist before trying new products if you have specific skin sensitivities or allergies.

This homemade lavender mint shampoo and body wash combines the cleansing properties of Castile soap with the soothing and refreshing scent of lavender and peppermint essential oils. Adding jojoba and vitamin E oils can help moisturize and provide nutrients to the skin. Adjust the amount and type of essential oils to your preference. Enjoy the naturally scented experience of homemade cleansing products!

Using customized, chemical-free products for your hair and body care routine provides various benefits contributing to your overall health and skin health. Here are some advantages:

1. Natural ingredients: Homemade products allow you to choose natural, gentle ingredients for your skin and hair. You can choose high-quality carrier oils, essential oils, and other natural ingredients known for their nourishing and beneficial properties.

2. Avoid harsh chemicals: Commercial hair and body care products often contain synthetic fragrances, preservatives, and harsh chemicals that can irritate and potentially harm your skin and overall health. Creating your products allows you to eliminate these chemicals from your daily life.

3. Personalized recipes: You control the ingredients in your homemade products so you can customize them to your specific needs and preferences. Whether you have sensitive skin, allergies, or unique hair care requirements, you can create a formula that works best for you.

4. Reduce environmental impact: Homemade products reduce the need for mass-produced, packaged personal care products. This facilitates a more sustainable and eco-friendly approach to self-care as you can use reusable containers and reduce packaging waste.

5. Cost-effectiveness: Making your hair and body care products can be cost-effective in the long run, especially if you already have essential oils and other basic ingredients. A little goes a long way so that a batch can last a while.

6. Aromatherapy benefits: Adding essential oils to your homemade products adds a pleasant aroma and potential aromatherapy benefits. Essential oils can promote relaxation, improve mood, and contribute to a more enjoyable self-care routine.

7. Customized scent: By choosing your favorite essential oils, you can create a custom scent that resonates with your preferences. This enhances the sensory experience of using the product and adds a touch of luxury to your daily routine.

8. Creative expression: Making your products allows you to express your creativity. You can experiment with different ingredients, recipes, and scents to make the process enjoyable and rewarding.

9. Transparency: You know exactly what's in your product, giving you

peace of mind that you're not exposing yourself to unknown or potentially harmful substances.

10. Satisfaction: A sense of satisfaction comes from making your products and taking an active role in your self-care routine. Using products that you make yourself can be incredibly satisfying.

It's important to note that while homemade products offer many benefits, it's also important to educate yourself on proper ingredient selection, dilution ratios, and potential sensitivities. Not all natural ingredients suit everyone, so be sure to do a patch test and consult a healthcare professional if you have specific concerns or skin conditions.

I. Soothing Lip Balm

Here's a simple recipe for a nourishing and hydrating lip balm using essential oils and natural emollients:

Element:
* 1 tablespoon beeswax pellets
* 1 tablespoon coconut oil
* 1 tablespoon shea butter
* 10 drops of your favorite essential oil (such as peppermint, lavender, citrus)

Guide:
1. melt beeswax pellets, coconut oil, and shea butter over low heat in a Pyrex container or double boiler. Stir gently until all ingredients are completely melted and well combined.

2. Remove the mixture from the heat and let it cool slightly for a few minutes.

3. Add the essential oil drops. Once the mixture has cooled slightly but is still liquid. Stir well to distribute the essential oils evenly.

4. Carefully pour the mixture into a small lip balm container or tube. If you are using a tube, make sure to pour slowly to avoid air bubbles.

5. Allow the lip balm to cool and set completely. This may take several hours.

6. Once the lip balm has been set, secure the container with a lid and label it with the date and type of essential oil used.

Usage:
Apply a small amount of lip balm to your lips whenever they feel dry or need moisture. The natural emollients in the balm will help nourish and protect your lips, while the essential oils provide a pleasant scent and potentially added benefits.

Note: Be careful when using essential oils on your lips, as they can be very potent. Make sure to use the proper dilution and choose essential oils that are safe for topical use and won't cause sensitivity.

Before applying lip balm to your lips, do a patch test to ensure you don't have any adverse reactions to the ingredients. If you have any allergies or sensitivities, it's best to consult a healthcare professional before using new products on your skin, especially around sensitive areas like lips.

There are several advantages to using homemade lip balm to keep your lips soft, moisturized and protected:

1. Natural ingredients: Homemade lip balm is made from natural ingredients like beeswax, coconut oil, and shea butter. These ingredients provide deep hydration without synthetic chemicals or additives that can irritate the delicate skin on your lips.

2. Customization: When making your lip balm, you have complete control over your ingredients. You can choose the oils and butter that best suit your skin type and preferences. You can also customize the scent and flavor by adding essential oils to create a lip balm that suits your taste.

3. Moisturizing: Beeswax, coconut oil, and shea butter are rich in moisturizing properties. They form a protective barrier on the lips, preventing moisture loss and keeping your lips hydrated for longer. This is especially beneficial in dry and cold weather.

4. Nutritious: Many natural ingredients in homemade lip balms contain vitamins and antioxidants that nourish and support healthy skin. Shea butter, for example, is known for its vitamin A and E content, which promotes healthy skin.

5. Protection: Natural ingredients in homemade lip balm can help protect your lips from environmental factors such as strong winds, cold temperatures, and UV radiation from the sun. This prevents your lips from getting chapped, dry, or sunburned.

6. Gentle formulas: Homemade lip balms are often formulated with mild ingredients less likely to cause irritation or allergic reactions. This makes them suitable for people with sensitive skin.

7. Economical: Making your lip balm can be cost-effective in the long run, especially when considering the ingredients' quality compared to some commercial products.

8. Sustainability: By making your lip balm, you use sustainable ingredients and reduce reliance on the single-use plastic packaging commonly found in store-bought lip balms.

9. Making experience: Making your lip balm can be a fun and creative DIY project. It allows you to try different oils, butter, and scents, giving you a sense of accomplishment and satisfaction.

10. Versatility: If desired, homemade lip balm can also serve as a basis for trying different flavors, scents, or tinted versions.

Remember that individuals may react differently to ingredients, so it's important to do a patch test before applying lip balm to your lips, especially if you have a history of sensitivities or allergies. If you are unsure about the safety of any ingredient on your skin, consult a healthcare professional before using this product.

J. Homemade Massage Oil

Here is a recipe for a relaxing and aromatic massage oil using essential oils and carrier oils:

Relaxing Lavender and Chamomile Massage Oil:

Element:

* 1/4 cup carrier oil (such as sweet almond, jojoba, or coconut oil)
* 8 ~ 10 drops of lavender essential oil

* 4 ~ 6 drops of chamomile essential oil

Guide:

1. Choose your carrier oil: Choose a carrier oil that suits your skin type and preferences. Sweet almond, jojoba, and coconut oils are popular massage oils because of their nourishing and gliding properties.

2. Prepare a clean bottle: Use a dark glass bottle with a dropper or pump for ease of use and to protect the essential oil from light and air.

3. Add the carrier oil: Pour the carrier oil into the bottle, leaving some space at the top.

4. Add essential oils: Drop lavender and chamomile oils into a carrier oil.

5. Cap and mix: Close the bottle tightly and shake gently to combine essential oils with carrier oil. This will ensure that the oil is evenly distributed.

6. Conduct a patch test: Before using massage oil on a larger skin area, conduct a patch test on a small area to check for any potential allergic reactions or sensitivities.

7. Heat the oil: When ready to use your massage oil, heat it slightly by placing the bottle in a bowl of warm water for a few minutes. This will enhance the comfort of the massage and help the oil diffuse smoothly.

8. Massage: Apply a small amount of massage oil to your hands and gently rub them together to heat the essential oil further. Then, apply the oil to your skin in circular motions or massage as needed.

9. Relax: Enjoy lavender and chamomile's calming and soothing aroma as you relax and let the massage oil work its magic.

NOTE: This massage oil is for external use only. Avoid contact with eyes and do not use on broken or irritated skin. If you have any allergies or medical conditions, please consult a healthcare professional before using essential oils.

Benefit:

* Lavender Essential Oil: Lavender is known for its relaxing and calming properties. It can help reduce stress and tension, making it a great choice for a relaxing massage oil.

* Chamomile Essential Oil: Chamomile has anti-inflammatory and soothing properties. It can help relax muscles and promote a sense of tranquility.

* Carrier Oil: Carrier oil provides glide for massage and nourishes the skin, leaving it soft and moisturized.

Use this massage oil to enhance the relaxation and overall well-being of your massage experience. Always ensure the essential oil you use is high quality and properly diluted before applying it to your skin.

Homemade massage oil has many benefits that can promote relaxation, relieve tension, and enhance intimacy during your personal or shared experience. Here are some of the main advantages:

1. Personalize: When making your massage oil, you can choose carrier and essential oils that resonate with you and your partner's preferences. This personalization can make the massage experience more enjoyable and tailored to your unique needs.

2. Natural Ingredients: Homemade massage oils are usually made from natural ingredients, such as carrier oils and essential oils. This may be a healthier and more nourishing option for your skin than commercial products containing synthetic fragrances and additives.

3. Relaxation: Many essential oils, such as lavender, chamomile, and ylang-ylang, have calming and soothing properties. These essential oils can help relax the body and mind and create a peaceful atmosphere during the massage.

4. Relieve muscle tension: Certain essential oils, such as peppermint, eucalyptus, and rosemary, have analgesic and anti-inflammatory properties. These oils can help relieve muscle tension and soreness and promote relaxation.

5. Increases intimacy: Sharing a massage experience with your partner can enhance emotional connection and intimacy. Touching and massaging each other creates a sense of intimacy and comfort.

6. Aromatherapy benefits: Essential oils used in massage oils can have aromatherapy effects. Inhaling pleasant aromas can trigger emotional responses, reduce stress, and elevate mood.

7. Sensory experience: Some essential oils, such as jasmine, sandalwood, and rose, are known for their aphrodisiac properties. Incorporating these essential oils into your massage oil can create a sensual and romantic atmosphere.

8. Stress reduction: Receiving or giving a massage can stimulate the release of oxytocin, a hormone associated with stress reduction and bonding. This can lead to an overall sense of well-being.

9. Skin nourishment: Carrier oils used in massage oils, such as sweet almond oil or jojoba oil, provide moisture and nutrients to the skin, making it soft and supple.

10. Communication: Sharing a massage experience allows open communication and the chance to prioritize each other's health. It is a way of showing care and affection through touch.

Remember, proper dilution and choosing the right essential oils are crucial to ensuring safety and effectiveness when making homemade massage oil. Always do a patch test and be aware of any allergies or sensitivities before applying the oil to larger areas of your skin. Open communication with your partner about their preferences and comfort levels is crucial to a positive and enjoyable experience.

We conclude the chapter by highlighting the versatility and creativity of DIY projects and recipes for men using essential oils. By participating in these programs, men can personalize their self-care routines, enhance their beauty practices, and create a harmonious and inviting environment. When making homemade products, following instructions, using quality ingredients, and prioritizing safety is important. Through these DIY projects and recipes, men can unleash their creativity, enjoy the benefits of natural ingredients, and enhance their well-being in a personalized and meaningful way.

Conclusion

Embrace the Power of Essential Oils

for Men's Health

This comprehensive book explores the power of essential oils in promoting men's health. From addressing common questions and misconceptions to delving into various benefits and uses, we've provided a wealth of information to help men harness the potential of essential oils in their lives.

By embracing essential oils, men can experience a wide range of benefits in all aspects of health. Essential oils provide natural and practical solutions, whether boosting energy and stamina, supporting muscle recovery, soothing joint and muscle discomfort, or meeting shaving and skin care needs.

Additionally, we discuss essential oils' role in promoting relaxation, focus, and mental clarity. From dealing with stress and anxiety to boosting confidence and motivation, essential oils can be valuable tools for managing emotions and enhancing overall mental health.

Going a step further, we also explore the impact of essential oils on male physical health and vitality. From balancing testosterone levels and supporting sexual health to addressing hormonal imbalances and symptoms, essential oils can support men's overall health and vitality.

This book emphasizes the importance of safe, correct use and selection of quality essential oils. By following essential oil safety guidelines and considering factors such as plant species, extraction method, and sourcing, men can ensure a positive and safe experience with essential oils.

Plus, we provide practical tips and techniques for maximizing the benefits of essential oils. From inhalation and topical application to blending and timing, men can incorporate essential oils into their daily routines and rituals to enhance their therapeutic benefits.

In summary, essential oils offer a natural and versatile approach to men's health. By embracing the power of essential oils and applying the knowledge and practices outlined in this book, people can experience the transformative impact of these aromatic wonders. Whether it's physical, emotional, or mental health, essential oils have the potential to support men on their journey to overall health and vitality. So, take the opportunity to harness the power of essential oils and open up a world of wellness to yourself.

About the Author

Li, Fuxian: Master of Bioinformatics, Ph.D. in Social Psychology. Senior essential oil physiotherapist in China, principal of plant essential oil training school. In the past 10 years, he has traveled to China and the United States, promoting traditional Chinese medicine aromatherapy, teaching hundreds of men to use plant essential oils to regulate their bodies, and helping to solve various problems commonly encountered by men. Through the summary of many cases, the solution of essential oil to men's problems in all aspects has been formed, which has been compiled into a book so that the majority of male compatriots can find a new, natural, and effective auxiliary healing method.

Cheng, Zhiqing: Senior Professor, Chief TCM Physician, Doctoral Supervisor of Zhejiang University of Traditional Chinese Medicine. The fifth batch of national old Chinese medicine experts academic experience inheritance work instructors, Zhejiang Province famous traditional Chinese medicine practitioners. Vice President of the Professional Committee of Plant Essential Oil Therapy of the World Federation of Chinese Medicine Societies. He is good at TCM diagnosis and treatment of coronary heart disease, hypertension, viral myocarditis, arrhythmia, heart failure, and other cardiovascular diseases, and has deep attainments in cholecystitis, cholelithiasis, spleen and stomach, urinary system, and internal medicine incurable diseases. In recent years, he has vigorously promoted and practiced aromatherapy in traditional Chinese medicine and has achieved good results.

Yu, Jiaqi: Chief Physician, Department of Urology, The First Affiliated Hospital of Zhejiang University School of Medicine. He is good at treating common diseases of urology and andrology, such as multiple kidneys, bladder, prostate cancer, tumors, etc. In the treatment of common and difficult diseases of the urinary system, some experience has been obtained, especially in the treatment of bladder tumors, prostate cancer, urinary tuberculosis, stones, and kidney tumors. There are many examples of the use of essential oils for men's unique health problems, and efforts are being made to promote them globally.

www.ingramcontent.com/pod-product-compliance
Lightning Source LLC
Chambersburg PA
CBHW052118270326
41930CB00012B/2675

9 781963 938005